M

Adele

**The Essential Medical Secretary**

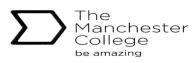

For Baillière Tindall:

*Publishing manager:* Jacqueline Curthoys
*Project manager:* Ewan Halley
*Development editor:* Karen Gilmour
*Project controller:* Derek Robertson

# The Essential Medical Secretary

## Foundations for good practice

Edited by

**Stephanie J Green**

Lecturer, Norwich City College of Further and Higher Education, Norwich

Foreword by
**Pauline Webdale**

Chairman of Council,
Association of Medical Secretaries, Practice Managers, Administrators and Receptionists

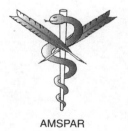

AMSPAR

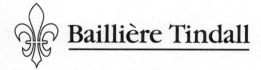

London Edinburgh Philadelphia Toronto Sydney Tokyo

Baillière Tindall
An imprint of Harcourt Brace and Company Limited
24–28 Oval Road,
London NW1 7DX, UK

Harcourt Brace and Company,
Robert Stevenson House,
1–3 Baxter's Place, Leith Walk,
Edinburgh EH1 3AF, UK

The Curtis Center,
Independence Square West,
Philadelphia, PA 19106–3399, USA

Harcourt Brace and Company,
55 Horner Avenue,
Toronto, Ontario, M8Z 4X6, Canada

Harcourt Brace and Company, Australia,
30–52 Smidmore Street,
Marrickville,
NSW 2204, Australia

Harcourt Brace and Company – Japan,
Ichibancho Central Building,
22–1 Ichibancho,
Chiyoda-ku, Tokyo 102, Japan

First published 1998

A catalogue record for this book is available from the British
Library.

ISBN 0 7020 2103 2

Printed and bound in Great Britain

# Contents

## Part 1
### The context of medical secretarial practice    1

**1. The development of the welfare state and the National Health Service**    3
*Veeren Rambohul*

Introduction; What do we mean by the welfare state?; Evolution of the health services; Key events in the post-1948 NHS; Reforms of the NHS – 1980s–1990s; Changes in related social services; Issues facing the welfare state in the 21st century; Changes since 1997; Conclusions

**2. The National Health Service today**    11
*Veeren Rambohul*

Introduction; Background of present management arrangements; Management at the national level; Managing the NHS at the local level; Issues facing the NHS; Conclusions

**3. The legislative context**    25
*Vincent Leach and Ingrid Anstey*

Introduction; The law and you; Statute law and common law; Criminal law; Civil law; Laws specific to health service procedures; The governing bodies; Charters and complaints; Employment law; The Disability Discrimination Act 1995; Conclusion

**4. Ethics and etiquette**    45
*Vincent Leach*

Introduction; Law and ethics; Ethical codes; Ethical principles; Ethical issues in the medical secretarial role; Etiquette; Conclusions

## Part 2
### Fundamentals of medical secretarial practice    59

**5. The qualities of the medical secretary**    61
*Jayne Pearce*

Introduction; Confidentiality; Cooperation; Commitment; Courtesy; Conclusion

**6. Communication**    75
*Sara Ladyman*

Introduction; General; Confidentiality; Verbal communication; The telephone; Visual communication; Written communication; Written correspondence; Internal/external systems to facilitate good communication; Conclusion

**7. Finance**    99
*Stephanie J Green*

Introduction; General practice; Private practice; Conclusion

**8. Information technology**    107
*Phillip Simons*

Introduction; The role of information in the NHS; Individual level; Local level; National level; The new NHS number; For hospital-based secretaries; General practice; Safeguarding the

Introduction; Drug names – generics and proprietaries; Reference sources; The Medicines Act 1968; The limited list; Drugs to be prescribed in certain circumstances under the NHS; Borderline substances; Misuse of Drugs Act 1971; Documentation; Repeat prescriptions; Dispensing of drugs; Summary of key issues; Conclusions

## *Appendices*

# Contributors

**Ingrid Anstey** BA(Hons) Law
Lecturer, Business School, Norwich City College of Further and Higher Education, Norwich

**Stephanie J Green** SRN CMB Part 1
Lecturer, Business School, Norwich City College of Further and Higher Education, Norwich

**Barbara Jones** DipPM MAMS
Practice Manager, Pen Y Bont Surgery, St Asaph, Clwyd, Wales

**Dilys Jones** AAMS CertEd
Lecturer, Business School, Norwich City College of Further and Higher Education, Norwich

**Sara Ann Ladyman** MAMS
Course Director, Talking Medical (Distance Learning), Gawcott, Buckingham

**Vincent Leach** MA MB ChB DRCOG MAMS LRPS
Chairman, AMSPAR Education Committee, Tavistock Square, London

**Grizelda Moules** MSc (Medical Informatics) MAMS DipTEFL FETC
Tutor, University of Bath, Claverton Down, Bath

**Jayne Pearce** MHSM MSAE MAMS DipMS
Chief Executive, AMSPAR, Tavistock House North, Tavistock Square, London

**Veeren B Rambohul** BA(Hons) MA IHSM
Lecturer, Business and Finance Department, Crawley College, Crawley

**Phillip Simons** BA MSc MHSM DipHSM
Administrative Assistant, Wessex Institute of Health Research and Development, University of Southampton, Southampton

**Tracey Sweet** MSc
Assistant Manager Support Services, Cornwall and Isles of Scilly Health Authority, St Austell, Cornwall

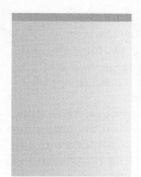

# Foreword

*Pauline Webdale*

Chairman of Council, Association of Medical Secretaries,
Practice Managers, Administrators and Receptionists

The world of the medical secretary is challenging and never mundane. Each day, sometimes each hour, brings something new to be dealt with.

It can be stimulating to be faced with these challenges, gratifying to gain experience and confidence over time, and satisfying to build up long-term relationships with patients and their families.

This role is truly at the sharp end of medicine and as well as any innate skills you may possess, continual learning and development will help bring new skills and enjoyment to the job.

It is probably no exaggeration to say that effective communication lies at the heart of most successful endeavours and nowhere is this more true than in medical practice. In our increasingly litigious society where people expect more, especially in speed of service and range of treatments, effective communication will make the team less vulnerable to legal challenges. Time spent providing a clear explanation or an apology for an unusual event or delay will go a long way to prevent misunderstanding and threatened legal action.

The 1998 White Paper, *The New NHS: Modern, Dependable*, heralds a turning point both for the National Health Service (NHS) and those of us who work within it. Replacing the internal market with integrated care will impact greatly on all our roles.

The 'team' concept, to which some only pay lip service, will need to become a reality in order to combine efficiency and quality with an emphasis on fairness and partnerships. This will be fundamental to the success of integrated care.

A modern and dependable NHS needs to be supported by accurate and current information. In recent years information technology has become too focused on supporting the transaction processes of the internal market. This has perhaps been at the expense of exploiting the potential of IT to support frontline staff in delivering benefits for patients.

The new drive for quality and efficiency will aim to make patients' records available electronically when needed, will use the NHSnet and the Internet to bring patients quicker test results, on-line appointment booking and up-to-date specialist advice. Knowledge about health, illness and best practice will also be available to the public through the Internet and the emerging public access media (e.g. digital TV). Finally, by developing telemedicine to ensure specialist skills are available to all parts of the country, equity will be assured.

There will be robust safeguards to protect patients' confidentiality and privacy, the aim being to create a powerful alliance between knowledgeable patients advised by knowledgeable professionals as a means of improving health and health care.

The role of the health authorities will also be different. They will be in a position to provide strategic leadership on the ground to the new Primary Care Groups. Having a stronger, clearer role will hopefully overcome the fragmentation which characterised the internal market. A true partnership approach will ensure all patients will benefit through coordinated, high quality and accessible services.

The NHS has reached a watershed which marks a clear direction to it becoming a modern dependable service. It must not mean wholesale structural upheaval which will generate cost and disruption which gets in the way of patient care. We have all seen too much of that sort of change and certainly have no appetite for more.

This tough and challenging programme will take us into the next century, working in a changed NHS in a changing world, where staff involvement will be emphasised. We owe it to ourselves to become well informed professionals, working to the clear high standards set by our professional body AMSPAR.

This book has many good qualities: it has a logical flow, is well written and is very comprehensive. Perhaps its best quality is that we are given a true flavour of the vast scope of the range of duties covered by the medical secretary. This book must be regarded as an essential working document which provides all the knowledge needed to supplement formal training and as a reference tool for updating as progress is made.

Finally, the value of this book as a training and management tool is very much in evidence. Both the newcomer and her more experienced colleagues can use it to obtain the necessary skills and expertise to meet the challenges ahead. This will enable them to develop their roles and, importantly, themselves to their full potential as key players in this emerging modern and dependable NHS.

Pauline Webdale, 1998
Chairman of Council, AMSPAR

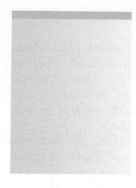

# Introduction

The National Health Service has undergone profound changes in recent years, and it is time that medical secretaries had a textbook which will reflect these changes and provide a foundation for their study and practice.

This book does not attempt to address subjects of straightforward secretarial or administrative practice. There are many other texts available which thoroughly cover these areas. Rather it concentrates wholeheartedly on the knowledge, skills and attitudes needed for the specific role and practice of the medical secretary. It identifies this role and especially the qualities necessary to work successfully as a medical secretary, as well as stressing the importance of teamwork in today's health services. It discusses the legal and ethical background of medical practice and examines the need for every member of staff in any area of medicine to understand the contemporary applications of fundamental and sometime ancient principles.

The book is divided into five sections. The first gives a background to medical practice in today's health services. It also addresses specific areas of organisation from the role of the Department of Health to the provision of care in the community. Particularly relevant legal and ethical considerations also have their own chapters, and particular emphasis is placed on etiquette.

Section Two discusses key aspects of medical secretarial practice common to both hospital and general practice. Chapters are included on the importance of the role within the team and the qualities required for effective and efficient practice. Communication skills are discussed in depth and chapters are included on the impact of IT and its role in practice. We have also included in this section a chapter on the various clinical aspects which the secretary needs to be aware of in both hospital and general practice. This is not to usurp any general role, but merely reflects the importance of acquainting readers with common pieces of equipment and their function. This section also addresses issues of finance in medicine, but acknowledges that this is an area of increasing specialist expertise, in which secretaries are becoming less involved.

Section Three provides information for the medical secretary working within the hospital environment with particular reference to other departments, record keeping and relevant procedures involving admissions, discharges and outpatient departments.

Section Four concentrates on the work of the medical secretary in general practice, identifying the roles of the primary health care team and explaining the day-to-day running of the general practice. It also includes a chapter which looks at important health and safety considerations in general practice.

Finally, the book includes an extensive range of appendices which contain a host of useful information not only for study but for job applications, career development and for reference when in practice.

## How to use this book

The book has been designed to help readers make the most of their studies and practice placements. Each chapter starts with clear objectives to enable the reader to anticipate its content. This is then followed by an introduction which provides a short overview of the chapter and its purpose for the reader. Some chapters also include a short list of documentation which it may be useful for the reader to obtain which are referred to within the chapter, e.g. a copy of a local practice charter.

Throughout, the chapters include reflection and discussion points where students are encouraged to reflect on particular points or problems highlighted within the text. This may be followed by an action point, where specific activities are suggested, encouraging readers to use their experiences in practice, or discuss issues with fellow students or other health care workers. Many chapters contain suggested further resources such as books or useful addresses. We hope this will prompt readers to read other publications and journals in order to keep their knowledge of their working environment up-to-date.

This book is designed specifically for students studying for diplomas in medical secretarial practice and as a useful reference for medical secretaries in practice, especially those who are considering moving from one area of practice to another.

# The Association of Medical Secretaries, Practice Managers, Administrators and Receptionists

The Association of Medical Secretaries, Practice Managers, Administrators and Receptionists (AMSPAR) was founded in 1964, initially as the Association of Medical Secretaries. Its primary task at that time was to promote recognition of the valuable role played by those working as medical secretaries, and to establish a nationally recognised professional qualification. Such was the success of the Association that it expanded both its membership and the range of qualifications during the 1970s, resulting in a change of the Association's registered name. A range of AMSPAR qualifications are now available at over 200 centres throughout the United Kingdom.

Today, the Association remains the only nationally recognised awarding body providing specialist qualifications for medical secretaries, receptionists and general practice managers. It has over 6000 individual members from all corners of the United Kingdom and a growing international membership. Further details of the Association's activities and membership opportunities are available from:

AMSPAR
Tavistock House North
Tavistock Square
London WC1H 9LN.

Tel: 0171 387 6005
Fax: 0171 388 2648

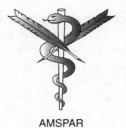

AMSPAR

# Part 1
# The context of medical secretarial practice

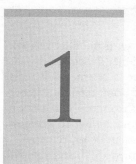

# The development of the welfare state and the National Health Service

*Veeren Rambohul*

## OBJECTIVES

- To explain what is meant by the term welfare state
- To describe the origins of the British welfare state, with particular reference to the development of the health services
- To examine the health and welfare reforms of the 1980s
- To provide an understanding of the issues facing the welfare state in the 21st century and an appreciation of the direction of recent government policies.

## INTRODUCTION

As we move into the third millennium, the British welfare state and the National Health Service (NHS) will be over half a century old. However, with the changes introduced in the 1980s and 1990s, it is becoming more and more certain that the British citizens of the year 2000 can expect a very different form of provision to that received by their forebears in the aftermath of the Second World War.

Medical secretaries will find the development of the NHS and welfare state quite enlightening, especially in seeing how various administrations have addressed problems in the management of welfare. The main theme of interest has always been, as now, the constant problems of pressing and increasing demands and how to tackle these in the face of new social pressures.

## WHAT DO WE MEAN BY THE WELFARE STATE?

The concept of the welfare state has evolved over a long period of time. It was around 1950 that it became acceptable to speak of the United Kingdom as having become a welfare state.

The *Encyclopaedia Britannica* defines the welfare state as follows:

> *A concept of government in which the state plays a role in the protection and promotion of the economic and social well-being of its citizens. It is based on the principles of equality of opportunity, equitable distribution of wealth, and the public responsibility for*

*those unable to avail themselves of the
minimum provisions for a good life.*

In 1942 the Report on Social Insurance and
Allied Services commissioned by the government
was published. This Report (which became known
as the Beveridge Report) recommended the provision
of comprehensive welfare benefits and services
to all citizens. It became the blueprint for the
post-war government to follow. It also became the
model for a number of countries and thus is a
major landmark in the development of the modern
welfare state. Sir William Beveridge, the author of
the Report, wrote:

*We should regard Want, Disease, Ignorance,
Squalor and Idleness as common enemies of
us all, not as enemies with whom each
individual may seek a separate peace, escaping
himself to personal prosperity, while leaving
his fellows in their clutches. This is the
meaning of social conscience: that one should
refuse to make a separate peace with a social
evil.*

One of the main features of the welfare state is
the provision of a comprehensive system of welfare
organised by the state. In the UK a series of
Acts were passed by Parliament at the time,
including:

1944    Education Act
1945    Family Allowances Act
1946    National Health Service Act
1948    National Insurance Act

The principle of the welfare state is based on the
notion of citizenship rights. In this context rights to
welfare should not be based on such qualifications
as working in certain industries, living in certain
parts of the country, or the social class or background
one belongs to. It means that any citizen,
regardless of his or her background, has the right
to avail himself or herself of the provisions made at
the time of his or her need. These provisions are not
meant to be charity, but a citizenship entitlement.

The state creates these rights through legislation,
and establishes obligations on its administration and agencies entrusted with the duty of making
these provisions available. Importantly, the
welfare state is redistributive in character. It redistributes
from the rich to the poor, from one generation
to the other, or collects from those in work to
compensate those not in work owing to sickness,
injury, disability, unemployment or retirement.

Students must guard against the belief that the
UK was the first country to become a welfare state.
Countries such as Denmark, Sweden and New
Zealand are deemed to have attained that status
several years before the UK.

**Reflection points**

◆ Think about the five social evils referred to
   by Lord Beveridge. What would you consider
   as being present day social evils. What might
   the state do to overcome these?

◆ Think about why the welfare state was set up.
   Are the reasons compatible with the
   aspirations of today's Britain?

◆ Which benefits would you like to see
   increased and which decreased or abolished?
   In considering 'deserving' and 'non-deserving'
   cases, assess whether your views have
   changed over time due to your own personal
   circumstances or to the influence of the
   media.

# EVOLUTION OF THE HEALTH SERVICES

Box 1.1 summarises the main stages in the development
of the health services until the inception of
the NHS in 1948. You may find it interesting to
trace how historical circumstances are reflected in
the health service we have today.

## Evolution of medical practice

The evolution of medical practice in this country
can be seen as a three-stage development.

## Box 1.1 Early history of the health service

| | |
|---|---|
| Pre-Tudor times | Monastic orders provided relief and care for the sick. The churches were also the main centres of teaching and learning. |
| Post-Reformation | Most of the established hospitals came into secular hands. By 1700 there were about a dozen voluntary hospitals, of which half were in London. Voluntary hospitals were managed by their own board of governors, and relied on rich benefactors, funds raised during 'flag' days, and on charges levied.<br><br>Initially, their aims were the same as the predecessor monastic orders but they soon started to exclude the destitute, sick children, pregnant women, the infectious and the mentally ill. Gradually, sick children and pregnant women came to be cared for in specialist voluntary hospitals. Although there was an expansion of voluntary hospitals in the 18th and 19th centuries, the vast majority of the sick, disabled and mentally ill were left to the Poor Law institutions. |
| Poor Laws | With the implementation of the Elizabethan Poor Laws, some of the workhouses set aside room and facilities for sick paupers. In time, sick paupers in the community could also attend. |
| 1808 | The first lunatic asylum for sick paupers was built out of public funds. The majority of mental institutions were built in the 19th century on the fringe of centres of population. These were passed to local county control in 1889. |
| 1834 | The Poor Law Amendment Act gave a boost to the expansion of Poor Law Infirmaries. With the curtailment of outdoor relief, more families had to enter the workhouses. |
| 1867 | An Act of Parliament enabled Infirmaries of a better standard to be built by local authorities. These soon adopted a similar model to the voluntary hospitals. |
| 1867 | Parliament directed local authorities to build Fever Hospitals. |
| 1897 | Qualified nurses started to be employed in workhouse infirmaries. |
| 1929 | The Poor Law Board was abolished. Control of workhouses and workhouse infirmaries was transferred to the County and Borough Councils. |
| 1939 | Emergency Medical Services were created as part of the war-time measures. |
| 1946 (Nov) | The National Health Service Act was passed. |
| 1948 | The NHS became operational. All hospital services came under a unified service under the Ministry of Health (voluntary hospitals were assimilated). As a compromise to pressure groups, the NHS was established with a tri-partite structure: |

1. the hospital and specialist services, managed by the hospital management boards and accountable to the Regional Hospital Boards

2. the general practitioner services (including GPs, opticians, dentists and chemists), answerable to local executive committees

3. community services, including district nursing, health visiting and environmental health, provided by local authorities.

## Before the 18th century

The first stage dates from before the 18th century when those providing medical services were physicians, surgeons and apothecaries.

The *physician* was a 'professional man' trained at a university (in those days Oxford and Cambridge and Edinburgh) who restricted his practice to a small wealthy clientele. An Act passed in 1511 attempted to limit the practice to qualified persons by controlling the number of 'quacks', who at the time outnumbered those who had any training. This Act empowered bishops to grant licences in their diocese and unlicensed practitioners had to pay a heavy fine. This proved not to be a very satisfactory arrangement, and in 1518 a group of physicians led by Thomas Linacre petitioned Henry VIII. The outcome of this was the granting of a Royal Charter setting up a Royal College of Physicians.

The primary functions of the Royal College of Physicians were to:

◆ license those qualified to practice
◆ punish those pretending to be qualified
◆ punish malpractice.

Although the College was not directly involved in providing pre-qualification training, it arranged lectures and seminars by the elites of the profession. Physicians thus practised as family doctors to those who could afford it and in hospitals, essentially the voluntary hospitals, the distinction between hospital doctors and general practitioners came later.

The *surgeon* was a 'craftsman', trained by apprenticeship. His work was supposed to be limited to surgical procedures, but many surgeons practised midwifery, kept shops and dispensed drugs. In 1461 the Company of Barber-Surgeons was founded, the title reflecting the origins from which the art of surgery has evolved! In 1540 the company gained royal approval, and certain rights and privileges were conferred, one of which was to be called 'Master'. In time, colloquial use changed it to 'Mister'. Hence in Britain a surgeon came to be called 'Mister' and not 'Doctor'.

The Royal College of Surgeons was formed later in 1800, but the social status of surgeons remained lower than that of physicians.

The *apothecary* was a 'tradesman' trained by apprenticeship, who was allowed to charge only for the sale of drugs prescribed by physicians. By the 17th century apothecaries were seeing patients and writing prescriptions, and, without acknowledging it, became the doctors of the middle and poorer classes. In 1617 a Society of Apothecaries was formed. Apothecaries were drawn mostly from lower middle class families and underwent a five-year apprenticeship training in the dispensing of herbs and drugs. In 1815 the Apothecaries Act gave the Society of Apothecaries the power to license and examine in medicine.

## From 1700 to 1858

The second stage of development dates from around the 19th century with the development of voluntary hospitals. The status of surgeons improved and some apothecaries began working in hospitals. At the same time it became increasingly important for doctors to hold a hospital appointment. In time this practice led to the distinction between hospital doctors and general practitioners, as more hospitals developed.

## After 1858

The third stage of development dates back to the 1858 Medical Act. This prepared the way for the common recruitment, training and registration of doctors, thereby removing the historical distinction between physicians, surgeons and apothecaries. Apart from the curricula, the shape of medical training has remained significantly unchanged since then.

Physicians had been able to combine working in the community and providing medical supervision to patients in the voluntary hospitals. Initially, the association with voluntary hospitals was more for prestige than for salaries. The association with hospitals was one way of building a reputation and securing a larger clientele outside. The more prestigious the hospitals (e.g. teaching hospitals) the better the prospects. Hence the development of Harley Street practices, where consultation surgeries still exist serving rich clients, in close proximity to the major London teaching hospitals.

The freedom to combine private practice with NHS work was a compromise reached after very intensive negotiations between medical interests and health ministers over arrangements for the 1948 NHS.

## KEY EVENTS IN THE POST-1948 NHS

Box 1.2 outlines the main developments in the NHS since 1948.

During the 1950s, 1960s and 1970s there was a general consensus that the welfare state should be supported and improved, especially in terms of access to services. There were also growing concerns about rising costs and how to manage budgets and resources within an increasingly complex system. However, the most significant reforms, and those which had the biggest influence on the

shape of today's health service, took place during the Thatcher government of the 1980s and 1990s. The 1980s saw a reappraisal of the role of the state and the successive Conservative governments effected radical changes to the way that state welfare was perceived and delivered. One of the most significant aspects was the creation of a 'mixed economy' in welfare. This meant that a mixture of state and private involvement was encouraged in a number of key areas. The most radical concept was the introduction of an 'internal market'.

## REFORM OF THE NHS – 1980s–1990s

The NHS was restructured in 1983, with the abolition of the Area tier of administration and the setting up of District Health Authorities. The most fundamental change came with the passing of the

---

**Box 1.2**  Major events in the NHS (1948–1998)

1948  NHS set up (see Box 1.1)

1962  Guillebaud Report. Allayed fears about rising costs. Introduced international comparisons. Percentage of gross national product spent on NHS in the UK significantly less than in other major developed countries.

1974  Reorganisation of the NHS. Introduction of Consensus Management. Local authorities (LAs) lose responsibility for community services, which are integrated with NHS at the local level. LAs retain responsibility for environmental health. Community Health Councils created for each District (Districts covered a population of approximately 250 000–400 000). Regional Health Authorities (14) created in England, and Area Health Authorities (AHAs) co-terminous with LA boundaries to manage services provided within each District. District management teams responsible for managing services within the District.

1983  Griffiths Report. Introduction of General Management. NHS restructured. AHAs abolished, District Health Authorities (DHAs) created.

1990  NHS and Community Care Act. Creation of the internal market, creation of NHS Trusts and GP fundholding scheme. New GP contract.

1994  Mergers of Regional Health Authorities (RHAs).

1996  Replacement of RHAs by regional outposts of NHS Executive. Mergers of DHAs with FHSAs (Family Health Service Authorities).

1998  The New NHS White Paper is launched, indicating the overhaul of GP fundholding, and the abolition of the so-called internal market, to be replaced by a system of integrated care based on a partnership between NHS bodies and other local agencies.

1990 NHS and Community Care Act. It was decided not to change the funding basis, but to look at further structural changes. Ministers became attracted to the ideas of Professor Alain Enthoven, an academic with interests in health service management, about the creation of an internal market within the NHS. Hence it was decided to redefine the management arrangements into two distinct groups of functions carried out by two separate groups:

*Providers* and *Purchasers*

All hospitals, community services units and general practices would become providers, who would negotiate contracts for their services with the purchasing Authorities. Authorities would be able to entertain bids for services from the private sector or from neighbouring NHS providers. In principle, funding from central government would be available to the purchasing Authorities based on population and adjusted for morbidity. Providers would still be expected to provide services for the local population but the old notion of District catchment boundary would no longer apply. Services would be 'seamless'.

Additional major changes brought about by the 1990 Act at this time were:

◆ the setting up of NHS Trusts. Hospital and provider units were able to apply to become independent of District and Regional Health Authority control and become NHS Trusts.
◆ group general practices that met the criteria for size could apply to become 'GP fundholders', which would allow them to manage 'funds' enabling them to purchase from hospital and community providers, services they required for their patients.

Responsibility for long-term care in the community was transferred to local authority Social Services. Thus Social Services, which already had the responsibility for providing residential homes, now became the 'lead' agency in the assessment and case management of the elderly, the mentally ill and those with learning difficulties who required care and were deemed ready to be transferred out of hospital into community homes. This latter change was due to the recommendations of Sir Roy Griffiths in his report *Caring for People* (HMSO 1989).

Throughout, the government encouraged the private sector to grow in the following main areas:

◆ private health provision, by subsidising health insurance
◆ private sector nursing homes, by supporting private nursing and residential care home by paying fees initially out of Social Security benefits and after 1994 out of Social Services funds subsidising health insurance
◆ Collaboration and partnership schemes between the private and state sector
◆ Further extension of competitive tendering and 'privatisation' of certain health-related services.

## CHANGES IN RELATED SOCIAL SERVICES

The local authorities had been responsible for the provision of:

◆ residential homes for the elderly
◆ residential homes for long-stay hospital patients who were deemed to be ready for discharge into the community
◆ day centres for various client groups
◆ domiciliary services such as home-help and meals-on-wheels
◆ social work.

The 1980s saw a squeeze on local authority funding as well as competitive tendering for all local authority services. Consequently, most of the local authority residential homes moved out of local authority ownership either through private sales or through management buy-outs.

The 1990 NHS and Community Care Act imposed the following obligations on the Social Services departments:

◆ lead agency responsibility in community care
◆ responsibility for assessment of need
◆ responsibility for care management in the community

◆ responsibility as from April 1993 for the funding of residential and nursing home places on the application of a means test.

### Reflection points

◆ Care in the community is an expression that covers a whole range of changes in the way that community services were provided, but what does it conjure up for you? How is it used in the media?

◆ Try to find out about different agencies which are involved in community care in your area. These will include housing and benefits agencies as well as health-related agencies. Try to distinguish between government-funded agencies and voluntary agencies.

## ISSUES FACING THE WELFARE STATE IN THE 21st CENTURY

The 1990s also introduced government policies geared towards improving service sensitivity to user needs. Initiatives in the NHS, as with other services, centred around improving customer/user/client/patient care. The government introduced the Citizen's Charter in 1992 and this initiative has been the formalised vehicle for setting standards that service users can in time expect to be maintained by public service providers. The Patient's Charter is being reviewed by the Labour administration although the importance of customer care is still being emphasised.

### Reflection points

◆ What new issues would you like to see covered in the Patient's Charter?

◆ As a medical secretary, you must be concerned about customer care. In addition to patients, who else might be regarded as your customers?

## CHANGES SINCE 1997

In May 1997, the general election brought the Labour Party to power after 18 years of Conservative government. The Labour Party has been perceived to be a 'friend' of the NHS and indeed this probably contributed to its popularity with the voters. In 1998, the government published its White Paper, The New NHS, outlining the changes it wants to make to develop the NHS over the next 10 years. Changes in policy regarding health and health promotion are also likely to continue to affect the way the health service develops, particularly in regard to general practice and primary care.

However, regardless of political changes, the challenges facing the welfare state remain as follows:

◆ meeting the needs of an ageing population
◆ the need for increases in health services to keep up with advances in medicine
◆ to reconcile the desire to reduce taxation and to meet increasing demands for services
◆ to ensure that resources are directed to end-users and not wasted on bureaucracy
◆ to ensure proper accountability of public expenditure and proper conduct in the management of public funds and services
◆ to ensure provision of services and assistance in line with the standards of a civilised and just society whilst avoiding abuses and disincentives
◆ to effect changes in the quality of services provided in line with the present user demands, and the perceived future needs of the economy and the nation
◆ to attract additional funding, and the pros and cons of turning to new and varied sources of funding, e.g. state, private and voluntary combined.

## CONCLUSIONS

As a medical secretary, it is important that you are aware of policy which affects the ways in which the organisation you work in is developing. This is true whether you are working in a hospital department or in general practice. Often policy can seem remote, but as a frontline employee in the NHS you are potentially a crucial member of the team in ensuring:

◆ quality to customers
◆ essential liaison between different members of health care teams as well as personnel from other agencies
◆ the provision of effective and efficient administrative support to the clinical team.

All of these are fundamental to the future of the NHS.

 **Exercises**

◆ Keep up to date with developments in health service policy by reading coverage in national newspapers. Try to obtain a copy of the executive summaries of government policy documents. They are available in libraries and from HMSO. The further reading suggested below may also be helpful in providing more detailed information about the history and background of the development of the welfare state and the health services.

◆ Discuss with colleagues what kind of help and advice you might be able to provide to a family who are now responsible for looking after a chronically ill relative in their home. How would you find out about the services which they will need to be aware of?

## FURTHER READING

Butterworth E, Holman R 1975 Social welfare in Britain. Fontana, London

Ham C 1992 Health policy in Britain. Macmillan, London

Ham C 1990 The new NHS. Radcliffe Medical Press, Oxford

Ham C 1994 Management and competition in the new NHS. Radcliffe Medical Press, Oxford

Hutton W 1996 The state we're in. Vintage, London

Johnson N 1990 Reconstructing the Welfare State ... a decade of change 1980–1990. Harvester Wheatsheaf, London

McKeown T, Lowe CR 1974 An introduction to social medicine. Blackwell Scientific Publications, Oxford, London

NHS Confederation 1997 NHS handbook 1997/98. JMH Publishing, London

Thatcher M 1993 The Downing Street years. Harper Collins, London

# 2

# The National Health Service today

*Veeren Rambohul*

## OBJECTIVES

◆ To explain the management structure of the NHS

◆ To describe the role of those responsible for managing the NHS

◆ To explain the arrangements for the delivery of health services

◆ To examine the main issues facing the NHS.

## INTRODUCTION

The National Health Service is the largest employer organisation in Europe, employing around one million people and spending around 6% of the UK's gross domestic product. It was designed when it came into being in 1948 to provide health care to all UK citizens free at the point of service. The service has been subjected to five major reorganisations over the last 25 years and some of these have been discussed in Chapter 1. However, the central principle of a service provided in large part from direct taxation to all citizens and virtually free at the point of use has survived through to the present day.

As a medical secretary it is very likely that you will work in some part of the NHS or be liaising with it. Therefore it is important that you appreciate how it has been set up and the services it comprises.

## BACKGROUND OF PRESENT MANAGEMENT ARRANGEMENTS

The present arrangements for the management and delivery of health services relate back to changes brought about by the 1990 NHS and Community Care Act, and the restructuring carried out in 1996 as recommended by the Functions and Manpower Review (1992). (For brief details of reorganisation before 1990 refer to the section on evolution of the health services in Chapter 1.)

The 1990 NHS and Community Care Act enabled the following changes to be brought about:

1. the separation of purchaser and provider functions within the NHS
2. the creation of Trust hospitals and other Trust provider units within the NHS
3. the creation of GP fundholders
4. the allocation of 'lead agency' responsibility for community care to local authority Social Services
5. streamlining the membership of Health Authorities.

The Act was based on two White Papers, *Working For Patients* and *Caring for People*. These measures were designed to take the quest for greater efficiency a step further by the introduction of an internal market within the NHS. Health Authorities and GP fundholders became purchasers of services. Providers of services, i.e. hospitals, community and primary care service providers, had to seek contracts from the Health Authorities and GP fundholders.

In 1992, amidst concerns about rising management costs in the new NHS, a Functions and Manpower Review was set up, and it recommended further streamlining of the management structure at the higher levels of the NHS. By 1995, the number of Regional Health Authorities was reduced from 14 to 8, and by 1996, Regional Health Authorities were dissolved and replaced by the Regional Offices of the National Health Service Executive (NHSE).

The organisation of the NHS is being reviewed as part of the White Paper published in 1998 and its future structure compared to the pre-1997 structure is illustrated in Figure 2.1. Further information can be found at the Department of Health's website on the internet: www.open.gov.uk

## MANAGEMENT AT THE NATIONAL LEVEL

The *Secretary of State for Health* is a cabinet minister entrusted with the task of formulating government policy on health. He or she has to operate both as a politician in meeting the demands of his/her party and its supporters, and as the head of a large state department. The specific role and duties include formulating health policies

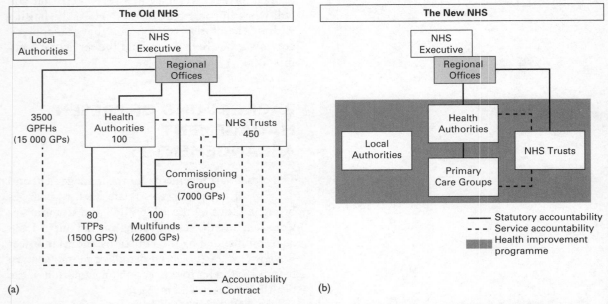

**Figure 2.1** The structure of the NHS (a) pre-1997 and (b) in the future. From Department of Health (1998) *The New NHS: Modern, Dependable*, HMSO, London, with permission. GPFH, GP fundholder; TPP, total purchasing practices.

and setting priorities and negotiating annual health service budgets in cabinet and with the Treasury. The Secretary of State for Health is assisted by four Ministers of Health, one in the House of Lords and three in the Commons. The performance of the Secretary of State is normally assessed on how effective he or she has been in gaining support for government policy inside and outside the service, and how changes brought under his or her Secretaryship are viewed. There is also now a Minister for Public Health whose remit crosses between various departments in addition to health, including the Environment and Education.

The *Department of Health* is the government department charged with assisting the Secretary of State and Ministers of Health in their state duties. The Department of Health is made up of three distinct groups:

1. The NHS Policy Board
2. The NHS Executive (NHSE)
3. Civil service administrative and support staff.

The *NHS Policy Board* is chaired by the Secretary of State and initially had a membership of around 15, including the Ministers of Health, the Permanent Secretary, the NHS Chief Executive, the Chief Medical Officer, the Chief Nursing Officer and a number of non-executive members with general management skills and experience. With effect from 1996 the chairmen of the eight Regions replaced the non-executive membership. The role of the NHS Policy Board is to strengthen the oversight of the NHS and its main concerns are:

◆ setting objectives and direction for the health service
◆ making strategic decisions
◆ approval of the overall budget and resource allocations
◆ receiving reports on performance and other evaluations from the service.

The *NHS Executive* is a small multi-professional management board led by the NHS Chief Executive. It has bases in Leeds and London. The membership includes the following:

◆ The NHS Chief Executive
◆ Director of Performance Management
◆ Director of Corporate Affairs
◆ Director of Finance and Corporate Information
◆ Director of Human Resources
◆ Director of Research and Development
◆ Medical Director
◆ Nursing Director
◆ Property Adviser.

The NHSE is responsible for planning and implementing the policies approved by the policy Board. The *NHS Chief Executive* performs the general manager function at the national level, is given authority to act on behalf of the Secretary of State and is the chief accounting officer for health service expenditure. Operating through the Regional Offices, one of the main responsibilities of the NHSE has been to oversee the development of the purchasing functions and to monitor NHS Trusts. The NHSE has been responsible for issuing guidelines for the development of the internal market. The functions of the NHSE therefore are:

◆ to act as the central headquarters of the NHS
◆ to develop the purchasing functions of the Authorities
◆ to monitor the performance of the NHS Trusts
◆ to establish with the Policy Board policies and priorities for the health service
◆ to allocate resources to the Health Authorities.

The *Chief Medical Officer* has a specific role in the publication of an annual report covering the state of the nation's health, and highlighting areas of medical and popular concerns. The Chief Medical Officer's recommendations are sought, particularly whenever the health of the general public is a matter of concern, e.g. controlling the spread of meningitis or BSE.

## NHS in Scotland

Prior to the 1990 NHS and Community Care Act, the health service in Scotland was provided and managed by Area Health Boards which were coterminous with local authority boundaries. There were no Regional Health Authorities. The Area Health Boards were responsible for the provision of primary and secondary care. This may account for the development of an excellent structure of health centres providing primary care.

The Area Health Boards were accountable to the Secretary of State for Scottish Affairs. With the reforms under the 1990 Act, the overall structure has remained, except for changes in the following fundamental areas:

◆ the creation of the internal market, i.e. separation of the purchasing and provider functions
◆ the creation of NHS Trusts with the responsibility of managing provider units
◆ the creation of GP fundholders.

In 1997 there were 47 NHS Trusts. A few directly managed units (DMUs) still existed due to the geography and small populations of the island health boards of Orkney, Shetland and the Western Isles. Scotland also differs from the rest of the UK in the sense that laws passed in Scotland are applied in the courts and in public administration.

## NHS in Wales

There is closer collaboration on health service management between England and Wales than there is between any of the other countries of the UK. Health and population statistics, for example, are published as population for England and Wales.

There are no Regional Health Authorities in Wales. District Health Authorities are directly accountable to the Welsh Office. The Welsh Common Services Authority (WHCSA) provides a range of specialist expertise in support of the operation and development of NHS Wales. Similarly, the 1990 Act introduced the internal market, NHS Trusts and GP fundholding in Wales. With effect from April 1996, five integrated Health Authorities were established, replacing the 17 Health Authorities and Family Health Services Authorities (FHSAs). The Health Promotion Authority for Wales provides national leadership, support and services for health promotion and disease prevention.

## NHS in Northern Ireland

In Northern Ireland there are also no Regional Health Authorities. There are four integrated Health and Personal Social Services Boards (Northern, Eastern, Southern and Western) responsible for health and social services. The reforms of the early 1990s introduced the internal market, NHS Trusts and GP fundholding. Consequently, by 1997 20 integrated Health and Social Services Trusts had been established as providers of services. A multi-fund involving 38 fundholding practices whose combined list size accounted for 27% of the population of the Eastern Health and Personal Social Service Board became operational in 1996.

## MANAGING THE NHS AT THE LOCAL LEVEL

As discussed in Chapter 1 and illustrated in Figure 2.1, health services at the local level are puchased by Health Authorities and GPs/primary care groups.

### Health authorities

In 1996, the District Health Authorities (DHAs) and the Family Health Services Authorities (FHSAs) were amalgamated more-or-less along the FHSA boundary lines, bringing the total number of Health Authorities to around 100. Core administrative functions of the FHSAs, such as maintaining patient registration and reimbursement of general practitioners, continued to be maintained under new 'core services agency' arrangements.

The Health Authorities are accountable to the Secretary of State through the NHS Management Executive's Regional Offices. They are held responsible for the implementation of national health policy. In particular, they are responsible for:

◆ assessing the health care needs of the local population
◆ meeting the assessed needs through the award of appropriate contracts to providers of services

◆ developing ways of meeting the needs of those who need primary as well as secondary care.

The aim of merging DHAs and FHSAs was to create an integrated purchasing authority which is then responsible with provider units for ensuring that local service needs are met. This process will in future be done in the form of long-term service agreements between Health Authorities, primary care groups and NHS Trusts. Working with local authorities, NHS Trusts and primary care groups, Health Authorities will take the lead in drawing up Health Improvement Programmes, which will provide the framework within which all local NHS bodies will operate.

## GP fundholders and primary care groups

The GP fundholding scheme was launched in April 1991. Initially the scheme was open to practices with over 9000 patients on their lists. This figure was reduced to 7000, then down further to 5000 in 1996. The scheme enabled large practices to receive funds for the purpose of purchasing health care for the patients on the practice list. The funding was allocated under four headings:

1. staff salaries
2. drugs and appliances
3. hospital services (including diagnostic tests, outpatient and certain inpatient services)
4. community nursing.

The freedom to purchase hospital services was limited initially to outpatient referrals, diagnostic tests and some elective surgery. Fundholders were also expected to maintain traditional referral patterns in the majority of cases. Referrals made outside those agreed with the Health Authorities were to be treated as extra-contractual referrals (ECRs).

Under new plans, primary care groups, comprising all local GPs (including previous GP fundholders and non-fundholders) together with other community professionals, especially nurses, will be responsible for commissioning services for the local community, working closely with social services. Primary care groups may become freestanding primary care Trusts. Pilot sites for primary care groups were set up in 1998.

The services which health authorities and primary health groups are purchasing are provided by:

◆ NHS Trusts
◆ general practice and primary care
◆ providers in the private and voluntary sector.

## NHS Trusts

Under the 1990 Act, the first wave of 57 Trusts came into existence on 1 April 1991. These covered a range of services, including acute hospitals, community services, mental health, learning difficulties and ambulance services. By April 1994, after the fourth wave, the majority of units (some 400) had opted out of Health Authority management and had become NHS Trusts. The remainder became Trusts by 1996.

The main powers and responsibilities of Trusts are as follows:

◆ to provide health services through contracts with Health Authorities and GP fundholders
◆ to manage NHS facilities vested in the Trust
◆ to generate income through commercial activities and private facilities
◆ to employ staff as necessary and determine their remunerations and terms of employment
◆ to provide education and training for NHS staff
◆ to determine its own management structure without needing approval from the Health Authorities, the NHS Executive or the DoH.

### Management of NHS Trusts

Trust Boards comprise a non-executive chairman and a chief executive together with up to five executive and five non-executive directors (Fig. 2.2).

The executive directors of a Trust hospital include:

◆ the Chief Executive
◆ the Director of Finance
◆ the Medical/Clinical Director
◆ the Head of Nursing

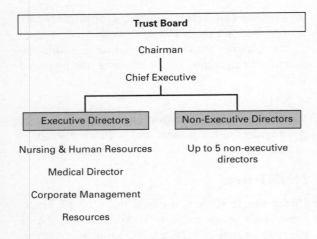

**Figure 2.2** The Trust Board. The tasks of the Trust are to determine overall Trust policies, monitor implementation of those policies and maintain the financial viability of the Trust.

◆ one other director (e.g. of Human Resources, Corporate Affairs, or Quality and Customer Services) or these roles can combined with any of the above.

The chairperson, and the non-executive directors, are not full-time employees of the Trust. These are individuals with particular skills and management experience established outside of the Health Service. Two of the non-executive directors have to be local residents, and the remainder are appointed by the Secretary of State. In cases where the Trust has responsibilities for medical training, one of the non-executive directors has to be a person from the relevant medical school.

Trusts have a duty to comply with public health and patient health and safety regulations. Thus they are expected to comply with guidance on the notification of defects, of adverse reactions to drugs, and of communicable diseases. They also have to participate in emergency and contingency planning.

Unlike private hospitals, Trusts have to respond to quality standards demanded by the Department of Health (DoH) under such initiatives as the Patient's Charter. They have to provide statistical information required by the DoH for the purpose of monitoring. Trusts have to allow access to DoH

and Home Office Inspectors, and to the Community Health Council.

## Trust management structure

The internal management of NHS Trusts may vary depending on the types of hospitals and services provided. Trusts have full autonomy in deciding on their management structure (Fig. 2.3). Most commonly, inpatient services in general hospital Trusts are grouped under specialties which are managed as *directorates*, e.g. medical directorate, child health directorate, etc. These may include one or several wards. Directorates are headed by a Clinical Director, who is assisted by a Senior Nurse and a Business Manager. The Clinical Director is a consultant within that specialty, with management responsibility to ensure that the directorate performs in accordance with plans and objectives agreed by the Chief Executive and the Trust Board. Directorates are given a budget to cover:

◆ staffing costs
◆ drugs and appliances
◆ funds to purchase other clinical support

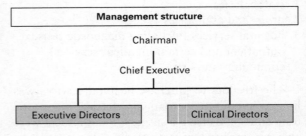

1. Executive Groups – Executive Directors, Clinical Directors and Chief Executive.

2. Operational Group – Executive Directors, General Managers, Service Managers.

**Figure 2.3** The management structure of a Trust. This Trust is divided into directorates, each responsible for carrying out a distinct area of service. Each surgical and medical directorate has a clinical director, who is a consultant in the relevant specialty. The support directorates, which provide support services to surgery and medicine, also have directors. In addition, each directorate has a service/business manager, and there are four general managers with overall responsibility for surgery, medicine, theatres and pathology.

services, e.g. diagnostic and paramedical services

◆ hotel services including domestic, catering and portering and linen services
◆ building and maintenance
◆ administrative costs and supplies.

Other clinical services, e.g. radiography, pathology, physiological measurement, paramedical services, are grouped under functional lines and set up as business units in their own right, with their own budgets and income from the services they provide to the inpatient directorates and to those outside the Trust.

All non-clinical services are organised along functional lines (e.g. estate services, medical records administration, portering services), with functional heads accountable to a Support Services Manager. Hotel services, such as domestic, linen and catering services (and portering and security more recently), have been subject to a programme of competitive tendering first introduced in 1983. All support services are expected to be managed along commercial lines in order to improve efficiency and cost-effectiveness. Trusts are expected to have more flexibility in introducing commercial and business systems prevalent in the business world.

## Community NHS Trusts

Community NHS Trusts provide such services as health visiting, school medical and nursing services, community chiropody, community dentistry, community nursing, child health, family planning, and well-women and well-men services. These generally have a directorate management structure, but directorates are formed along lines of geographical sectors, and directors may not necessarily be from the ranks of doctors. Community NHS Trusts also exist for mental illness and learning disability services. These have internal management arrangements which combine geographical sectorisation and specialty divisions.

### Reflection point

◆ What other kinds of Trusts have you come across? Try looking in your telephone directory under health services and see how many and what kind of trusts are listed there.

Ambulance services and blood transfusion services were previously managed by Regions for groups of user Districts. Ambulance services have been allowed to set themselves up as NHS Trusts. The Blood Transfusion Service has been reorganised under a new Blood Transfusion Authority.

## Ambulance services

Ambulance services are required for the transportation of emergency and urgent cases to hospital, and for inter-hospital transportation. They are also required for a large number of non-emergency cases, e.g. non-ambulant patients being discharged, or being transported to and from outpatient and day hospital attendances. There are around 37 ambulance services in England, 5 in Wales, 1 in Northern Ireland and 1 in Scotland. By 1997 all of these had become NHS Trusts or had become part of a larger Trust.

### Reflection points

◆ If you are working in a Trust or have been involved with a Trust as part of your work experiences, try and find out about its management structure. Many trusts produce brochures explaining their structure. Compare your findings with the roles and functions outlined above.

◆ Try and identify which services have been subject to competitive tendering (e.g. linen services or cleaning). Try and find out whether this has been successful or whether any problems have been experienced.

Non-emergency journeys make up around 80% of all journeys. For instance, during the 1995 financial year the ambulance services in England undertook 3625 million emergency and 14 210 million non-emergency journeys.

Concerns about the ambulance services have in the past been focused on the following:

1. status of an emergency service
2. operational cost-effectiveness
3. response times.

The Patient's Charter requires that, in 95% of cases, emergency ambulances should reach patients within 14 minutes in urban areas and 19 minutes in rural areas. A review of standards in 1996 recommended that more meaningful standards be developed. In the case of the ambulance service the recommendation is that in immediate life-threatening cases response should be within 8 minutes, both in urban and in rural areas.

The ambulance services have undergone considerable changes in the 1980s and early 1990s. A variety of measures have been introduced to improve efficiency.

◆ ambulance controls are fully automated
◆ emergency ambulance vehicles are equipped and manned by specially trained crews with paramedical skills
◆ volunteer drivers and vehicles are used for non-urgent 'hospital transport'
◆ a variety of vehicles, e.g. helicopters, high-speed cars and motorcycles are used to improve response time.

Emphasis is on stabilising the patient on arrival and preparing for transportation to the appropriate service.

Requisitioning an ambulance for a patient in contact with the NHS requires authorisation from the doctor and should specify the type of ambulance required (sitting cases, stretcher, escorted or sole traveller, etc.).

The ambulance service is required to respond to all 999 calls made by members of the public. All calls are logged automatically. In April 1997, four ambulance services (Essex, Derbyshire, Berkshire and West Midlands) were identified as advanced sites for the introduction of 'priority dispatching'.

Subsequently it is expected that all ambulance controls will be able to prioritise 999 calls.

## The blood transfusion service

The national blood transfusion service began in 1946. Currently the service in England is managed by the National Blood Authority (NBA), which was created in 1993 to replace the Central Blood Laboratories Authority and the National Directorate of the National Blood Transfusion Service.

The NBA has become responsible for 15 Regional Transfusion Centres (RTCs) since 1994. The objectives of the NBA are to:

◆ maintain and promote blood and blood product supply based on a system of voluntary donors
◆ implement a cost-effective national strategy to ensure adequate supply
◆ meet national needs
◆ ensure high standards of safety and quality
◆ ensure cost-efficient operation of the Blood Centres, the Bio-Products Laboratory and the International Blood Group Reference Laboratory as parts of the national service.

Under plans approved in 1995 to reorganise the blood service, there are now three geographical zones with administration centres in Bristol, Leeds and Colindale (North London). Bulk processing and testing is being consolidated in 10 centres but the 15 centres retain various functions in addition to storing and supplying functions. A national computer system has been introduced to improve organisation of donation, inventory and stock control.

The NHS uses around 5000 litres of blood a day and demand has been rising by around 4% each year. Only 5% of the population are donors, hence the NBA's struggle is constantly to recruit and retain more donors. Blood also has a relatively short shelf-life, and also needs to be compatible with the recipient's own blood group. There are four main blood groups A, B, O and AB, with either rhesus-positive or rhesus-negative type. Group O negative is a universal type and can be given in an emergency to anyone. In the UK the majority of people are of A and O blood groups.

A major change in blood transfusion therapy has been 'component therapy', enabling patients to be supplied with the specific blood product they require. There are a number of different blood products as follows:

◆ *Red blood cells* contain haemoglobin, which carries oxygen around the body. These are used in cases of anaemia and during operations. Red blood cells have a shelf-life of 35 days.

◆ *White cells* are essential for fighting infections and are given to patients who for one reason or another have insufficient amounts or who are unable to produce their own.

◆ *Platelets* are essential in the clotting process and are used in the treatment of leukemia. Platelets last for 3 to 5 days only.

◆ *Plasma* is a liquid with many useful components including factor VIII, needed for treatment of haemophilia, human albumen used in the treatment of severe burns, immunoglobulins used against infectious diseases like measles and hepatitis.

The Blood Centres are reimbursed by the hospitals for the products ordered and used.

**Reflection point**

◆ How does the blood service manage when supplies are low? Have you been aware of advertising either locally or nationally for blood? Make sure you know what your blood type is and be aware that it is enormously important that individuals volunteer to give blood.

## General practitioner services

General practitioners in the UK are independent contractors who provide services through contracts of services held with the NHS. As such, they are not employees of the NHS, but self-employed professionals, a significant number of whom work as partners in group practices. Among the ranks of general practitioners are included the following:

◆ 30 000 family doctors or GPs
◆ 15 000 dentists
◆ 11 000 opticians
◆ 10 000 retail pharmacists.

Since 1948 contracts for these were administered by organisations directly responsible to the Ministry of Health. Initially these organisations were called Executive Committees, subsequently renamed as Family Practitioner Committees in 1974, then renamed Family Health Services Authorities in 1991. The essential functions of these had been:

◆ to assess the health needs of their local population
◆ to maintain a register of patients on GP lists
◆ to reimburse practitioners for work done
◆ to assess the needs of the local population
◆ to develop services in collaboration with other Health Authorities and general practitioners
◆ investigate complaints relating to breaches of the contracts of service
◆ to implement health policies as issued by the DoH.

In the 1990s FHSAs were given a more proactive twin-role of enabling their local populations to obtain the services they needed and assisting practices to develop services to the standards demanded. In 1996 FHSAs and DHAs were amalgamated, thereby unifying the Health Authorities' purchasing, planning and monitoring functions.

GPs had previously been paid by a combination of capitation fee (i.e. based on the number of patients on the GP's list) and a number of fees for items of service. GPs were also entitled to claim reimbursement for practice expenses such as renting of premises, employment of receptionists, cleaning, heating, lighting. In 1990 new contract terms were introduced, including 'target payments'. For details of the 1990 contract see Box 2.1.

Full details of remuneration and reimbursement can be found in the 'Red Book' (see Chapter 7).

The general practitioner services have been the traditional area where successive governments have introduced charges. Currently charges are collected from patients for the following:

| Box 2.1 | Main changes in GPs' contract (1990) |
| --- | --- |

1. Doctors should be available for at least 26 hours a week

2. Target payments introduced for immunisation and cervical screening programmes thus replacing item of service fees previously applied in these areas

3. A new postgraduate education allowance introduced

4. GPs will receive supplements to reflect the 'Merit Award' system for hospital consultants

5. A special allowance introduced for GPs who teach students within their practices

6. Higher rate for GPs who do their own night visits

7. Removal of restrictions on the type and number of staff that can be employed in a practice

8. Arrangements for women GPs unable to return to full-time work

9. Regular health screening to be provided by GPs for the over 75s

10. More health promotion clinics to be provided for which special payments can be claimed

11. Payments for minor surgical procedures, e.g., removal of warts.

◆ each item on GP prescription dispensed
◆ eye tests and dispensing of spectacles
◆ dental care received.

Children, pregnant women, nursing mothers and the poor on income support are exempted from most of these charges. Those with chronic conditions are also entitled to discounts on prescription charges.

GPs hold a central role in primary care. It is estimated that on average 4.4 visits per year are made per person to GPs. On average the GP list size is around 2000 patients per GP. Practices may be based on private premises owned or rented by the practice or in health centres designed and built by Health Authorities to accommodate as required the full primary care team. GPs work closely with other members of the 'primary care team' to provide a range of preventative and curative services. These days most practices have health visitors attached to them. Other professionals working closely with them include district nurses, community midwives, community psychiatric nurses, chiropodists, therapists and social workers. (The primary health care team is discussed further in Chapter 15.) In order to provide a more comprehensive service in the surgery, practice nurses are employed to undertake a range of duties such as health education, health checks, counselling as well as nursing procedures. Services provided by GPs are listed in Box 2.2.

GPs have been encouraged to expand the range of services they provide, by undertaking some of the minor procedures which before were

| Box 2.2 | Services provided by GPs |
| --- | --- |

◆ Diagnosing and treating common illnesses

◆ Referrals as required to the hospital and specialist services

◆ Certification of incapacity and fitness for work

◆ Health check-ups

◆ Cervical smears

◆ Health promotion clinics

◆ Family planning clinics

◆ Immunisation

◆ Maternity services

◆ Minor surgery

◆ Counselling

◆ Medical examinations at a charge for a number of personal purposes. e.g., insurance, seat belt exemptions, etc.

◆ Complementary therapies, e.g. acupuncture, homeopathy

dealt with by the accident and emergency (A&E) departments of local hospitals. Most large practices now employ practice managers to assist the GPs in managing the 'business' of the practice. Additionally, considerable investment has been made in computer systems to improve the information gathering and processing to ensure that claims for work done are accurate and verifiable. Practices are encouraged to produce practice brochures and information leaflets to inform local residents about the range of services they provide.

The reforms in the 1990s were designed to strengthen the role of GPs in the NHS. GPs as the key members of the primary care team act as gatekeepers in the majority of cases for patients requiring secondary and tertiary care. GPs play a key role in making decisions about the referral of their patients to hospital consultants, and to specialist units. The 1994 *Towards a Primary Care-led NHS* policy document made it clear that GPs will play a crucial role in this area – not only in providing individual care but also by extending their influence in the purchasing process. Additionally, working with other community professionals, they will be likely to be involved in increasing the types of services which they can offer.

A fuller discussion of the main issues for medical secretaries working in general practice is provided in Part 4.

### Reflection point

◆ From your work experience or personal contact, find out what services are offered by different GPs in your area. Try and get the opportunity to ask members of staff how these services have been developed or extended over the last ten years. You may come across rural practices that are operating as satellite outpatient departments, working with visiting consultants. Try to find out more about these new flexible arrangements.

## The private sector

The private sector has been a small but important part of health care in the UK. In the 1980s, with the application of tight finance in the NHS and various incentives given by government, the private and voluntary sector received a major boost. By 1990 it was estimated that the private and voluntary sector provided up to 15% of all health care beds in the UK.

The private sector is made up of private hospitals and facilities (which include profit-making and non-profit-making organisations) and private health insurance. It provides an alternative to the NHS for those willing and able to pay. It is intended to offer its patients greater choice, a generally better standard of hotel services and less worry about waiting for operations. In some cases it complements existing NHS services by providing services at a charge which the NHS is unwilling or unable to provide (e.g. some types of cosmetic surgery).

Before the 1980s, the major providers of private inpatient services in the UK were the non-profit hospitals (e.g. Nuffield, BUPA); in 1979 these made up 72% of the sector. In the 1980s a number of for-profit companies expanded (e.g. AMI, Human Inc., Charter Medical), increasing the number of private hospital beds to near saturation point by the end of the decade, with reports of companies making losses due to overprovision.

The most dramatic increases of the 1980s had been in the private nursing and residential home beds. These increases had been due to:

◆ a government squeeze on NHS and local authority spending
◆ a guarantee of social security support for patients discharged to private homes
◆ pursuit of long-standing policy of transferring care for the mentally ill and those with learning difficulties to the community, creating demands for nursing home places
◆ implementation of hospital closure programmes.

Private nursing homes may also be run by voluntary organisations with charity status.

## The voluntary sector

The voluntary sector has existed by the side of the NHS in order to provide services and undertake research into particular conditions which the NHS has not been able to provide. The majority of these rely on voluntary donations, and contributions from statutory bodies. The Marie Curie Foundation and the Macmillan Foundation are voluntary organisations which provide community nursing services for patients with cancer. St Christopher's Hospices are hospice services for the terminally ill funded by the voluntary sector. These organisations are all run as charities, relying on fundraising to pay for the services they provide.

Considerable criticisms were aimed at the National Lottery when it was first launched for adversely affecting the voluntary organisations that support health services. It is expected that in time more community-based projects will be supported by National Lottery funds. The government has indicated that lottery money will be used to fund health projects such as developing health advice and fitness centres.

It is also likely that reduced resources within the NHS mean that the voluntary organisations will be relied upon more and more to fill the gaps.

### Reflection points

◆ Discuss with colleagues what kind of services might be funded via the lottery and why.

◆ Find out about voluntary services available in your area by consulting the telephone directory. For example, is there a hospice in your area?

# ISSUES FACING THE NHS

## Funding

The cost of the NHS has been a major preoccupation for all governments. Box 2.3 lists the measures that governments have taken to try and control the cost to the taxpayer.

---

**Box 2.3** Government measures to control costs in the NHS

◆ Introducing charges for certain services

◆ Applying strong budgetary control

◆ Implementing cost reduction and efficiency measures

◆ Introducing an 'enterprise culture'

◆ Introducing business management

◆ Introducing an 'internal market' and competition

◆ Creating incentives for the private and voluntary sector

◆ Shifting some of the service burden to the voluntary sector

◆ Creating incentives for private health insurance

---

The increases in management costs that the new NHS has seen have been justified on the grounds that the NHS had been previously 'undermanaged'. Measures announced in 1992 aimed to reduce the increase in management manpower by streamlining top-level management. Under the Labour government, commitment has been made to reduce drastically the cost of management bureaucracy within the NHS and to divert these funds to direct patient care. The first measure in this respect has been the suspension of the next wave of GP fundholding in 1997 and diverting the management costs involved into specific areas of patient care.

Whatever measures are taken, demand for limited resources will continue to grow and resource-constraints will continue to be the biggest influence on the health service.

## Consumer focus

One of the worrying observations of the reformed NHS is that several of the Trusts have not been able to meet the performance standards set out under the Patient's Charter. There has also been severe criticism of the way that some of the Charter targets have been trivialised, namely the introduction of so-called 'hello nurses' in A&E departments instead of genuine improvement of waiting time in the department. New charter standards and developments in both national and local accountability to patients and other users of services will be a major influence on services.

## The primary care-led NHS?

Maintaining a balance between preventative and curative care (balance between primary, secondary and tertiary care) and between the acute/glamorous/high-tech and the so-called 'Cinderella' services (mental health/care of the elderly) has been a major concern. Additionally, the government is committed to encouraging prevention through the promotion of healthier lifestyles. Public health and the primary-care-led NHS are two challenges for services which are likely to influence future developments.

## CONCLUSIONS

This chapter has outlined the present structure of the NHS, and has given some indication of how it is likely to develop in the future. Changes in the way in which local health services are delivered are likely to have a significant impact on the way that GP practices work and therefore it is important to keep abreast of developments. Furthermore, an understanding of how services are accountable will help all medical secretaries to appreciate the importance of their role and function in the effective delivery of quality health services.

### Exercises

◆ In addition to the further reading suggested below, it is also recommended that you keep up to date with current affairs as they relate to the health service and, if possible, seek further information through one of the health service related journals such as *The Health Service Journal*, which is available from most good newsagents.

◆ When you are at work or on a practice placement, ask to see any information relating to the management structure and roles, such as the Trust handbook or practice leaflet.

## FURTHER READING

Drury M, Hobden-Clarke L 1994 The practice manager. Radcliffe Medical Press, Oxford

Ham C 1994 Management and competition in the new NHS. Radcliffe Medical Press, Oxford

Ham C 1990 The new NHS. Radcliffe Medical Press, Oxford

HMSO 1998 The new NHS – Modern. Dependable (White Paper). HMSO, London

HMSO 1988 Our healthier nation (Green Paper). HMSO, London

Johnson N 1990 Reconstructing the Welfare State – a decade of change 1980–1990. Harvester Wheatsheaf, London

NHS Confederation. 1997 NHS handbook 1997/98. JMH Publishing, London

NHSME 1994 Towards a primary care-led NHS. NHS Management Executive

# 3

# The legislative context of medical secretarial practice

*Vincent Leach and Ingrid Anstey*

## OBJECTIVES

- To outline the basic principles of laws and rights
- To describe the issues involved in trespass and negligence
- To explain the laws that are specific to health service procedures
- To consider how to deal with complaints
- To examine the main aspects of employment law.

## INTRODUCTION

All citizens of the state are subject to the law. There are additional rules and regulations for workers in health care. This chapter gives a brief overview of the different types of law and how they affect the health service, your fellow health professionals and your role as a medical secretary. On completion of this chapter you should have some knowledge of the law as it affects health care workers and be aware of some of the legal pitfalls which may be met. If a legal opinion is required the appropriate authority must be consulted.

Before reading this chapter you may find it useful to:

- look for some pamphlets on health and safety at work
- obtain any instructions that are available concerning complaints at your place of work
- obtain copies of the Patient's Charter, your Health Authority charter standards, your practice charter, even if not employed in general practice.

## THE LAW AND YOU

The advances in modern medicine, and the increased knowledge of medical matters via the media, have increased people's expectations of health care. When these expectations are not achieved, there is an increasing tendency to complain and to go to law to claim compensation. Consequently, it is essential that all workers in health care have some knowledge of the legal framework within which they work, and the legal pitfalls they may meet. Although legal matters are primarily the responsibility of the health care professionals, as an essential member of the health care team, the medical secretary has a responsibility to ensure the efficient management of the team, and to look after the interests of colleagues and people using the service.

## Civil liberties and rights

All laws develop originally from the law of rights, which has a long history going back to Magna Carta in England, the declarations of the French Revolution and of the American Independence. Essentially these are:

◆ the right to life
◆ the right to freedom, including freedom from interference, and freedom of movement
◆ freedom of speech and right of assembly
◆ equality under the law and the right to a fair trial
◆ the right to privacy
◆ the right to health and happiness, including a standard of living to achieve health and well-being
◆ the right to own property.

These have been incorporated in the United Nations Declaration of Universal Human Rights. They might be called the fundamental human rights, but there are additional civil rights, which might vary in different countries. In the United Kingdom we have civil rights such as:

◆ the right to free health care
◆ the right to free education
◆ the right to have clean air and water.

From these rights laws have been enacted and breaking these laws may bring about penalties. It should be noted that as yet the European Convention on Human Rights has not been incorporated into English law. However, as a member of the European Union, we are subject to the Treaty of Rome and to the European Court of Justice.

## STATUTE LAW AND COMMON LAW

There are two sources of law:

◆ statute law, which relates to laws as laid down in Acts of Parliament
◆ common law, which relates to how these laws are modified in courts of law. Statute law will be taken over common law in any conflict between the two.

Both statute law and common law divide into criminal law and civil law.

Statute law is laid down by Parliament in Acts of Parliament.

### Reflection point

◆ Take a few minutes to think of some laws that have been laid down by Parliament and are therefore statute law. There are plenty, covering, for example, traffic offences, wearing seat belts, dangerous drugs. What is the most recent law that you are aware of?

Common law is the way that the law is modified and evolves. This is by cases that have been sent to court and interpretations made of statute law and previous cases. This is especially so where a case has gone to the Court of Appeal and the House of Lords. The House of Lords in its judicial capacity is the highest court in the country. The House of Lords will give a judgment where there is a significant point of law at stake. Tony Bland was severely brain damaged in the Hillsborough disaster. He was in a persistent vegetative state (PVS). The House of Lords decided that his life was of no value to him and that hydration and nutrition could be withheld. This ruling was necessary to prevent his doctors being charged with murder because they caused his 'death' by starvation. Certain cases may also go to the European Court of Justice.

# CRIMINAL LAW

Criminal law is punitive law initiated by the state against an individual. Some examples of the matters covered by criminal law include:

◆ to protect persons and animals from violence and cruelty
◆ to protect vulnerable members of society against abuse of person and property
◆ to prevent offence to others, for example public nuisances
◆ to protect property, for example against theft and damage.

A health care worker is just as liable to prosecution for theft as a burglar entering your home. There are occasions when the apparently innocent action of a secretary may be misinterpreted. For example, taking the possessions of a person in hospital for safe keeping may be misconstrued and accusations laid against the secretary. This is perhaps more likely when dealing with a confused or forgetful person. Always follow the correct procedures, including signatures where necessary, to prevent this unfortunate mishap. Administering an injection without consent could lead to a charge of assault. Carelessness during an operation causing the death of a patient could lead to a charge of manslaughter, as this would constitute gross negligence.

---

**Reflection point**

◆ From your experience think of examples where actions may be misconstrued or where if things go wrong there may be a criminal offence. Think about the following example: You are working as a ward clerk. It is a busy day with new patients arriving for admission and other patients being discharged. You notice that lockers are not being checked because of the speed of turnover – what might the consequences be? What if you notice a nurse taking a watch and some money from an elderly patient's locker. In what ways could you interpret this act? What sort of procedure should be carried out here?

---

Intentions may be critical in deciding whether or not there is legal culpability. For example, in the terminally ill cancer patient the only way of controlling the pain might be with a very high dose of morphine which could prove to be fatal. In this case, the intention is clearly to control pain and not to kill and death is the unintended, possibly unfortunate, side-effect.

Taking a person's property and putting it in a safe for safe keeping might be acceptable, if the person could not give consent. But, putting the property in your locker for safe keeping could easily be open to several interpretations. If the property was found in your home, your good intentions would be very difficult to prove. So the facts of a case may be used to infer intentions even if the act was intended innocently.

# CIVIL LAW

Civil law covers situations where individuals seek recompense for a harm that has been done to them. Civil law defines the rights and duties of individuals to one another and provides a system of remedies such as actions to award damages to compensate the wronged individual. Civil courts do not punish the wrongdoer, they only assess the level of damage and the compensation which must be paid. If a wrong act is committed under civil law it is known as a tort, as opposed to a crime, which is a wrongdoing committed under criminal law.

These torts include the following categories of special interest in health care:

◆ trespass
◆ negligence.

## Trespass to the person

### The law

Trespass to the person is also known as battery. Battery is defined as intentional physical contact with another person in a way which is known to be objectionable to that person. Trespass is an extremely important and complex concept in the medical context and the following points will indicate why.

◆ Not all touching is trespass, but if physical contact is deemed to be offensive, aggressive or invasive it could be considered to be trespass.

◆ Trespass does not have to result in actual physical harm in order to be battery. Just touching somebody could be considered trespass if it were done in an offensive or aggressive way.

◆ If *consent* to be touched is granted then there is no claim for trespass or battery. Consent is discussed in detail below, but it should be noted that it can be either expressed or implied, and oral or written.

◆ Trespass to the person also includes assault and false imprisonment.

There are exceptions in the law, for example in cases where people may need to be restrained in order to avoid being a danger to themselves or to others. No battery is committed where such acts are based on lawful authority.

## The medical context

All forms of physical treatment require the patient's consent. Medical treatment can be considered battery without this consent. For consent to be valid:

◆ the patient must be informed, i.e. an explanation by the medical practitioner as to the general nature and purpose of the proposed treatment.

◆ the patient must be competent, i.e. they must be capable of understanding what is being proposed

◆ the patient must be willing; their consent is not valid if it has been coerced, or induced by mistake.

## Consent

Consent is a subject that presents legal and ethical problems. Essentially it is a legal matter first and foremost. There can be difficulties deciding when consent has been given to prevent a charge of trespass. One of the main issues is that consent has to be *informed*; what constitutes informed consent?

Consider the following situations.

◆ If a person has a learning handicap or is mentally ill what level of information is required?

◆ In the case of children at what age may they be considered competent to make a decision?

◆ Was enough information given for the person to be able to understand the possible consequences of the investigation or treatment? What information should be given about side-effects before a drug is prescribed? Consultations would be excessively long if every possible side-effect had to be discussed in great detail before writing a prescription.

Some exceptions are listed below.

◆ In some circumstances a court may compel treatment, say, in the case of a child who needs a blood transfusion and the parents are Jehovah's Witnesses and refuse treatment. An application could be made for the child to be made a ward of court and then the court may give permission for the treatment to go ahead.

◆ A special case is where a person is mentally ill and is treated against his will. The Mental Health Act will be discussed in a separate section.

◆ Before operations it is usual for the patient to sign a consent form for a particular operation. If the surgeon finds a different condition or an additional condition, what is he or she to do?

◆ There can be implied consent: holding out one's arm for a blood sample to be taken may be construed as consent.

The legal principles allow that young people can agree to medical treatment, without the consent of their parents, provided they can understand the nature and the consequences of the treatment and the consequences of not having the treatment. A more difficult situation is where a young or incompetent person refuses life-saving treatment. Young or incompetent persons may be judged not to understand the consequences of their decisions and others are obliged to make the decision for them. Sometimes where there is conflict only a court of law may make the decision.

## Relevance to the medical secretary's role

As a secretary, you may be involved in ensuring that consent has been given before a procedure is performed.

> **Reflection points**
>
> ◆ You are working in a GP practice where minor surgery is carried out regularly under local anaesthetic. Is it necessary to have written consent?
>
> ◆ While you are in work placements check the procedures for obtaining patient consent and which members of staff are involved in this. How old must you be to sign your own consent?

As you will have seen from the examples and reflection points given above, consent is a very important concept to understand. It particularly relates to two duties you may be performing as part of your role.

**Chaperone duties.** You may be required to 'sit in' while the doctor or nurse treats or examines the patient, to witness the examination and what has taken place. Medical practitioners are presented with a particular problem where a patient's competence may be in question, for example:

◆ teenagers unaccompanied by their parents
◆ patients with mental disorders
◆ elderly patients.

In the event of the trespass or battery allegation, you may therefore be required to give evidence.

**Consent forms.** Patients are required to complete consent forms before operations. A sample consent form is illustrated in Figure 3.1. You may be asked to get the form signed. This is a very important task, and you must be careful that the consent given is valid. If in doubt, or if the patient is in doubt, you must refer back to the relevant medical staff. The consultant may need to discuss the proposed operation with the patient again. It is

not your role to discuss the patient's concerns with him or her. All decisions on matters of consent must be made by relevant clinical professionals as they are ultimately accountable for decisions of this kind.

## Negligence

Negligence is perhaps the most common tort or wrongdoing that confronts the individual working in a health care setting.

### The law

In law, negligence means failing to take reasonable care to avoid acts or omissions that you can reasonably foresee would be likely to injure another person. Injury in this context is taken to mean failure to achieve a desired outcome; such as a live birth or successful operation or other treatment. Failing to take reasonable care could be failure to examine properly, failure to carry out appropriate investigations or carrying out medical or surgical procedures incompetently. There are two points which need to be kept in mind when considering negligence:

◆ the fact that the harm is foreseeable gives rise to 'a duty of care' towards the person
◆ there must be actual harm done.

### The medical context

All health care professionals have a duty of care towards the patients they treat. The standard of care expected of them is that of the reasonably skilled and experienced medical person, i.e. a doctor or nurse must exercise the medical skills that would be expected of any competent doctor or nurse.

A doctor, nurse or any other health care professional breaches this duty if:

◆ They fail to inform the patient of any risks that might reasonably be anticipated as a result of the proposed treatments. (Note: if a patient, having been informed, then agrees to the treatment, he or she has consented to the risks involved and therefore cannot complain if they occur.)

**SAMPLE CONSENT FORM**
For medical or dental investigation, treatment or operation

Health Authority ..................................................    Patient's Surname ................................................

Hospital ...............................................................    Other Names ......................................................

Unit Number .......................................................    Date of Birth .....................................................
Sex: (*Please tick*) Male    Female

**DOCTORS OR DENTISTS** (*This part to be completed by doctor or dentist.*)

*See notes on the reverse*

**Type of operation, investigation or treatment for which written evidence of consent is considered appropriate**

I confirm that I have explained the operation, investigation or treatment, and such appropriate options as are available and the type of anaesthetic, if any (general/local/sedation) proposed, to the patient in terms which in my judgment are suited to the understanding of the patient and/or to one of the parents or guardians of the patient.

Signature ....................................................    Date ...................................................................

Name of doctor or dentist ..............................................................................................................

**PATIENT/PARENT/GUARDIAN**
1. Please read this form and the notes overleaf very carefully.
2. If there is anything that you don't understand about the explanation, or if you want more information, you should ask the doctor or dentist.
3. Please check that all the information on the form is correct. If it is, and you understand the explanation, then sign the form.

I am the patient/parent/guardian (*delete as necessary*).

I agree
- ◆ to what is proposed which has been explained to me by the doctor/dentist named on this form.
- ◆ to the use of the type of anaesthetic that I have been told about.

I understand
- ◆ that the procedure may not be done by the doctor/dentist who has been treating me so far.
- ◆ that any procedure in addition to the investigation or treatment described on this form will only be carried out if it is necessary and in my best interests and can be justified for medical reasons.

I have told
- ◆ the doctor or dentist about the procedures listed below I would *not* wish to be carried out straightaway without my having the opportunity to consider them first.

..................................................................................................................

..................................................................................................................

Signature        ...........................................................................................................

Name              ...........................................................................................................

Address           ...........................................................................................................

(*if not the patient*)  ...............................................................................................

**Figure 3.1**  A sample consent form.

◆ The treatment itself is carried out in such a way that it falls short of what is to be expected from a competent health professional.

◆ The standard of treatment falls below what would be consistent with current practice, i.e. medical knowledge or the use of equipment or drugs must be up to date and generally used and accepted by the medical professional as a whole. Competent health professionals are *not* required to provide innovative treatment.

In general practice, it is the GP and in the hospital, the Health Authority who are legally responsible for the conduct of all their employees. This is known as vicarious liability and it means that they are liable for any negligent acts of other professionals working for them. However, all team members have a requirement to fulfil their individual duties adequately.

Sometimes, however, employees can also be responsible for their negligent acts along with their employer. Under the Occupiers Liability Act 1957, both GPs and Health Authorities have a duty of care towards visitors to ensure their safety whilst on their premises. Note that there is a higher duty of care towards children, and special care must be taken to ensure that they come to no harm. As a medical secretary, you may be responsible for ensuring that equipment and drugs are well out of reach, and that the premises that you work on are kept safe and clean. (See also Chapters 10, 15 and 17 on general practice and safety in the clinical environment.)

### Relevance to the medical secretary's role

You may feel that the question of negligence is a matter for the health care professionals and outwith the role of the medical secretary. It must be emphasised again that the secretary is an essential member of the health care team.

Legal responsibility for the patient does not begin or end with the medical treatment required. GPs and local health authorities have a duty to ensure that all aspects of patient care are competently handled, and this includes the relevant paperwork and all communication with patients.

---

**Box 3.1**  Administrative tasks that medical secretaries may be responsible for

◆ Patient phone calls
◆ Front desk attendance
◆ Registering new patients
◆ Admitting patients into hospital
◆ Processing clinical data
◆ General clerical tasks
◆ Emergency appointments
◆ Keeping accurate medical records

---

If you were to send the wrong notes to theatre, a person may have the wrong leg amputated. A misspelling in a discharge letter may mean the GP prescribes the wrong medication. Omitting to send a referral letter may mean a person needing urgent treatment suffers unduly or even dies. An X-ray is useless unless the clinician receives the result at the right time. The clinical notes are essential to ensure the clinician has all the relevant facts of a case. The notes are of no value if they are lost in transit between one department and another.

Legally, medical secretaries also have a requirement to fulfil their individual duties adequately. Surgeries and hospitals may list administrative tasks which staff can refer to when necessary (Box 3.1). An agreed standard policy will exist for many of these duties.

As a medical secretary you have a crucial role in many of these tasks.

*There is only one golden rule – if in any doubt consult you employer or superior.*

## LAWS SPECIFIC TO HEALTH SERVICE PROCEDURES

There is a whole range of laws and regulations covering health care. The following sections deal with some of the most important for you to know about as a medical secretary and your role in ensuring that the proper procedures are observed.

# Pregnancy

## The law

In pregnancy, the woman's GP owes her a duty, not only to safeguard her own well-being, but to ensure the healthy development of the baby. In the event, however, that there is a conflict between the mother's health and that of the unborn child, the doctor's primary consideration must be for the mother, but he or she is expected to minimise the risks of harm to the fetus as well.

In childbirth, it is a criminal offence for anyone other than a registered practitioner or midwife to assist at a birth except in an emergency. Although the mother is lawfully entitled to give birth alone, she risks prosecution for gross negligence manslaughter if the baby subsequently dies. The key points to note are:

◆ Doctors/nurses can be liable for negligence where incompetence harms either the mother or the child.
◆ Consent must be obtained from the woman for any invasive antenatal treatments. Consent is implied, however, for any treatment which takes places during the birth itself.
◆ Any refusal of treatment must be respected, unless in order to save lives doctors must risk committing battery. Their defence would be that it is a necessity, or that the woman is deemed incompetent to refuse.

## The medical secretary's role

GP surgeries commonly have an antenatal programme consisting of a series of check-ups, tests and examinations. The relevant forms generally include Item 1: A maternity care sheet and Item 2: A maternity care pack. The two main administrative duties are:

◆ ensuring the forms are correctly completed, particularly information relating to midwifery services, and sections of the forms relating to patient details for blood tests, other clinical tests and screening
◆ making sure appointments are made and are being kept. This is particularly relevant to midwife bookings.

On hospital admission, it is important to check:

◆ that medical records contained in the pregnancy pack are present
◆ that the patient has been informed of the hospital facilities
◆ that all admission forms are complete and correct
◆ that medical staff have received all clinical and personal data.

If on admission a patient informs you that she objects to certain medical procedures being used (for example the use of particular drugs during delivery), you must ensure that the medical staff know of this so that they can discuss this further with the patient if necessary.

# Termination of pregnancy

## The law

The Abortion Act of 1967 introduced lawful termination, but it contains strict provisions as to when such a termination can be performed, and by whom.

The key points to note are:

◆ special rules apply in emergency cases
◆ fathers have no legal rights to prevent termination
◆ medical staff can be exempt from participating in a termination if they have expressed their conscientious objection to such procedures
◆ the termination must be carried out in a place specified by the law, i.e. a registered clinic or hospital.

## The medical issues

The Abortion Act states that a termination is lawful when two registered medical practitioners are of the opinion that the particular case meets at least one of the following criteria:

◆ there is a risk to the woman of physical or mental injury (before 24 weeks)
◆ there is a risk of grave permanent damage to her physical or mental health.

Decisions based on these criteria are not restricted to clinical assessment alone but can include environmental factors too. Other criteria include:

◆ the risk of loss of life is greater if the pregnancy is continued than if it is terminated.
◆ there is a substantial risk that the child born would suffer from such physical or mental abnormalities as to be seriously handicapped (this judgment may not be based purely on the medical assessment). Other adverse risks can be considered if the pregnancy continues, for example, the mother's ability to cope with, and adequately care for, existing children, especially if a severely handicapped child is born.

### The medical secretary's role

Once more, it is essential that the administrative duties around termination are carried out competently and accurately. This includes:

◆ Ensuring appointments are correctly made. This is particularly important when the length of pregnancy is an issue, and where the patient may require counselling.
◆ Checking consent forms are currently completed and signed.

## Procedures on the death of a patient

### The law

In law there is a distinction made between natural death in ordinary circumstances and exceptional death, where death has occurred through unnatural causes or in exceptional circumstances or both.

Procedures regulating a normal death are contained in the Births and Deaths Registration Act 1953. Procedures regulating exceptional deaths are contained in both the 1953 legislation and the Coroners' Act 1988. Box 3.2 lists the deaths that are reportable to the coroner.

Note also the Human Tissue Act 1961. This regulates organ donation, post-mortem and bodies donated for teaching purposes.

| **Box 3.2** Deaths reportable to the coroner |
| --- |
| 1. Deceased not attended by doctor in last illness |
| 2. Deceased not attended by doctor in last 14 days of illness |
| 3. Cause unknown |
| 4. Death unexpectedly sudden |
| 5. Death due to disease or poisoning |
| 6. Unnatural courses (rare diseases) |
| 7. A violence (accidents, murder, manslaughter, infanticide) |
| 8. Neglect |
| 9. Abortion |
| 10. Suspicious circumstances |
| 11. In police custody or prison |

### The medical context

There is a standard procedure in the event of a normal death. The doctor issues a death certificate which is sent to the registrar and retains a counterfoil certificate. The informant (normally a relative or hospital secretary) notifies the registrar of the deceased's details, applying if relevant for permission to cremate the deceased as well.

Documents required for cremation include an application form (obtainable from the registrar or funeral director/undertaker) confirming the deceased's consent and that death is due to natural causes. Other forms that are required include:

◆ medical certificate from deceased's GP, disclosing any interest in the deceased (e.g. the deceased's estate)
◆ medical certificate issued by an independent senior practitioner, or pathologist in the event of a post-mortem.

The registrar enters the death on the register and issues a disposal certificate. The procedure in the event of an exceptional death is as follows. The doctor issues the certificate, initialling Box A that he is reporting to the coroner and sends this to the registrar. The informant sends details to the registrar. The coroner receives the GP's or hospital doctor's report by phone and the official report from the registrar and he or she can either:

◆ take no further action and report to the registrar, who will then enter the death and issue a disposal certificate
◆ order a post-mortem and take no further action – again reporting back to the registrar
◆ order an inquest.

The inquest in an investigative process is aimed at establishing (usually publicly) the cause of death. The verdict can include: death by misadventure, unlawful killing and natural causes. The coroner reports back to the registrar who enters death in the register and issues a disposal certificate.

### The medical secretary's role

Generally speaking, there are few administrative duties required. However, you may be expected as a hospital secretary, in the event of the deceased having no one else, to act as official informant. In this case you should refer to the instructions on the right hand side of the medical certificate, ensuring that you supply the registrar with all the details of the deceased which are required. This includes if possible the deceased's medical card. Alternatively, you may be asked by the bereaved and possibly bewildered relatives to assist in collating and completing the required paperwork.

Finally, the GP or hospital may, in the event of a coroner's inquest, be asked to give medical evidence. You must ensure that all the deceased's medical records are available and up to date. You should also be aware that if the doctor decides in the circumstances of a normal death to arrange a post-mortem by a pathologist you may be required to record the relatives' consent, and prepare the post-mortem report.

## Sickness certificates

### The law

Provision has now been made for patients to complete their own medical certificates, along with the continued practice of using a GP's certificate when required.

### The medical issues

For the first 7 days of illness the patient completes a sickness certificate for:

◆ illness lasting up to 7 days on the seventh day
◆ illness continuing over 7 days immediately.

For any illness that does continue after the seventh day, the GP is required to complete the relevant certificate if in his opinion the patient is unfit for work:

◆ for illness up to 2 weeks
◆ for illness up to 6 months.

### The medical secretary's role

As these certificates are available from surgeries, staff will be required to issue patients' forms for them to complete. Ensure that patients know that the completed certificate must be sent to their local Department of Social Security (DSS) office. You may also be required to assist the doctor in issuing other reports for various purposes including insurance policies.

## The Mental Health Act 1983

### The law

The Mental Health Act 1983 (section 1:2) defines mental disorder as 'mental illness, arrested or incomplete development of mind, psychopathic disorder and any other disorder or disability of mind'.

### The medical context

The Act distinguishes three specific mental disorders:

◆ psychopathic disorders
◆ severe mental impairment
◆ mental impairment.

Patients who voluntarily admit themselves for hospital assessment or treatment are recognised by the act as informal patients, and are free to discharge themselves at any time.

Patients who are compulsorily admitted are either:

◆ detained temporarily – for emergency assessment (72 hours) or for assessment (28 days).
◆ detained on a long-term basis – for treatment initially for a 6-month period subject to reviews.

In cases of compulsory admission:

◆ the patient's mental disorder must be of a nature or degree that makes hospitalisation appropriate
◆ admission is required for the health and safety of the patient or the protection of others.

In cases of psychopathic disorder and severe mental impairment, there must be

◆ evidence of abnormally aggressive or irresponsible conduct
◆ an existing treatment available.

## Admission procedures for treatment

For voluntary patients the procedure is as for admission with physical illness. Compulsory admission requires an application to the hospital by an approved social worker or nearest relative, and a recommendation by two medical practitioners. The following points are also relevant:

◆ the social worker can obtain a displacement order from the county court displacing the nearest relative in the event of incompetence or unreasonable objection to compulsory admission
◆ the recommendation and application legally authorises the hospital manager to detain the patient
◆ court orders are also available in the case of convicted offenders to admit them for psychiatric treatment if the judge considers this appropriate.

## Consent to treatment

As discussed, the general law states that a competent adult has an absolute right to refuse even life-saving treatment. Under the Mental Health Act, voluntary patients retain this right absolutely and all patients retain the right to refuse treatment for physical ailments. Non-consensual treatment administered to compulsorily detained patients is therefore limited to their mental disorder only. The Act specifically safeguards against non-consensual psychosurgery, hormone or electroconvulsive therapy (ECT).

Doctors retain the common law protection of treatment compulsorily administered in the patient's best interest. Additionally, non-consensual but urgent treatment can be administered under certain provisions of the Act.

## Discharge procedures for compulsorily detained patients

The Act authorises certain persons to discharge patients who have been detained compulsorily as follows:

◆ registered medical officer
◆ hospital manager
◆ nearest relative
◆ mental health review tribunal.

Specific procedures are available for reviewing the position of compulsorily detained patients.

## The medical secretary's role

It may be the duty of a medical secretary to fill in relevant documentation for any of these procedures. As always, accuracy is essential. You may also be asked to act in the role of chaperone in some of the situations described above.

## THE GOVERNING BODIES

In addition to the laws of the land, both doctors and nurses are also regulated by their governing bodies, which have statutory power to regulate these professions and to ensure that practitioners who are in breach of these rules are not able to practise. They have a very significant role in protecting the public.

## General Medical Council (GMC)

To function as a medical practitioner of whatever type it is necessary to obtain registration by the GMC. Hence the phrase 'Registered Medical Practitioner'. The GMC has a mixture of medical and lay members, has been set up by Act of Parliament and is concerned with the standards of medical education, and the ethical and professional standards of practising doctors. Doctors who act in an unprofessional way due to ill health may be suspended until they have been adequately treated. If the offence has been a criminal or other serious unprofessional offence, suspension from the medical register may be permanent.

## The United Kingdom Central Council (UKCC)

For nurses, midwives and health visitors the governing body is the United Kingdom Central Council (UKCC). The UKCC has a similar statutory regulatory role to that of the GMC. It is responsible for maintaining the register of professionals who are permitted to practise as nurses and regulates the boundaries of nursing practice. It also provides guidance on ethical issues.

The comparable organisation for medical secretaries is AMSPAR (the Association of Medical Secretaries, Practice Administrators and Receptionists), although it does not have statutory powers over its membership.

Although the issues covered by the UKCC and the GMC may not be directly applicable to the work of a medical secretary, nevertheless all workers in health care have to work in the environment set by the law and the statutory bodies.

# CHARTERS AND COMPLAINTS

Laws are just one aspect of the rules and regulations that protect patients and govern professionals' behaviour in the health service. Another aspect is that patients and other users of the health service have certain rights, such as those covered by the Patient's Charter. This next section looks at these rights, and more importantly at how to deal

with the complaints which may emerge if patients do not feel they have received the respect or treatment they are entitled to.

## The Patient's Charter

The Patient's Charter, which was introduced in 1992, sets standards and encourages people to complain if those standards are not reached. It lays down guidelines for acceptable standards of care to be delivered to patients and their families in all areas of the NHS. It covers waiting times in open waiting areas, acceptable waiting times for surgery or first appointments, the right to emergency treatment and for referral for a second opinion in consultation with a patient's GP. The Charter also gives information about community services, ambulance, dentistry and pharmaceutical services, and has a separate section on the rights and standards that patients should expect from maternity services. The aim is to promote high standards of health care in the UK and underlines the fundamental values of the NHS, alongside the rights of the patient.

**Reflection point**

◆ The Labour government is reviewing the Patient's Charter in order that it should reflect not only patient's rights but also their responsibilities. Look at a copy of the Patient's Charter in an area where you have worked. Can you see how it might change in order to reflect patients' responsibilities?

The Department of Health sets guidelines and standards through initiatives and circulars. Health Authorities, hospitals and GP practices have been encouraged to set up their own charters. In general practice there may be an undertaking to offer emergency appointments immediately or at least on the same day, depending on the degree of urgency, and that no appointment is delayed more than 48 hours.

**Reflection points**

◆ Have you seen (1) your own GP's practice charter; (2) your local hospital's charter?

◆ Do you think charters have improved services? Have they made providers more accountable? Do they inform the general public of their rights or simply increase expectancy? If you get the opportunity it would be useful to discuss this with colleagues, and with other health care professionals.

## Coping with complaints

The first person receiving a complaint is very often the receptionist/secretary. The way the initial complaint is handled can make the difference between a moan or grouse, seeking information and a complaint.

Very often the complainant is merely seeking information as to the reason for a delay or why something appeared to go wrong. Very often the most aggressive complainant is the most frightened or the most upset. Responding by aggression, sarcasm or belittling the complainant makes the aggression worse and verbal abuse may develop into physical abuse. Keeping calm and being prepared to understand the other person's point of view and problem will take the heat out of most situations. Make sure that the complainant understands that the complaint will go to the appropriate authority.

## Complaints in hospital practice

In hospital practice there will be procedures for dealing with complaints and a 'Consumer Relations Officer' who will have the authority and the knowledge and expertise to handle the problem. A sample complaints form is illustrated in Figure 3.2.

A complaint may be referred to the consultant concerned so that the complainant may be offered an explanation or possibly an apology. A com-

plaint about administration, say delay in waiting rooms, may be referred to the manager of the unit. A complaint concerning clinical competence will usually be referred to a panel of doctors and lay persons. Many complaints will go straight to hospital management from the person involved, from a solicitor or from the local Community Health Council. There will normally be an internal mechanism for handling complaints. This mechanism varies from hospital to hospital.

**Reflection point**

◆ Many Trusts have a 'complaints, suggestions or compliments' brochure – what are they trying to suggest here? Try to obtain a copy and find out who is involved in any procedures – which of the above three are going to require procedures?

## General practice complaints

In general practice there should be a procedure for handling complaints and this became obligatory from 1 April 1996. If it is a complaint over appointments or obtaining repeat prescriptions, the appropriate person to handle the complaint may be the practice manager. On clinical matters the medical partners should handle the complaint. The ultimate responsibility lies with the medical partnership and the involvement of a partner is often essential.

If the complaint cannot be satisfactorily dealt with at practice level then the complainant, who may not be the patient, may take the complaint to the Health Authority. Box 3.3 lists ways in which the complaint might be settled.

## The Health Service Commissioner (the ombudsman)

Essentially the ombudsman is the final appeal when other mechanisms have failed to produce a fair result for a complainant. All other mechanisms for complaining, outside the law, must have

**HELP US TO *HELP* YOU**

**HOW TO 'COMPLAIN, MAKE SUGGESTIONS OR COMPLIMENT US'**

*The Newtown Health Care NHS Trust is committed to looking at ways to improve our service to you. You can help us by telling us what you think of the services we provide, good or bad.*

- If you have any suggestions, comments or complaints to make about the services we provide, and the way we provide them, we would be happy to hear from you. We value your comments and can use them when making changes to our services.
- You can use this form to write your comments or complaints on.
- If you need any help or advice to fill in this form, the ward or department staff would be pleased to help you.
- You may wish to contact the Community Health Council for free Independent Advice.

*Community Health Council, Mid-Town Road, Newtown NT2 2PG. Telephone 01999 624 610*

**YOU CAN MAKE YOUR COMPLAINT BY FOLLOWING THESE GUIDELINES**

1) If something happens which causes you concern, we would like to try and put it right straight away. Our staff will make every effort to address your concerns and sort out your problems. If they cannot help, they will arrange for you to speak to someone who can.
2) If your complaint is not resolved at that stage you may wish to see your Consultant or the Senior Manager for the area concerned.
3) If you are still dissatisfied and wish to make a formal complaint you should contact the: Customer Services Manager, Newtown Health Care NHS Trust. Telephone 01999 287 571.

**Our standards for dealing with formal complaints are:**

- You can expect us to write to you within 2 days to tell you we have received your letter or call.
- You can expect us to send you a full written response within 28 days.
- If for any reason we are unable to complete the investigation within 28 days, we shall write to you and offer an explanation for the delay.

*You may receive a call from someone at the Trust at a later date asking if you were happy with the way in which your complaint was dealt with. You are not obliged to comment on this if you do not wish to.*

DATE OF EVENT _____

Suggestion ☐  Comment ☐  Complaint ☐
(Please tick)

_____

_____

_____

_____

_____

Your name (please print)
_____

Address: _____

_____

_____

Telephone No.
Today's Date
Names of anybody else involved
_____

_____

*You can hand this complete form into any of our wards or departments or alternatively send it to:*

**Figure 3.2**  A sample complaints form.

**Box 3.3** Settling general practice complaints

◆ The complaint might be settled by an officer of the Health Authority pointing out that it is not an appropriate case.

◆ The complaint will be assessed by the chairman of the complaints committee as to whether or not there is a case to answer.

◆ There may be reference to an informal procedure where the complainant and doctors concerned meet with a panel and try and reach a compromise and understanding.

◆ If this fails or if the parties would not agree to an informal hearing, then there is a reference to the service committee.

◆ The service committee consists of lay persons and doctors with a lay chairman. It is a tribunal and not a court. Statements are not taken on oath. The standard of proof is that of 'probability' and not that of 'beyond all reasonable doubt' as in a criminal court of law. Each side may be helped by a lay person. Often the doctor is helped by a colleague, usually a representative from the Local Medical Committee. Often the complainant is helped by a representative from the Community Health Council. Neither side may have legal representation.

◆ If either party is dissatisfied with the outcome of the hearing, then they may appeal to the Secretary of State for Health. In that case a formal appeal panel sits and re-tries the case, taking evidence on oath, and each side may employ lawyers to present their case.

◆ Under certain circumstances the case may be referred to the GMC by the committee.

◆ The complainant may go to law and sue for negligence whether or not the doctor is found in breach. There may be a complaint to the GMC whether or not there is a complaint in law or a finding of breach of terms of service by the service committee.

been used. The ombudsman has powers similar to a High Court and can require documents and persons to assist his investigations but his investigations are carried out in private. In general he will not investigate if there are ongoing legal or disciplinary investigations.

Originally the ombudsman was only concerned with maladministration within the NHS. Examples of maladministration are:

◆ bias, neglect, delay, inattention, ineptitude, perversity, turpitude, arbitrariness, rudeness
◆ unwillingness to treat the person as a person with rights
◆ failure to answer reasonable questions
◆ showing bias because of colour, sex, or any other grounds.

The ombudsman will have the power to investigate complaints of a clinical nature once other disciplinary or legal investigations are complete.

### The medical secretary's role

The primary reason for complaints and resultant lawsuits is often not medical injury itself, but the failure of communication. Medical secretaries are an essential and vital link in that chain of communication. The handling of a complaint, the handling of a difficult or aggressive person may make a great difference to the outcome of the complaint, saving stress upon the health care team and also on the complainant. Going through a complaints procedure is just as stressful to the complainant as to the doctor. The best prevention against complaints is to show that you are treating the other person with respect and understanding and above all that you care.

## EMPLOYMENT LAW

There are also laws that you need to be aware of in your role as an employee within the health service. Employment laws cover the duties and rights of both employers and employees and are derived through common law and statutory provision, i.e. have been passed by Parliament. The principal legislation regulating employment is the

Employment Rights Act 1996. An employment contract is an agreement between employer and employee which contains general terms and conditions, namely:

◆ conditions of pay, including holiday benefits and sick pay
◆ hours of work.

## The law

Within 2 months of starting work, a statement of particular terms must be sent to the employee, including:

◆ job description
◆ notice requirements
◆ disciplinary procedures (and grievances)
◆ length of contract
◆ holiday entitlement.

Certain rights and responsibilities affecting both employer and employee have either been incorporated, or implied, by law into all usual employment contracts. Employees' rights include:

◆ receiving notice
◆ redundancy pay
◆ maternity leave
◆ protection from discrimination or unfair dismissal
◆ conditions of pay including pension schemes and authorised deductions (National Insurance and PAYE)
◆ protection from discrimination under the Equal Pay Act 1971; Sex Discrimination Act 1975 (as well as the Treaty of Rome article 119 and the EU equal pay directive, and equal treatment directive).

Duties to be met by either employer or employee include:

◆ conduct which ensures *mutual* trust and confidence
◆ confidentiality (not disclosing employers' confidential information elsewhere)
◆ obeying employers' responsible and lawful orders
◆ using reasonable care and skill in carrying out employment

◆ providing as an employer a safe and healthy working environment for staff; this duty is regulated by the Health and Safety at Work Act 1974 and by later supplemental regulations.

### Relevance to the medical secretary's role

When taking up employment as a medical secretary, you need to check that you receive your initial contract or letter of appointment, and the statement of particular terms applicable to your role, within 2 months of starting work. You should note all the terms carefully, particularly the job description. If this includes any duties you are not prepared to undertake, you need to make this clear immediately. An employee who refuses to fulfil all *contractual* obligations may not be able to claim unfair dismissal.

Employees' rights are incorporated by law into the contract and cannot be excluded. Note, however, that these rights can only be exercised after a period of continuous employment. Check this with your practice or hospital manager or official trades union representative. Note that you are legally entitled to join a trades union, or to refuse to do so, if you wish. You are by law protected from verbal and physical harassment during your work. If such an event occurs, it must be reported immediately to your employer or trades union official.

## Health and Safety at Work Act 1974

The 1974 Health and Safety at Work Act does not only apply to shops and factories. It lays down an approach to occupational health, safety and welfare and it applies to many premises that are not covered by previous legislation, including laboratories, hospitals and general practice surgeries. Although the occupiers of these premises already owed their visitors the common duty of care, as laid down in the 1957 Occupier's Liability Act, this duty only required reasonable precautions to be taken for their well-being.

The 1974 Act lays down duties on employers (including the self-employed) to provide and maintain a safe place of work. Its aim is to make all employers and employees aware of the need for safety at the place of work. The main requirements are that:

◆ all facilities are suitable, clean and safe
◆ equipment used is safe with adequate protection provided where necessary
◆ hazardous substances are controlled and safely handled
◆ refreshment breaks are allowed where rest periods are essential in the operation of certain equipment.

## The medical context

The Health and Safety Act is very important in terms of working conditions within the health service. Further regulations of relevance in hospitals and surgery premises are the Control of Substances Hazardous to Health Regulations (COSHH) introduced in 1988 and the regulations introduced by the EC in 1993 (see also Chapter 17).

In general practice, it is the practitioner who employs the staff; in the hospital, staff are employed by the Health Authority. Particular areas of concern exist in a surgery or hospital regarding health and safety. These include:

◆ handling hazardous substances, including medications, patients' samples, instruments
◆ use of X-ray equipment and other potentially dangerous equipment
◆ use of VDU screens
◆ dangerous or difficult patients
◆ maintaining a particularly thorough standard of hygiene.

Your employer is obliged by law to provide a healthy and safe environment. You should check the surgery's or hospital's standard policy on this, especially as regards handling potentially dangerous equipment or substances (see also Chapter 17). Most noticeably, there should be a policy about the handling of needles and sharps which covers methods of handling them and action in the event of injury. There should be a written policy statement to provide as safe and healthy working conditions as possible and to enlist the support of employees to achieve this objective. In addition, employees have a duty to take reasonable care to avoid injury and harm to themselves and their colleagues, and not to misuse equipment and clothing provided for their safety. There should be an accident book to record all accidents to members of staff or visitors. Employers should offer hepatitis B and other immunisations where appropriate.

It should be noted that employers are only responsible for injuries which occur in the course of an employee's contractual duties. They are not responsible for any activities on your part that result in injury that are not part of your contractual duties.

## Whitley Council

The Whitley Council has been involved in setting pay scales within the NHS since 1947. Its remit includes:

◆ 'To secure the greatest possible measure of cooperation between management and staff of the NHS with a view to increasing efficiency and ensuring the well-being of those employed in the services'.
◆ 'To provide machinery for the negotiations of pay and conditions of service' (General Whitley Council).

The Council has several functional committees covering many professional, administrative and clerical grades of staff. The Whitley Council also has a very important function of hearing appeals if employees are aggrieved by a disciplinary action by an employer. Trust hospitals and GPs are not obliged to pay Whitley scales. These developments are gradually reducing the effect of the Whitley Councils. There are some advantages in having an

**Reflection point**

◆ Because of the Whitley Council, you should be able to have some idea of the salary scales, and conditions of service, which are recommended within the NHS so that you can compare with the salary and job description you are being offered.

independent system of arbitration to settle disputes and a national standard does reduce the risk of exploitation.

## Discrimination and harassment

Employment law also links to Acts which cover racial and sexual discrimination. These Acts prevent an employer discriminating against an employee and ensure equal pay. An employer may not discriminate against an employee on the grounds of gender (including marital status), race, religion, nationality, ethnic group or disability.

## Sexual harassment

The Sex Discrimination Act does not specifically mention sexual harassment but it has been interpreted in common law that an employer discriminates against a woman on the grounds of sex if he treats her less favourably than he treats or would treat a man and that the woman suffers a detriment. Significant awards have been made in the courts. In addition, such actions may be construed as constructive dismissal by an industrial tribunal.

Examples of some actions that may constitute sexual harassment include:

◆ unwanted and unnecessary physical contact
◆ demands for sexual favours with a prospect of promotion or other favours
◆ suggestive, lewd, gender-related remarks and innuendoes which are derogatory and offensive
◆ sexual assault.

It is possible for men to suffer from sexual discrimination and harassment in the same way as women.

# THE DISABILITY DISCRIMINATION ACT 1995

## The law

Disability is defined as 'a physical or mental impairment which has a substantial and long term adverse effect on a person's ability to carry out normal day-to-day activities'. The Act makes it illegal for providers of goods, facilities or services to discriminate against people with disabilities. It is also unlawful for an employer of more than 20 people to discriminate against a person with disability, because of their disability. Employers have to make reasonable arrangements to enable people with disabilities to be employed.

## The medical context

Hospitals, Health Authorities and possibly some larger practices may have to, for example:

◆ alter premises
◆ modify procedures
◆ supply additional training and training manuals
◆ provide a reader or interpreter.

Health care is a service and a person with disability must be offered the same services as anyone else and would include such examples as:

◆ wheel chair access is an obvious necessity as is the provision of lifts and hand rails
◆ facilities for interpreters for the hard of hearing
◆ sighted persons available for reading forms and documents
◆ access for guide dogs for a blind person.

The Act means that if someone is disfigured it would be wrong to insist that they sit in a room by themselves whilst waiting for attention. If they prefer to sit by themselves that would be a different matter.

A deaf person may be holding up a queue; it is wrong to ask them to step aside to let other people come first. However, if a person is jeopardising the service for others then the provider would be justified in not providing the same service. Examples could be a person with a disability endangering themselves or others, or disrupting the service for others by unruly behaviour.

As a secretary you cannot be expected to know all the regulations concerning employment. It is important that you know they exist for your protection and the protection of others. If you are unsure, or if you think something is unfair or dangerous, seek advice from your manager, union official or employer. If your employers do not recognise trades unions, the Citizen's Advice Bureau or a solicitor may be your only way of getting advice. For members of AMSPAR there is a legal helpline.

## CONCLUSION

This chapter has provided an outline of the principles of the laws which affect the health service and also some details about particular laws you need to be aware of as a medical secretary. These include:

◆ the legal responsibilities of other members of the health care team
◆ your responsibilities as part of the health care team to ensure that patients' rights are protected
◆ your role as a medical secretary in ensuring that the proper procedures are observed when dealing with legal duties
◆ the importance of dealing with complaints appropriately when patients believe their rights have been breached
◆ your rights as an employee within the health service.

The chapter has demonstrated some of the problems and difficulties of working in health care and how, unwittingly, it is possible to fall foul of the law. Fortunately, there are many sources of advice, including AMSPAR, the Local Medical Committee, and hospitals and Trusts with in-house expertise. There is also one golden rule for all workers in health care: if in any doubt, consult the appropriate authority.

### Exercises

◆ Obtain a recent copy of Medeconomics, which goes to every general practice and gives the current Whitley scales with a brief outline of the responsibilities of each grade.

◆ During placements, try to find an opportunity to discuss legal problems with a practice manager or GP. What do they think are the key issues for medical secretaries?

## FURTHER READING

BMA 1992 Rights and responsibilities of doctors. BMJ, London

BMA 1993 Medical ethics today. BMJ, London

Brazier 1992 Medicine, patients and the law. Penguin, Harmondsworth

Dyer C (ed) 1992 Doctors, patients and the law. Blackwell Scientific Publications, London

GMC 1995 Duties of a doctor. GMC, London

Gostin L 1983 A practical guide to mental health law. MIND Publications, London

Health and Safety Commission. Guidance on the recording of accidents and incidents in the health services.

Health and Safety Executive. Essentials of health and safety at work.

Kennedy I, Grubb A 1994 Medical law, 2nd edn. Butterworth Heinemann, Oxford

Knight B 1992 Legal aspects of medical practice, 5th edn. Churchill Livingstone, Edinburgh

McLean SAM 1989 A patient's right to know. Dartmouth, England

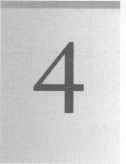

# Ethics and etiquette

*Vincent Leach*

**4**

## OBJECTIVES

◆ To consider the relationship between law ant ethics

◆ To outline some important codes of ethics

◆ To describe the main ethical principles

◆ To examine ethical issues in the medical secretarial role

◆ To consider some aspects of etiquette in the medical context.

## INTRODUCTION

*Law tells us what we must do.*
*Ethics tells us what we ought to do.*
*Etiquette tells us what we should do.*

We have seen in Chapter 3 that many problems in law have an ethical basis or content. Ideally, laws should reflect the moral and ethical standards of the age. Sometimes law is ahead and sometimes behind the ethical and moral standards of the country or generation concerned.

At the end of this chapter you should have a basic idea of medical ethics, and some of the problems brought about by modern technological medicine and resource allocation and limitation. It is essential that all workers in health care have a general idea of the ethical framework in which doctors and nurses operate.

In addition, there is a discussion of etiquette and how we should treat colleagues and the users of the health services. Professional etiquette is a complex issue for health care professionals, and in this chapter we will be looking at how medical secretaries must be aware of both medical etiquette and their own professional code of conduct which is set down by AMSPAR (Association of Medical Secretaries, Practice Managers, Administrators and Receptionists).

## LAW AND ETHICS

The rapid advance in medical technology can create ethical problems ahead of legal directives. For example, advances in genetic screening may mean that future problems such as heart disease or cancer can be detectable. This could mean that getting insurance or a mortgage becomes more difficult or more expensive. You may be aware of debates over in-vitro fertilisation, surrogacy and the prolongation of the lives of severely malformed babies. The management of patients in persistent vegetative state (PVS) has become a major topic since the death of Tony Bland following the Hillsborough disaster. Euthanasia is a subject which is often discussed in the media.

As a medical secretary you may feel these issues are not of direct interest to you. However, they are becoming matters for great public debate in the media and elsewhere, and everyone should take an interest in these topics in a democratic society. Many secretaries now work in accident and emergency departments, intensive care units, special care baby units, and even on general wards, where these problems are almost daily occurrences. It is important that as a key member of the health care team you are aware of the ethical dilemmas of modern medicine, and have some understanding of the difficulties of working as a health care professional. It is important that you realise that the actions of a secretary can ease or worsen the problems. As in legal matters, it is essential that you have some knowledge of medical ethics and the framework of modern medicine. People will ask you questions, so being aware of the problems surrounding some of today's issues will help you to avoid possible errors and pitfalls. As always, if in doubt ask the appropriate authority.

## ETHICAL CODES

You will understand that doing the right thing is not always a case of not acting illegally. Ethics is the word used to describe the philosophical study of right and wrong. Later in this chapter, we will be looking at some of the frameworks and principles of ethics. Firstly though, it is helpful to look at an example of an ethical code in medical practice. The most well known example of this is the Hippocratic Oath. This is an example of a code of ethics and it provides guidance to help

doctors know how they should behave, and reassure their patients that they will be treated as well as possible.

## The Hippocratic Oath

The Hippocratic Oath, probably written in the 5th century BC, is the most famous ethical code and is still taken by some, but by no means all, medical students today. The version shown in Box 4.1 has been updated and is taken from the International Code of Medical Ethics. It is known as the Declaration of Geneva. It is a more modern version of the Hippocratic Oath and was originally written in 1948 but revised in 1968 and 1983.

It is difficult, if not impossible, to establish hard and fast rules to cover all eventualities and

---

**Box 4.1    The Declaration of Geneva**

◆ I solemnly pledge myself to consecrate my life to the service of humanity.

◆ I will give to my teachers the respect and gratitude which is their due.

◆ I will practise my profession with conscience and dignity.

◆ The health of my patient will be my first consideration.

◆ I will respect the secrets which are confided in me, even after my patient has died.

◆ I will maintain by all means in my power, the honour and the noble tradition of the medical profession.

◆ My colleagues will be my brothers.

◆ I will not permit considerations of religion, nationality, race, party politics or social standing to intervene between my duty and my patient.

◆ I will maintain the utmost respect for human life from its beginning even under threat and I will not use my medical knowledge contrary to the laws of humanity.

**Reflection points**

◆ Read this code carefully. Think about how it affects your role as a medical secretary working alongside medical professionals.

◆ Are these principles being adhered to worldwide? Look out for examples of debates about medical issues in the media and discuss them with your colleagues or other students.

◆ The World Medical Association is an organisation which debates ethical dilemmas in medical developments. Try and find out more about its impact on ethical thinking.

---

**Box 4.2** The AMSPAR Ethics Code

A secretary must:

◆ At all times observe strict confidentiality. Anything learned from a patient, a medical practitioner, patients' records or correspondence must never be disclosed to any unauthorised person.

◆ Never discuss any personal and confidential matters relating to patient or practitioner or criticise his/her employer or another doctor's behaviour or treatment.

◆ At all times use discretion when talking about the medical practitioner to any person.

◆ At all times confine his/her functions to those covered by the job description.

◆ Never assume responsibility for assessing the patient's clinical condition and initiating prescriptions.

◆ Strive at all times to foster good relations between doctor and other members of the health team.

◆ At all times behave in a manner calculated to maintain respect and confidence of patients and demonstrate a high standard of professional conduct.

---

situations in modern medicine. Modern medical ethics reflect the influence of different religions and beliefs, and try to establish principles in societies where religious beliefs have been rejected by many individuals. Often ethics tend to come down to individual conscience and beliefs. Laws are not necessarily the basis of medical ethics but laws should reflect current feelings and opinions. Medical ethics are often based on principles rather than fixed rules and laws.

## The AMSPAR Code of Ethics

In studying this chapter it might be of value to consider each topic in relation to the AMSPAR Ethics Code for medical secretaries (Box 4.2). You will see that the Code reflects the Declaration of Geneva but is particularly applicable to the secretarial role within the team.

**Reflection point**

◆ Compare the AMSPAR Code to the Declaration of Geneva as set out in Box 4.1. What similarities and differences can you see?

## ETHICAL PRINCIPLES

### The principle of duty

The technical word for this is deontology. Duty implies there are certain inviolable rules which should be adhered to. The traditional rules are religious laws. The Ten Commandments from the Old Testament, and part of the background of Judaism, Christianity and the Muslim religions, are a good example; you shall not kill, commit adultery, steal, and you shall respect your parents, and so on. Buddhism has the Noble Truths, which are similar rules. Rules such as these imply there is an inherent right and wrong and that we all have a sense of right and wrong.

**Reflection points**

◆ Consider 'you shall not kill'. Visualise circumstances in which it would not be ethically wrong to kill another person.

◆ Are there occasions when to steal might be ethically acceptable?

◆ Is it always ethically correct to tell the truth?

The difficulty with hard and fast rules is that there are always worthy exceptions. Obviously it would be considered appropriate to kill in self-defence. Unless a pacifist, it would be correct to kill in wartime in defence of one's country. A vegetarian might extend the principle to animal life. It is possible to do great harm if we always told the truth without considering consequences. An example is how and when we give bad news to a person, say, who has cancer.

## Do no harm

The technical word is non-maleficence. There is a long tradition from the Hippocratic age, when the saying was 'Above all do no harm'. In former times, when medicine did not do much good, it

**Reflection points**

Nowadays, it seems straightforward to assume that modern medicine always does 'no harm' but consider the following issues:

◆ Mr Black is having treatment for raised blood pressure. The treatment makes him lethargic and impotent. Is this doing harm?

◆ Some inoculations have been linked to cases of brain damage in children. How many cases of brain damage are acceptable to prevent the mass of children getting whooping cough?

◆ Every year there are a considerable number of suicides from paracetamol overdose. Should paracetamol be banned?

was possible, in fact likely, that procedures such as bleeding and purging did far more harm than good.

In modern times it is difficult to practise medicine at least without the risk of doing harm. If drugs did not have side-effects, if every operation was successful, in other words if risk could be entirely removed, then the principle could be universally applied. The best one can achieve is balancing the risks against the possible benefits. A doctor should always try to *act in the best interests* of his or her patient. A secondary consideration is the best interests of society; for example, whether people suffering from epilepsy should be allowed to drive.

### The medical secretary's role

These are also important issues for the medical secretary. Cases of doing harm may legally be cases of negligence. For example, a wrong prescription may do great harm, but the reason for the wrong prescription may be delivery of a wrong message, such as a typing error, by the secretary. Accidents in the operating theatre may arise because of administrative and clerical errors. Errors in diagnosis and treatment are obvious instances of harm being done. There is a much more subtle form of harm, but no less serious, arising out of poor communications. Giving a person bad news requires great skill and understanding. It must be admitted that not all health care professionals have the appropriate skills. As a medical secretary you must not give clinical information without being absolutely certain that you have the authority. There is great danger in, innocently, giving the results of tests or examinations without first consulting the health care professional concerned. Imagine how much harm may be done if, even with the best of intentions, a secretary makes comments such as 'Don't worry, this doctor is very good at treating cancer'.

The most important point to remember is that you must consult relevant health professionals regarding the correct procedure in situations such as this. Most general practices have a policy to help cope with these kinds of problems. Always check with a senior member of the administrative

◆ to prevent disease
◆ to ease symptoms including the symptoms associated with dying
◆ to help people to live as full a life as possible despite the presence of disease or handicap.

**Scenario**

Consider what you should do in the following situation. Discussing this scenario with colleagues may be useful.

Mrs White rings up for the result of her cervical smear. What would you say (a) if the smear is negative, (b) the smear shows abnormal cells?

It may well be that arrangements have been made in a particular department, and with particular patients, that negative results may be given by the secretary. The fact that the secretary will not give the result, but hedges, may in itself cause alarm and panic. For a woman to be told she has abnormal cells in her smear immediately makes her think she will die with cancer of the cervix. Abnormal cells may be due to infection and not all significant abnormalities develop into true malignancy.

**Scenario**

These principles seem straightforward, but consider the following scenarios.

◆ If a patient is suffering from terminal cancer would it be of benefit to resuscitate him after an overdose?

◆ A patient has had a severe stroke, is paralysed, cannot speak, and is distressed by a catheter. Because he cannot swallow he is fed through a gastrostomy (an artificial opening through the abdominal wall). The GP has been called because the patient has developed pneumonia. Should the GP treat the pneumonia?

staff on their protocols when you require a work placement or start a job. Above all, it is not the duty of the secretary to give clinical information without being satisfied that it is the wish of the health care professional.

**Reflection point**

◆ Think about which sections of the AMSPAR Code are relevant to this issue.

## Do good

Beneficence is the technical word, to do good is perhaps the purpose of medicine above all others. It has been said that the motto of the NHS is 'To give years to life, and life to years'. Examples of beneficence in this context include:

◆ to preserve and prolong life
◆ to recognise and cure disease

## The principle of consequences

In considering whether or not an act is ethical it may be judged by its outcome, and the technical word for this is consequentialism. Is the consequence of an act good or bad? Is the action in the person's best interests? Does the action increase the happiness of the person? Does the action benefit society as a whole? Does the action increase the happiness of society as a whole?

Thus you will see that only considering consequences may lead to further ethical dilemmas and conflicts. A Jehovah's Witness would not accept blood transfusion even at the risk of death. Many people believe that life must be prolonged at almost any cost, even at the cost of prolonged suffering. Many believe that life must be prolonged in persistent coma (PVS), or severe dementia, even at great cost to the resources of the health services.

To try to resolve some of these dilemmas other principles have been devised.

### Reflection points

◆ A simple example is building a by-pass. This may improve the lifestyle of the inhabitants of a village as whole. But if you run a village shop, would you be so keen if you might lose trade?

◆ A more complex example is using animals for testing. Do you think that the benefits to individuals or to society as a whole justify experiments of this kind? You may feel differently depending on whether the tests are aimed at finding a cure for cancer, or just another type of cosmetic.

## Respect for the individual

We all expect to be treated as individuals and not be arrested without having performed an illegal act. Respect for the individual is so important that a separate section is allocated to this principle and will be dealt with in the section on etiquette. The principle of respect also involves the principle of respect for autonomy, which literally means self-rule. This covers the capacity to think and to act independently and freely, and includes:

◆ autonomy of thought – the ability to think for oneself, having likes and dislikes, having beliefs and the ability to make judgments
◆ autonomy of will – the ability to make decisions for oneself
◆ autonomy of action – the ability to perform acts voluntarily.

A very important issue which is related to respect for individuals is informed consent. We discussed consent in Chapter 3 in its legal context. Informed consent is an important principle in modern medicine. As discussed in Chapter 3, treatment without consent may be considered in law to be an assault.

## Paternalism

The opposite of respect for autonomy is paternalism. The traditional medical model is paternalistic.

Having made a diagnosis, a doctor was expected to give instructions as to what the patient should do to cure the disease, 'Doctor knows best'. This attitude was acceptable when the doctor was much more highly educated than most of his clients. With increasing education people have greater knowledge of medical facts and want to know more about their condition, treatment and the consequences of different treatments or of no treatment. Acting in the best interests of the patient, it might be necessary for a doctor not to give all the relevant information and make the decision for his or her patient because the patient is incapacitated by confusion, or extreme pain. It may be that some people cannot make decisions for themselves.

A great problem is deciding if a person is capable of making decisions and therefore autonomous. A person of sound mind may refuse any treatment even if this leads to death. There have been cases of anorexia nervosa (also known as 'slimmer's disease') where individuals have refused treatment and died. A major difficulty is deciding at what age children may be considered as autonomous and free to make decisions about their health care. Similar problems occur in cases of mental illness and dementias.

## Justice and fairness

A very important ethical principle is that of justice. In an ideal world 'to each according to his need' would be the universal principle. In all health care systems there are constraints due to limitation of resources. Even if all the finance was available there would still be limits on, say, the number of hearts or kidneys available for transplantation.

One school of thought states that all human beings are of equal value. The decision should be made on the basis that all lives are of equal value. The following quotation is from the Talmud, a Jewish legal text.

*He who destroys a single life is charged as if he destroyed a whole world and whoever rescues a single life is credited as if he saved the whole world.*

**Reflection points**

Consider the following mental exercise. Imagine there is one kidney available for donation. In the ward are the following individuals:

◆ A child

◆ A child with learning disabilities

◆ A mother with two children

◆ A man of 60.

To whom would you give the kidney? Would it make any difference if the normal child was an orphan? Would it make any difference if the mother was an alcoholic who neglected her children? Would it make any difference if the man was a famous scientist near to finding a cure for cancer? Consider the resource constraints within the NHS. Have they had any influence on how decisions about who to care for are made?

The above example is a purely theoretical exercise but it does demonstrate the problems in allocating resources between paediatrics, care of the mentally ill, and care of the elderly, as examples. Whether the problem is infertility or serious life-threatening disease, every sufferer from any particular condition and every worker in the field wants the maximum resources for the condition.

**Reflection point**

◆ Is it also unfair if the high profile of some conditions means that they get more resources than other low profile conditions? What difference is it likely to make if a famous person supports a particular cause such as AIDS? Which causes might not attract so much media interest and do they suffer as a result?

For justice and fairness:

◆ All people must have an equal consideration and assessment of their wants and needs.
◆ Having assessed the problems, decisions must be made as to what options are possible on the basis of potential benefits.
◆ What should be done, and what is best for the patient, considering the patient's priorities?
◆ Decisions must be made according to what is available within a particular health care system.

However, it is not the responsibility or role of the secretary to make judgments or make comments about these matters. If there appears to be an injustice then the person should be referred to the appropriate authority for consideration of his or her case. A citizen has the right to expose injustice and illegal practices to the legal authorities and to the press and media. If injustice is apparent then a secretary's employers should be consulted first. If satisfaction is not received then the secretary perhaps has a moral right to publicise this injustice – whistleblowing – but this will be at some personal risk.

## ETHICAL ISSUES IN THE MEDICAL SECRETARIAL ROLE

A later chapter (Chapter 5) is devoted to the qualities of the medical secretary. The practical considerations of how we promote ethical behaviour, as we will discuss in this section, are the foundation for a good medical secretary. You will also find that places of work, whether hospital or general practice, will have developed their own policies to ensure correct working practices and an efficient form of care for the patient. Medical secretaries, along with other members of the team, need guidelines in order to be effective. The following sections deal with the most important principles in terms of the role of the medical secretary:

◆ confidentiality
◆ discrimination.

## Confidentiality

We have discussed the principle of non-malefi-cence, of not doing harm. The medical secretary is in a position to do most harm by breaching confi-dentiality. Sometimes the breach may be innocent, sometimes in good faith, but it may be damaging nonetheless. Confidentiality of patient informa-tion means that only the person concerned has the authority to give permission for any information to be given to a third party.

### Reflection point

◆ Consider what you would do under these circumstances:

A man rings to ask if his wife attended clinic or surgery. A mother rings up to ask if her 14-year-old daughter is on the pill. A policeman asks if someone with particular injuries or identification marks attended accident and emergency or surgery.

Some requests may appear to be reasonable and innocent. They may appear to be in the best inter-ests of the person concerned. There may be strong and cogent reasons why a wife may not wish her husband to know she is attending her doctor because she has gone to discuss her husband's mental state or drinking habits. The reasons for an action are a matter of confidence between the per-son and his or her health care professional and are nothing to do with anyone else. Even the name and address of a person may be of great signifi-cance. It is not uncommon for a woman to be frightened that her estranged husband should find out where she is living.

A doctor may break the confidentiality rule if he or she considers it to be in the person's best interests. As a secretary you may be involved in these and similar actions, say, in contacting the police or the Driver and Vehicle Licensing (DVLC) so that your employer can give the infor-mation. In all instances seek guidance. As indi-cated in Chapter 3 it is the doctor's, not the secre-tary's, responsibility to divulge information. This might be in the person's best interests or in the interests of society as a whole. It may well be the doctor's decision to notify the DVLC when an epileptic continues to drive. If a serious crime has been committed then information may be given to protect society. In either case the doctor may have to justify his or her action in a civil court or in front of the GMC.

### Reflection points

◆ Consider how you would feel if the next time you went to your doctor, you discover that your next door neighbour is the new secretary at the practice? How might someone who was HIV positive feel in the same circumstances?

◆ Look round your office or surgery; can you see areas where confidentiality might be breached?

Examples of office procedures which might compromise confidentiality include:

◆ Several people at the reception desk at the same time and able to hear each other's conversation.
◆ The telephone within earshot of other people at the desk.
◆ Case notes, pathology laboratory, and X-ray results lying around in full view.
◆ Free access to the computer with patients' data. Check that passwords are safeguarded and used correctly. See also Chapter 8 on using computers.
◆ Fax machines placed in public areas. Make sure that if you are sending confidential information by fax that it will arrive at the right number and only be read by the correct health care professional.
◆ Calling across the waiting room. For example, it would not be appropriate to call out

messages about people's prescriptions, such as 'Your prescription for the pill is ready'.
◆ Putting confidential material in a waste bin; it should be shredded.

With the use of passwords and encryption of transmitted data, and protection from the Data Protection Act, it might be felt that everything possible has been done to protect confidential information within a computer system. The weak link in the chain is the human being. It is no use having sophisticated techniques if a secretary can be persuaded to hand over information by payment of a bribe or promise of favours, even though this is illegal.

In some instances confidentiality is broken by law. There is compulsory registration of births, marriages and deaths. Wills become public knowledge. Income tax inspectors have access to our earnings. Doctors have to notify certain infectious diseases.

For the benefit of their patients, doctors share information and pass it on to each other.

◆ When a person first registers with a GP information is passed to the person doing the registration. This is passed to the Health Authority and details sent to the central register.
◆ Records are sent from the old GP to the Health Authority, then to the new authority and finally on to the new GP and the secretarial staff. At all the different stages lay people are handling confidential information.
◆ When a person is referred to hospital, personal details are included with clinical information.
◆ Secretaries concerned with costing and purchasing have access to the clinical details.
◆ Results of tests and X-rays pass through non-medical hands.

There is a great deal of information going around the NHS and other agencies, much of it within easy access of those who do not have the right to know. You are the guardian of much of this information. Do not be tempted to look up details about your family, friends or acquaintances out of mere curiosity. In some organisations this

would be an act warranting instant dismissal. All health care information should only be seen by those 'who need to know'.

Always be vigilant about confidentiality. If you see places where there may be breaches discuss the matter with your manager or employer. Always be on your guard. If in doubt, seek guidance. If you are aware that confidentiality might be threatened, check what the health professional intends. Confidentiality is referred to in four out of the seven clauses of the AMSPAR Code of Conduct, which emphasises just what a crucial aspect of your practice it should be.

## Discrimination

In Chapter 3, we discussed some of the legislation which aims to prevent discrimination, but discrimination is also an ethical issue. When we were discussing justice and fairness earlier in this chapter, it was emphasised that everyone has equal rights to medical treatment regardless of their race, gender or religious beliefs. Equally, these should be recognised and respected. As a medical secretary it is essential that you do not discriminate against anyone in the line of your work. Discrimination is illegal and unethical and is in breach of professional conduct.

**Reflection point**

◆ You may think that discrimination is only an issue about race, but there are many ways in which people are discriminated against. Women, children, old people, people with mental illness, those who are HIV positive can all be victims of discrimination. Think of ways in which access to health care services might discriminate against different kinds of people.

Discrimination can be overt; for example, a receptionist could refuse someone access to the doctor because she didn't like the way he looked. However, most discrimination is covert and sometimes people are unaware at a conscious level that their behaviour or actions are unjust and unfair. For example, many practice leaflets and notices might only be available in English and therefore information is unlikely to be readily available to people whose first language is not English.

Most hospitals will have a written policy regarding discrimination and some Trusts may have Equal Opportunities personnel. Try and find out what is the policy in your work area and read any leaflets that are available. Always be vigilant about your own attitudes, and try and be aware of how discrimination arises, and can therefore be countered.

# ETIQUETTE

There are books of etiquette showing how to address a bishop, a knight or how to lay a dinner table. This section is more to do with how we treat each other and show each other respect irrespective of race, creed or social standing.

Many contacts with the health services are over the telephone or over a reception desk. The initial contact may be the first contact with the NHS, the hospital or the practice. The manner of the introduction may colour the rest of the consultation or affect the attitude of the person on admission. Telephone and other techniques of handling people will be dealt with in Chapter 5. However, it is worth repeating that you should always be polite, give your name and ask in what way you may help. Do not keep people waiting too long without acknowledging their presence and apologising for any delay; preferably give some explanation for the delay.

## Reflection point

◆ Next time you ring up an organisation listen to the telephone technique. Are you treated as a person? Is the approach brusque or condescending? How long are you kept waiting, did you get irritated and frustrated?

Titles may be important to some people. It is worthwhile finding out if a person prefers to be referred to as Ms, Miss or Mrs. Some people prefer to be referred to by first name, other people will find this too familiar and be offended. Some people will prefer an even more formal approach and wish to be called sir or madam. The correct approach you will only find out by experience and be prepared to alter your approach if it seems to be causing offence. Use the more formal approach first, using the more informal when the barriers have been broken down. Among colleagues the same techniques apply. An office manager may prefer to be called by his or her first name. Some doctors and employers may prefer the intimacy of first names.

There is often confusion, especially in hospitals, as to the correct title for a member of the medical staff. The rule is that surgeons are called mister and the rest are called doctor. Most medical practitioners have separate degrees in surgery and medicine. Some countries, such as the USA, have a combined degree of MD and all are referred to as doctor. If you are in contact with an American surgeon he or she will be referred to as 'doctor'.

## Manners and attitudes

The use of the correct title is relatively unimportant. What is important are manner and attitude. In the section on autonomy we discussed how all people are entitled to respect, purely as human beings, irrespective of age, sex, colour, ethnic or religious group or social or economic class. It is one of the fundamental principles of the NHS that all should be treated equally according to need. The scruffy unkempt man in front of you may be a wealthy farmer not a tramp. Even if he is a tramp his medical needs could be very great and should be considered impartially. Appearances may be very deceptive. Attitudes may also be deceptive. The most aggressive person may be the most frightened person. The aggressive person under the influence of drugs or alcohol may well be pacified by a calm approach, by proper etiquette, and by not responding with aggression.

### Reflection point

◆ Next time you go into a bank, building society, travel agent or other business, observe techniques. How are customers treated? Are different customers treated with different levels of respect and etiquette?

Tact and diplomacy are required in handling all people, but especially those who are acutely or even terminally ill. Tact is required in handling those who are concerned about their loved ones or have been bereaved. Treat all how you would prefer to be treated under those circumstances. Try and put yourself in their position. Above all, the AMSPAR Code states that you must 'At all times behave in a manner calculated to maintain respect and confidence of patients'.

### Reflection point

◆ Refer again to the AMSPAR Ethics Code given earlier in Box 4.2. Which parts of the code are specific to medical etiquette? Why is it necessary for AMSPAR to make this statement? Consider these statements when reading this section.

## Medical etiquette

There are also issues of medical etiquette which are very relevant to your role as a medical secretary. Medical etiquette is primarily concerned with how health care professionals treat each other. As a secretary you will be involved in these matters.

In general, except in an emergency, it is not ethical for a doctor to see another doctor's patient without the consent of the doctor. This is the basis of the referral system within the NHS and in private practice. The GP is the holder of the total patient record and responsible for continuity of care. This is of great value within the NHS and does not apply in many other health care systems around the world. If a doctor has seen a patient of another doctor then he or she should inform the patient's doctor about the diagnosis and action taken. If one doctor refers to another all relevant information must be made available. It may be a secretary's task to collect and send this information. A secretary could be of great help in checking that the necessary notifications and letters have been sent.

## Professional criticism

It is not ethical for one doctor to criticise the actions of another. Therefore, it would not be ethical for a member of his or her staff to criticise another doctor. Criticism is sometimes indirect. A hospital doctor may say to a relative, 'We could have done more if the patient had been referred earlier'. There may be an implied criticism of the GP whose management of the case may have been quite correct. Even if the management had not been correct it is not for another doctor to criticise and possibly be the instigation of a complaint. By inference, it is not correct for a member of staff to criticise another professional. This is not objecting to 'whistleblowing' or advocating a professional closed shop. In your role, you must beware of repeating comments you may have heard outside the practice, or of becoming involved in discussions with anyone about the practice of the people who work there.

This is also referred to in the AMSPAR Code: 'At all times use discretion when talking about the medical practitioner to any person'. This obviously refers to criticism as discussed above, but it also covers praise as indicated in the next section.

## Advertising

Doctors do not advertise in the commercial sense. It is acceptable for doctors to give information in a practice leaflet or to notify colleagues that they are available for consultations. To suggest or even imply an excellence or superiority over colleagues is not acceptable. This principle extends to your role as a medical secretary and it is not acceptable for you to recommend any doctor or health professional to anyone in a way that might compromise other professionals.

### Reflection points

◆ You work for a private doctor and someone wishes to see your employer without a reference from another doctor. What should you do?

◆ A person starts to criticise a doctor who is not your employer. You know some of the criticisms may have some justification. Discuss how you would handle such a situation with your colleagues.

## Personal prejudices

Doctors must not let their own beliefs or views on a patient's lifestyle, culture or beliefs affect their judgment and any treatment given or arranged. If there is conflict because of personal beliefs between a patient and the doctor then the doctor should inform the patient of his or her right to see another doctor. This might apply when there is a request for contraception or termination of pregnancy, contrary to the doctor's own personal values. It is essential that the beliefs and opinions of any members of staff are not permitted to interfere with everyone receiving the appropriate medical care to which they are entitled. The doctor/patient relationship is built on trust. Comments and actions by other members of the health care team can damage or even destroy that trust and do irreparable harm to the patient.

## Continuity of care

Doctors are responsible for making sure there is continuity of care for their patient. In hospital this may mean a junior is responsible for the day-to-day management of a case, but the ultimate responsibility rests with the specialist. This is especially relevant to your role as a medical secretary as you may have to be aware of who is on call for emergency admissions and who is deputising for the doctor concerned. In general practice, a partner or deputising service might be on call. You may have to find a locum for your employer. It is essential that you are aware of the deputising arrangements within a practice, whether a general practice or within a suite of specialists. The medical secretary's role is to ensure that relevant information is relayed to guarantee continuity of care.

## CONCLUSIONS

To be an effective member of a health care team it is essential to know something of the ethical framework within which health care professionals have to work. Increasing demands, new techniques and resource limitation are altering the framework almost daily. Be prepared for new ideas and attitudes, but remember that the basic principles that we have discussed in this chapter should always inform the way you think and act in your role as a medical secretary. Above all, treat people as you would wish to be treated yourself.

### Exercises

Try and discuss some of the issues and reflection points raised in this chapter with colleagues and friends. Look out for cases which are reported in the media and discuss them too. Try and get as many facts as possible and try, as far as possible, to remove bias and prejudices when thinking or discussing the problems.

◆ Make a list of all the ways in which confidentiality can be breached. Think about the physical layout of work areas. Think about access.

◆ Think about the different forms of patient notes and information there may be – how do we safeguard them?

◆ Is there a practice/department policy laid down for these areas of work, such as confidentiality or discrimination? Where do you find it?

# FURTHER READING

Beauchamp TL and Childress JF 1989 Principles of biomedical ethics. OUP, Oxford. *This is perhaps the next textbook for anyone wishing to study medical ethics in more detail, but not light reading.*

BMA 1993 Medical ethics today. BMJ Publishing, London. *This gives the BMA opinion on most subjects and very useful for reference.*

Cohen SL 1993 Whose life is it anyhow? Robson Books, London. *This is a very readable account of some of the problems encountered in intensive care units.*

Gillon R 1986 Philosophical medical ethics. John Wiley, Chichester

GMC 1995 Good medical practice. GMC, London

McDowell J, Stewart D 1988 Concise guide to today's religions. Scripture Press, England

Phillips, Dawson 1985 Doctor's dilemmas. Harvester Wheatsheaf, London. *This is probably the most readable book on medical ethics.*

# 2

## Part 2
## Fundamentals of medical secretarial practice

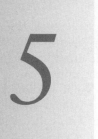

# 5

# The qualities of the medical secretary

*Jayne Pearce*

## OBJECTIVES

◆ To provide a broad overview of the role of the medical secretary

◆ To assist the reader to evaluate personal strengths and weaknesses

◆ To outline appropriate coping strategies

◆ To stimulate debate and discussion

◆ To promote professional behaviour and supply a code of conduct

◆ To encourage self-development.

## INTRODUCTION

What do we mean by 'qualities'? The dictionary definition states a quality as being 'a characteristic, something that is special in a person or thing'. The contents of this chapter will examine a range of key characteristics of direct relevance to the work of a medical secretary. We present a combination of personal qualities and professional skills, all of which are desirable in a medical secretary. The chapter does not aim to provide an exhaustive list but rather a summary. From the premise that we all have highly individual characteristics, we will aim to highlight those of most value to the medical secretary in the workplace. Whilst reading, use the reflection points and scenarios to evaluate your own qualities. Identify any areas of weakness and list your strong points.

Working as a medical secretary can be a most rewarding and challenging experience which allows the individual to become a valued member of the health care team. It is essential for all medical secretaries to become aware of their potential in order that they may contribute effectively to the care of patients and achieve job satisfaction. All employers will require a medical secretary to perform a wide range of routine functions competently and efficiently. Improving your performance and capabilities will identify you as a valuable asset to the team.

The majority of the qualities outlined in this chapter can be brought together under four general titles: confidentiality, cooperation, commitment and courtesy – the 4Cs.

## CONFIDENTIALITY

The delicate relationship between patient and doctor is based on a foundation of confidentiality and trust. Medical ethics and etiquette are fully discussed in Chapter 4, which demonstrates that the provision of health care is dominated by a code of ethics. The medical secretary must uphold this code and maintaining confidentiality is an essential requirement. The Association of Medical Secretaries, Practice Managers, Administrators and Receptionists (AMSPAR) publish an Ethics Code which all members must observe. The first point of this code states that any information learned from a patient, the patient's record, a medical practitioner or correspondence must never be disclosed to any unauthorised person.

The medical secretary should never initiate unauthorised release of information and must remember that the prime objective is to provide a service to each individual patient. This may create difficulties when dealing with a patient's relatives who may be distressed, anxious and in need of information. As a medical secretary, you will frequently be the first point of contact for many of these callers and you will need skills to cope effectively.

### Scenario

You receive a telephone call from the wife of a patient. The family are well known to you. You also know that the husband has elected not to reveal the extent of his illness to his family at present. The family have observed his decline and are very distressed to not have any definite information. His wife asks if you know about her husband's illness. She explains her worry and is obviously in a very emotional state. She asks you directly to reveal his diagnosis. She also says, 'I don't know what to do. Why can't you help me?'

What is your initial reaction to this caller? How will you answer her question? What type of assistance might you be able to provide?

This type of conversation will be a common occurrence in any health care environment. Your initial reaction should include attentive listening, noting the salient points of the conversation and empathising with the caller. What it should not include is any indication of the patient's condition or other personal information. This caller is looking for information, which you are unable to supply. The conversation should be related to the medical practitioner who will decide what further action is required. Most of all, this caller needs to be listened to in a kind and respectful manner but the patient's right to privacy must be maintained.

### Reflection point

◆ Identify two more examples of situations where you will be required to maintain confidentiality whilst dealing with enquiries from relatives. What external factors may compromise confidentiality in the workplace?

You have a duty to protect any patient-related information in your care. You should become aware of the external factors which may compromise confidentiality.

### Computers

Most hospitals and practices will use computers to store patient information and the subject of information technology is covered in Chapter 8. You will probably use a word processor to produce clinic letters, summaries and reports. During the course of your work, you may be called away from your word processor at short notice to deal with other enquiries and events. You may be in the middle of a lengthy document. When presented with urgent interruptions you should, if possible, save the unfinished document and file it before leaving your office. Alternatively, the information can be protected by turning off the screen so that visitors to the office will not be able to see it.

## Written information

Despite the introduction of computers, the majority of patient information is still received and stored on paper. These documents are confidential and should always be treated with care. Incoming correspondence should be placed inside a file or folder before being distributed to the medical staff or other team members. If you are called away whilst using patient records, you should cover letters or close the medical notes before leaving them unattended.

## Telephone

The telephone is widely used in all health care environments. If conversations conducted via the telephone may be overheard by others, you need to be aware of a possible breach of confidentiality. When speaking to patients ensure that your responses are appropriate if you are not alone. This is particularly relevant if you are working in a reception area as members of the general public may be queuing at reception to make appointments, collect prescriptions or ask for information. If you find yourself in this position, you should avoid using the patient's full name, address or telephone number as these may provide bystanders with enough clues to identify the person. If the call is a routine enquiry, this should not present you with too many difficulties. However, if the call requires more in-depth discussion, it would be preferable to transfer it to another telephone or to telephone the caller back to ensure a reasonable degree of privacy.

You must also be cautious when telephoning a patient as they may be at work or have visitors and may feel unable to speak to you openly. Under these circumstances an individual may appear uninterested, uncommunicative or obstructive. It should become part of your routine to check that the patient feels able to have the conversation before you continue.

## Messages

Leaving a message presents a further risk to confidentiality and should be avoided if at all possible.

However, if you are contacting someone as a matter of urgency, restrict your message to your name, organisation and telephone number and ask that the person contacts you. Answerphones are now commonplace both in the workplace and in many homes. Be aware that you can never be sure that only the patient will hear the message.

## Facsimile machines

As with answerphones, the fax has become a common method of communication. It is inappropriate to send any patient-related information via a fax as you do not know where the receiving machine is situated or who has access to the printout. Remember too that it is always possible that the fax may be routed to a wrong number.

## Careless talk

General discussions with work colleagues about patients should be avoided. Discussing patients with anyone outside the workplace is unacceptable under any circumstances. However, discussing individual patients' needs with colleagues is frequently necessary but should be undertaken at appropriate times in appropriate surroundings. You should ensure that the conversation cannot be overheard by anyone other than the members of the team who are involved in that person's care. If circumstances arise where you need to exchange information in front of others, do not identify the patient by name. It may be possible to use other general identifiers, such as 'The lady you saw first thing this morning telephoned to say ...' or 'Your patient with the tumour from yesterday wants to talk to you again'. Each situation should be judged individually and if there is any doubt, wait for a more suitable opportunity.

## COOPERATION

The following phrase is frequently used in job advertisements: 'must be willing to work as part of the team'. What exactly does this mean? The concept of an effective team is based on cooperation and communication. A team cannot be effective if its members do not cooperate to achieve their objectives and if communication is poor. The criteria for being a good team member are not easily measured but certain key characteristics can be found in all efficient teams.

## Communication

The sharing of knowledge and information with other team members is a prime factor in effective teamwork. The medical secretary will often find herself at the centre of a health care team with responsibility for ensuring accurate and appropriate communication of information (Fig. 5.1).

The constituent members of a team will be determined by the individual patient's needs. Throughout the period of care, information will be exchanged between members of the team and this will often be facilitated by the medical secretary.

### Scenario

One of the medical staff has requested that you arrange a team meeting to review the case of Mrs Sanders. This will be the second team meeting relating to Mrs Sanders. Consider what you need to do. Devise an action plan to follow. What information needs to be communicated? How will you achieve this?

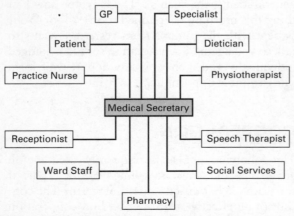

**Figure 5.1** The medical secretary and the health care team.

Team meetings of this nature are common in both general practice and hospital departments. You should have considered the date, time and venue in the first instance. Once these details have been finalised, information regarding the meeting needs to be conveyed to each team member, either in writing or by speaking to those involved. The information needed by the team at this stage can be referred to as the what, why, where and when. What is the meeting for? Why is it being held? Where and when will it take place? Notes taken at the first team meeting should be available at the second meeting along with the patient's medical records, including any relevant X-rays and investigation results. You should ask the person convening the meeting whether any further action is required in advance. Refreshments may be required, particularly if the meeting is to be held at lunchtime or early evening. Keep a record if any team member is unable to attend. Check who will be available to take notes at the meeting or whether you will be required to attend.

You can see that you will be the key organiser of this meeting and that good communication practice is vital in this situation.

### Scenario

At the case meeting, you were requested to take notes. A list of action points were identified for immediate attention. The physiotherapist had been unable to attend. The team leader is going away for 2 weeks and asks you to ensure the necessary follow-up action is initiated and to prepare a brief report to be available on his/her return.

What will be your first priority following the meeting? Identify all the tasks to be completed and devise an action plan to follow, giving yourself a timescale.

## Trust

All members of the team must feel able to trust their colleagues to carry out their duties and responsibilities in a competent and acceptable manner. Teamwork breaks down when trust is absent from the relationships. Trust will be earned by demonstrating your reliability and organisation skills. In the case of Mrs Sanders' case meeting, the medical secretary was responsible for organising the meeting and for ensuring that all the appropriate personnel were informed. The team leader trusted that this task would be completed effectively.

The first priority following the meeting will be to prepare minutes/notes for circulation. In this case you should have considered the possibility that one of the action points identified at the meeting involves the physiotherapist. It would then be appropriate for you to contact the physiotherapist as a priority. An action plan can be written in a number of formats but a simple outline is provided in Box 5.1.

Action plans provide you with an easy reference guide for any task you are responsible for. You can check your progress without having to read through all the documentation and they will enable you to communicate the requirements to other team members more effectively. By following your action plan you will be able to provide the team leader with an informative report on the situation on the day he/she returns from leave. Your trustworthiness will have been effectively demonstrated. Being an active team member will enhance your feelings of job satisfaction as you will know that your contribution is valued and beneficial to patient care and support. Being a willing and able member of the team will identify you as a valuable asset to the organisation.

## COMMITMENT

Anyone who contributes to patient care and support should invest a level of commitment in the role they perform within the organisation; in other words, giving priority to the needs and wants of the organisation. The following characteristics are desirable in all medical secretaries and demonstrate commitment.

### Reliability

As previously discussed, the medical secretary will often work at the centre of patient care. As a result, colleagues, patients and external agencies will rely upon you to carry out your duties both competently and promptly. Being reliable means always taking appropriate action when asked, completing work within accepted deadlines and responding to enquiries as soon as possible. People who are invariably late, who do not meet deadlines, who do not respond to requests within acceptable time periods and who do not complete a task without being reminded are generally viewed as unreliable.

| **Box 5.1** Example of an action plan | |
|---|---|
| **ACTION REQUIRED** | **DEADLINE** |
| Read notes and pass on relevant action points to physiotherapist | Within 1 day |
| Prepare minutes | Within 3 days |
| Circulate minutes | Within 5 days |
| Request feedback on action taken by team members | Within 10 days |
| Prepare brief report for team leader | Within 14 days |

 **Scenario**

You work in a large practice in a team of three medical secretaries. Each secretary looks after a named team of medics. Each secretary is required to provide cover if a colleagues is absent. You have slipped into a habit of poor time-keeping which results in the others providing cover for you on a regular basis.

What effect might this have on the service received by your patients? What effect does this have on your colleagues? What effect does this have on you? What action might you take to change the situation?

## Precision

As a medical secretary, one of the most valuable attributes you can possess is that of precision. This ability should be applied to every aspect of your work. One area of obvious relevance is the production of typed documents where precision will lessen the amount of time spent on corrections. Even the most accurate touch-typist can make errors. Proof-reading of all documents before presentation is therefore essential. Do not rely solely on the spell-check facility on your word processor as this will not identify words which have been correctly spelt but used out of context. It will not check your use of grammar or punctuation. An effective, but time-consuming, proof-reading technique is that of reading the text out loud. Errors or omissions become more obvious when heard. Another useful tool is to read each sentence backwards, as this concentrates your attention on each word rather than on the overall meaning of the text.

Your work will require you to keep a variety of records, both manual and computerised. It is essential that you enter information accurately and check the details before closing a file or record. In a hospital, patients are allocated an identifying number at the point of registration. When accessing a system to find a patient record number, you will rely on the patient's surname, first name and date of birth. If the patient's surname is spelt incorrectly, the system will not be able to find the file. Apart from being time-consuming, this can result in the patient being registered twice at the same centre and being allocated a second case notes number. If this error is not spotted at an early stage, it is possible for a patient to have two separate sets of medical records in circulation at the same time.

Another aspect to remember is that the information held on the hospital Patient Administration System (PAS) will be used to invoice the purchasing authority for treatment given. If the information is inaccurate, the purchaser will not be able to relate the invoice to the patient registered at the practice. The result will be further, unnecessary correspondence to resolve the issue, creating avoidable delays. The importance of accuracy cannot be over-emphasised.

As previously discussed, you will be using the telephone a great deal during your work. Most telephone conversations will require you to receive and record information for future reference. Your method of recording this information must be reliable and accurate, as you may be receiving urgent investigation results, prescribing or medication information, or other clinical details. You will also receive cancellation of appointments and changes of address.

### Scenario

Mrs Jenson telephones you to give her new address and telephone number. She has already moved but forgot to notify you in advance.

Other than the new address and telephone number, what other details should you request from the caller? Which records will need to be updated?

The most essential information you need is the caller's full name and correct spelling. On the telephone what sounds like Jenson could in reality be Genson, Jensen or Jemson. If you omit to take the caller's first name, you could find yourself faced with an extensive list of Jensons to search through. It would also be a useful precaution to check the caller's date of birth to be sure of accurate identification. When you have taken the new address and telephone number, read the information back to the caller to check it is correct. A change of address needs to be entered on the computerised patient record, the medical notes and on any other medical records which are kept within your organisation.

## Effective use of time

As a medical secretary you will experience fluctuating workloads. You will be required to adopt appropriate time-management techniques to cope. Learning to control how your time is used and identifying problem areas will help you to achieve more in the time available. Time is your most precious resource and you must learn to use it effectively. There will be occasions when you are required to work to a specific deadline and you should learn to plan accordingly.

## Scenario

At the end of the day, you receive a lengthy medical report with the request to complete it by 2.00 p.m. the following day for the patient to collect. You go to work early the next day to type the report and arrive at 7.45 a.m. The normal working day starts at 9.00. On arrival you open the post which includes a letter your team has been waiting for. The rest proves to be routine correspondence only. At 8.00 you start the medical report. At 8.30 one of the doctors arrives for a social chat and a coffee. He leaves at 8.50 a.m. You have only completed one third of the report. Five minutes later your office colleagues arrive and the normal daily flow of telephone calls and tasks begin. At 11.30 you return to the medical report. You realise that you will have to work through lunch in order to complete the report on time.

Was the extra time used effectively? If not, why? Was the report given priority? What external factors influenced the use of time? How might these have been managed better?

Clearly, the objective of completing the report before the busy day began was not achieved. In this situation the post could have been left unopened until the normal start of the day as nothing was achieved by dealing with it at that time. The medical report was not treated as the first priority. The interruption by the doctor could have been dealt with by explaining why you were there so early and stating that you could not stop at that time. When colleagues arrived you could have explained the urgency of the situation to them and ask that your telephone calls be covered for a short period of time. Exercising control in

this manner would have ensured the objective was achieved.

## Setting priorities

An ability to organise your daily workload will assist you in maintaining control. You will be asked to complete a wide range of tasks during each working day. It is important to realise that tasks will carry differing levels of urgency. If you work solely for one person, prioritising the tasks will prove relatively simple. However, most medical secretaries work for more than one person, all of whom will provide work requiring immediate or priority attention. Your dilemma will be what to address first. Priority setting is a skill we all use in our everyday lives and it is an organisational skill which can be developed.

## Scenario

You work for two consultants, who share a team of junior staff. You have returned to work following 3 days' leave. Your in tray contains the following:

◆ six messages: three from patients, one from your manager and two from drug company representatives

◆ an audio tape from one of your consultants marked urgent

◆ a file of incoming mail

◆ a note from your other consultant asking you to locate some X-rays for a patient scheduled for surgery that afternoon.

Consider this list. Decide the priority of each, giving an explanation for your decision.

When deciding the priority of a task, ask the following questions:

What do I know?

Is there an obvious deadline?

Which has the most immediate need?

You may have decided that finding the X-rays should be your first priority. You know the patient is due to go to theatre in the afternoon so you have a specific deadline. Alternatively, the urgent audio tape may have been your first priority as you have no knowledge of the contents and the doctor concerned thought it important enough to be marked urgent.

The incoming mail is clearly of secondary importance in this situation. This is a routine task and there is no set deadline. The list of messages will need to be examined and placed in order of priority, depending upon the content of each message. You might consider that the three patients have the most immediate need of your attention over your manager and the drug representatives. Alternatively, the message from your manager may need to take precedence.

If you organise your tasks in this manner you will ensure that you meet urgent needs and deadlines whilst making the best use of your time.

## Accepting responsibility

As you progress within your post, you may be presented with situations which require a greater degree of responsibility. These situations should be viewed as opportunities to develop new skills, to use your existing skills and to demonstrate your value to the practice or department. When busy, it is tempting to view additional responsibility with a negative attitude, considering only the impact this may have on your current workload.

### Scenario

A new clerical assistant has been appointed. Your manager asks you to plan an induction programme for this person.

Devise a list of topics around which an induction programme could be constructed. What personal skills will you use by accepting and completing this task?

An induction programme should be specific to the environment and the post of the new member of staff. Your list should have covered the following areas:

◆ familiarisation with premises and facilities (e.g. toilets, kitchen, canteen, fire extinguishers)
◆ introduction to existing staff and description of roles
◆ supplying written protocols or procedures (e.g. fire drill, health and safety regulations, timetables)
◆ training on telephone, fax and copier operation
◆ introduction to filing systems
◆ provision of internal staff list and telephone directory
◆ training on computer systems.

To perform this task competently you will require effective written and verbal communication skills, time-management techniques, good judgment for priority setting and assessing the needs of the new member of staff, and the department.

It is appropriate at this point to warn you about the pitfalls of accepting too much responsibility. Always ensure that the task allocated falls within your area of skill and knowledge. Never be afraid of asking for further guidance or assistance from your manager, experienced colleagues or the medical team. Although you should be willing to become involved in new ventures, beware of allowing yourself to become overburdened with work within set deadlines.

## COURTESY

In this section we will consider those qualities which govern your relationships with people. Your interpersonal skills describe your reaction to and interaction with others. As a medical secretary you will be dealing with people from all sections of the community. Your colleagues and clients will demonstrate a variety of differing cultural attitudes and beliefs, come from varied social and economic groups, may suffer difficult domestic backgrounds and circumstances. The cornerstone of good interpersonal skills is to afford all people equal respect, care and consideration.

## Your colleagues

As previously discussed, the medical secretary will often work at the centre of a multidisciplinary team of health care staff. You will have contact with many types of personality: some pleasant and helpful, others brusque or obstructive. You should demonstrate a professional attitude to all colleagues regardless of their position or status within the organisation. Acknowledge that each person has a contribution to make. Do not judge your colleagues by your own morals or beliefs. You should show tolerance and control in the face of adversity. You should never allow personal feelings to influence your professional relationships.

## Your clients

Your clients will include patients, relatives, external agencies and other health care workers. Always remember that you are representing your employer when dealing with clients. The service you provide will influence the client's opinion not only of you, but of the medical team and the whole organisation as well. You should display a helpful and pleasant disposition at all times. You must be non-judgmental, non-discriminatory and approachable. In medicine it is common to hear the term 'patient advocate'. A simple definition of this phrase is that an individual will act as a supporter or ally of the patient. The medical secretary will act as a patient advocate in many situations, particularly when a patient is trying to communicate information or requests to members of the medical team. You will be relaying information on behalf of the patient.

### Reflection point

◆ Think of an acquaintance whom you do not particularly like. Try to analyse why this person provokes this reaction in you. Then think of someone you do like and identify why you like this person.

In the main, your reaction to a person is based on your own standards of attitude and behaviour. There will be specific qualities that you admire and habits that you find irritating. In your personal life you can choose the people you spend time with. In your professional life, this choice is not always available to you. You will be required to work and have contact with people you do not like or admire. However, these personal feelings must be put to one side in order that you can perform your role effectively.

### Scenario

You work in a deprived inner city area. One of your patients is a known drug user, with a reputation for aggressive behaviour, who attends the local secondary school. He attends without an appointment and demands that you make arrangements for him to see a doctor today.

Describe how you will deal with the situation and what factors might influence your handling of the request.

On a personal level, you may hold strong anti-drug convictions which make you dislike this person. You may even have a child relative who attends the local school who has had an experience with this person which has coloured your view. In this scenario, your first priority would be to establish whether or not the patient needs an urgent appointment and to provide this patient with relevant information in a professional, non-judgmental, manner.

## Assertiveness

Assertion can be described as the process of standing up for your own rights whilst respecting the rights of others by expressing yourself in direct, honest and appropriate ways. The aim of assertiveness is to satisfy the needs of both parties in any given situation. Assertiveness will assist you in coping with difficult situations at work such as:

◆ feeling anger or frustration
◆ disagreeing with seniors
◆ dealing with irate patients
◆ responding to unreasonable requests.

Your ability to be assertive should not be confused with being aggressive. Nor is it the opposite of being polite. Assertive behaviour is a skill which can be learned and improved. Being assertive will result in your becoming more effective in your job and will also improve your self-confidence. You will be taking responsibility for your behaviour, which will in turn allow you to become proactive rather than reactive.

### Scenario

Your manager telephones you to say that a colleague has been sent home ill and asks that you cover the reception desk for the afternoon session. You are working on a lengthy report for one of the medical team to take to an important meeting this evening.

**What is your response to your manager?**

An assertive response would be, 'I appreciate the problem but at present I am typing a report which is required for the meeting this evening and will not be able to help until it is finished'. A non-assertive response would be, 'Well, I am in the middle of this report but I suppose I could work on it over lunch instead'. An aggressive response would be, 'You must be joking, I've got this report to do and I can't possibly spare any time for you'.

The non-assertive response will leave you with difficult deadlines to meet, a feeling of frustration that you have been 'put upon', and anger with yourself for not fully explaining your own situation. The aggressive response will earn you a reputation of being unhelpful and obstructive and will leave you feeling very defensive.

To be assertive you must believe the following statements:

◆ I am in control of my behaviour
◆ I can change my behaviour
◆ I am responsible for what happens to me
◆ I can learn from any situation.
◆ I can take the initiative to reach objectives.

We have examined the role of assertion in refusing requests but assertiveness will be equally helpful to you when making requests.

When you wish to make a request, be straightforward. Do not apologise for making the request. Be direct, precise and provide a reason for the request. You must learn not to take a refusal personally by accepting the other person's right to say no.

## Handling aggression

Dealing with aggressive or abusive people can be emotionally unsettling and lead to an undesirable confrontational exchange. When faced with an aggressive patient it will help you to remain assertive by remembering the following:

◆ their behaviour may be affected by pain or discomfort
◆ their behaviour may be the result of frustration
◆ their behaviour may be the result of severe anxiety
◆ their behaviour may be due to a recognised neurological or psychiatric disorder.

### Scenario

You are manning the reception during a clinic. Owing to a shortage of medical staff the clinic is running behind schedule and several patients have been waiting for more than one hour. A patient approaches the desk wanting to know why he is being kept waiting so long. His voice is raised and he appears very tense. He unjustly accuses you of allowing other patients to go ahead in the queue and calls you inefficient.

**What is your initial reaction? What is your response to the question?**

In most cases, the individual will not be attacking you on a personal level but you are supplying an easy target.

It is particularly difficult to deal with an aggressive patient in front of other people in an unusually stressful time. In a situation such as this, it is wise to take a pause before offering your response. Use an assertive tone of voice but do not retaliate or show anger. Do remember to put the patient's needs first. Be calm, concerned and confident when you respond. If you are unable to provide the patient with an adequate explanation, seek further information or advice from someone more senior. Put yourself in his shoes and imagine how you would feel under similar circumstances. Add to this the possibility that he is ill or in pain and you can see why he is demonstrating aggression towards you, as the person representing the organisation.

## Handling stress

It needs to be acknowledged that stress is ever present in our lives and is inevitable during times of increased pressure in the workplace. Stress is a normal human reaction to difficult situations and is sometimes described as the 'fight or flight' response. A small amount is beneficial but too much stress can be detrimental to your health, state of mind and performance.

There are a variety of causes of stress in the workplace, some of which are listed below:

◆ long hours without proper breaks
◆ complex or time-consuming tasks
◆ rapid changes within the organisation or management structure
◆ unrealistic deadlines
◆ inadequate resources
◆ lack of communication
◆ fear about job security
◆ fear of being perceived as unable to cope
◆ developing new skills
◆ continuous interruptions.

You must become familiar with your own stress threshold and learn to recognise signs and symptoms which may be related to stress. Some of these are listed below:

◆ anxiety
◆ pounding heart
◆ inability to relax
◆ sweating
◆ indigestion
◆ depression
◆ weariness
◆ restlessness
◆ insomnia
◆ despondency
◆ moodiness
◆ moaning
◆ short temper.

In addition to the physical signs, you should be aware that your work performance could also be affected in the following ways:

◆ indecision
◆ poor time management
◆ absenteeism
◆ lack of humour
◆ low productivity
◆ increased frequency of errors
◆ apathy/disinterest
◆ poor presentation of written work.

There are a number of steps we can all take to combat the effects of stress. One of the most important is improving your physical health and lifestyle. You should be aware of the dangers of smoking, drinking alcohol, lack of sleep and erratic eating habits. Pay attention to your diet and ensure you are providing sufficient amounts of appropriate fuel for your body. Taking regular exercise and being aware of your level of fitness will also help you to fight stress.

Relaxation techniques can be learned and employed as part of your normal lifestyle. Regular exercise is an excellent way to relax and promote well-being. Other physical activities may prove more rewarding to you as an individual, such as dancing, gardening or DIY. It is your responsibility to ensure that you always maintain an acceptable balance between work activities and leisure time. If your workload is consistently too large, admit that you are only human and seek further advice or help.

---

**Box 5.2** CARL

◆ **C**ommunicate – recognise your limitations and ask when you need help

◆ **A**ssert yourself – avoid conflicts and frustration

◆ **R**ecognise stress – identify and tackle sources at an early stage

◆ **L**ifestyle – take responsibility for your health and protect your leisure time

Learning to recognise excessive stress can be turned to your advantage. Examine the situation and identify the main source of stress, and then tackle the situation directly. Your assertiveness skills will help you in this task.

You might find the checklist in Box 5.2 useful: Adopt CARL as your coping strategy, or develop your own personal code, and take it with you into all working environments.

## CONCLUSION

This chapter has illustrated many of the personal skills and qualities that are desirable in an effective medical secretary. The scenarios and reflection points serve as exercises for you to highlight your own strengths and weaknesses and will provide you with ideas for future self-development. We have illustrated ways in which the role of a medical secretary may become extended, with time and experience, allowing opportunities for complete involvement as a member of the team. The patient is at the centre of everything you do as a medical secretary and this should remain your main priority at all times.

The skills you bring to your work will enhance the service provided to each and every patient, provide your medical team with professional, efficient and reliable support and supply you with a great sense of job satisfaction and achievement.

**Exercises**

◆ Imagine you have been shortlisted for your first post as a medical secretary, having successfully attained your AMSPAR qualification. Bearing in mind the contents of this chapter, what questions do you think the interview panel might ask you? Make a list of possible questions and plan an outline of your answers. How will you influence the panel to appoint you over other, equally qualified, individuals? What will single you out as the obvious person for the job?

With a colleague from your study group, take turns to be the interviewee and interviewer. Use the questions you have devised on each other, without giving any prior warning as to what those questions might be. Decide on a scoring system and interview each other for approximately 10 minutes. Following this, compare notes and offer constructive criticism on each other's performance and presentation. Finally, you must decide whether or not you would have employed each other, based on the interview performance.

◆ You are an experienced medical secretary who has been employed in the same area/department for many years. The good news has just been announced that funds have been approved to increase the levels of staffing. The existing staff have long worked under difficult conditions with heavy workloads and your manager has invited you to contribute your views at a team meeting to discuss what the staffing priorities should be. Your workload is too large for one person and there are several areas of responsibility you would like to take on, but simply have not had enough time to do so in the past.

How will you approach this situation? What kind of information and evidence will you present in order to influence the decision-makers to include additional secretarial assistance in the recruitment programme?

How will you present this information? Plan your reasoning and ensure that you reflect the needs of the patients in your notes.

◆ As a result of the announcement of an imminent local rationalisation of services, there is much speculation about the future of your hospital. Staff morale has fallen to a low ebb. Your manager comes to you to ask for your assistance in helping to allay staff fears about their future and ensure the team continues to function effectively.

How will you react to this request? What information will you ask for? What suggestions would you make to your manager with regard to improving staff morale? How will you respond to colleagues who voice their fears to you directly? Examine the issues surrounding this situation.

## FURTHER READING

Pringle M (ed) 1993 Change and teamwork in primary care. BMJ Publishing, London

Black K, Black K 1995 Assertiveness at work. McGraw-Hill, Maidenhead

Haynes ME 1992 Make every minute count. Kogan Page, London

Brem C 1995 Are we on the same team here? Allen & Unwin, Sydney

Sommerville A 1993 Medical ethics today: its practice and philosophy. BMJ Publishing, London

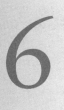

# Communication

*Sara Ladyman*

## 6

### OBJECTIVES

◆ To consider the overriding communication issues such as confidentiality affecting the medical secretary

◆ To focus on verbal communication: active listening, availability of information, checking skills, recording and relaying messages, suggestions for and emphasis on telephone technique, including useful proformas and reflection points

◆ To focus on visual communication: dress code and body language

◆ To focus on written communication: details of medical record content and secondary files, best practice for typewritten correspondence, managing workload, examples of labelling and proforma letters and prioritising work

◆ To conclude with an examination of internal and external systems which can facilitate good communication, for example tracking systems, short bibliography of useful books for the medical secretary, information dissemination, the mail, fax and e-mail.

## INTRODUCTION

This chapter is concerned with communication skills. A wide range of communication skills are essential to enable you to be an effective member of the team providing patient care. Your role is to relieve your medical team of the administrative workload and the communication skills you use will necessitate verbal, visual and written competence. We will be looking at each of these areas in this chapter. You will find it helpful to obtain a copy of the Patient's Charter.

## GENERAL

To communicate effectively with patients and members of staff you will need to assess systematically the needs of the patient and others, planning the response that best meets the individual's specific need.

All staff and patients with whom you come into contact should be treated politely, respectfully and in a helpful manner, regardless of their social standing, nationality, appearance or age. You should familiarise yourself with the Patient's Charter and the rights of patients. In particular, patients have a right to see or speak to their doctor and you must not interfere with this right but facilitate this communication by the active management of your doctor's time, assessing which administrative queries can be resolved by yourself and come within your responsibilities, and which messages must be passed on to the doctor for action, and prioritising these accordingly. You should read Chapter 4 on ethics and etiquette, which explores this area in greater depth.

# CONFIDENTIALITY

Patients have a right to confidentiality and there are some general guidelines you should be aware of. These are outlined below.

You must not disclose anything learned while at work with anyone and you should not pass comment on the ability of any doctor or nurse, and should never place them in an awkward or difficult situation.

You must not release any information about patients, not even to the police or a solicitor or insurance company acting on behalf of a patient.

Requests for information must be passed to the patient's doctor and the doctor will only release information with permission, usually in writing, from the patient. There are some exceptions, for example certain notifiable diseases where the public health could be put at risk. There will, however, be clearly defined procedures laid down for disclosure of information to the appropriate bodies.

## Informing patients of test results

You must not give any results to patients. In the majority of instances patients have to be given an appointment with the doctor to receive results and the appropriate advice and you should familiarise yourself with your organisation's policy and procedures and act appropriately. You should inform the doctor who last saw the patient of any request from the patient for results and he/she will advise.

In the unlikely event that you are asked by the doctor to contact a patient with a result it must be delivered only to the patient or to the parent of someone under 14 years of age, and no one else.

If a relative or the parent of someone over 14 years of age asks for results, or indeed wishes to discuss their relative, you must politely explain that the patient must make an appointment for the results or contact the department themselves. You should not discuss one patient with another.

Ordinarily you should be able to provide information about chemists, dental surgeons, opticians and other local practitioners but you must not channel patients to one particular practitioner. There should be a list available so the patient can make a choice.

---

**Box 6.1  Confidentiality**

*Do:*

◆ clarify who is calling and why

◆ only give authorised information direct to patient or guardian

◆ take telephone number and call back if in any doubt as to legitimacy of caller and double check information before doing so

◆ observe medical etiquette

◆ seek advice from medical or senior staff if unsure whether or not to pass information on.

*Do not:*

◆ disclose anything learned at work

◆ pass comment on ability of staff to patients or recommend doctors

◆ release information to a third party unless you have received a written request and acquired written consent from doctor and the patient

◆ leave messages on answerphones, and if you do, leave only minimum details, preferably just your name and the number to contact you on

◆ inform patients of results

◆ discuss one patient with another.

---

Personal responsibility: if you become aware of problems, for example GP or patient dissatisfaction arising because of a lack of appointments for patients, you should inform your manager or consultant so that remedial action may be taken.

Some dos and don'ts for confidentiality are listed in Box 6.1.

# VERBAL COMMUNICATION

Your work will include receiving and relaying oral and written messages between members of your medical team and patients, doctors, departments and organisations internal and external to your hospital or surgery. Remember that the tone and intonation of your voice can positively or

| Box 6.2 | Medical etiquette |
| --- | --- |
| GPs | Address the GP as 'Doctor...' followed by his or her second name, e.g. 'Doctor Smith'. |
| Consultant physicians | Called 'Doctor' followed by their second name, e.g. 'Doctor Smith'. |
| Consultant surgeons (male) | Referred to as Mister followed by their second name, e.g. 'Mister Smith'. |
| Consultant surgeons (female) | Miss, Ms or Mrs followed by their second name, e.g. 'Miss Smith'. |
| Professors | Called Professor, e.g. 'Professor Smith'. |

negatively affect the person to whom you are speaking and care should be taken.

It is important to observe medical etiquette when speaking with doctors and nurses. The guidelines given in Box 6.2 will assist you; however, if in doubt it is best to ask.

A consistent and precise approach to taking and relaying messages is essential for the accurate and prompt resolution of queries. There are a number of different tools you can use to facilitate good communication and these are outlined below. We will make particular reference to communication with patients.

**Reflection point**

◆ As a medical secretary you are one of the 'windows' of the hospital and what you communicate and how you communicate will colour the view patients and other staff have of your department and hospital.

## Listening skills

It is important to listen to patients and others wishing to leave a message. Active listening requires you to:

◆ focus on what the patient is saying
◆ repeat back what has been said to you to ensure understanding
◆ moderate your voice levels to protect confidentiality
◆ allow the patient to say everything they have to say, e.g. to describe full symptoms and their duration, spelling of medication and so on
◆ use positive language – rather than saying, 'No, you cannot see the doctor today', say, 'Yes, you can see the doctor but I am afraid he is very busy today and has no free appointments. Let us see when he/she can see you'.

**Reflection point**

◆ What are some of the distractions which can get in the way of active listening and how can you minimise these?

In addition to the message you should always record the following information from the caller:

◆ full name
◆ date of birth and/or hospital number
◆ contact telephone number
◆ address (if applicable).

Always check any details that are unclear, even if the person leaving the message expresses irritation. It is far better, often critical, to check details at the time of the message rather than take down incomplete or incorrect details which then require further action.

## Availability of information

As well as receiving a full message it is important that the doctor has as much information to hand as possible in order to decide on action to be taken.

As a general rule, any message regarding a patient should be accompanied by the patient's medical records, which may necessitate a trip to the medical records store. This ultimately avoids unnecessary delay as the doctor will undoubtedly ask to refer to the medical records and may need to record in them any action taken.

## Checking skills

We have mentioned the need to check your correct understanding. A useful tool to check a spelling alphabetically is the international alphabet (Box 6.3). It is advantageous to learn this.

Read the message back to the caller to make sure you have the correct information, even if you feel confident that you have all the facts. Always note the date and time of the call.

## Recording and relaying messages

A spiral bound notebook is an essential tool for effective message management. Messages taken on scrap paper can easily be mislaid whilst a notebook provides a lasting record for future reference and messages taken in chronological order and dated can be more easily prioritised for action.

Messages can be relayed either verbally or in writing, depending on their nature and urgency, and you will need to familiarise yourself with the times you can expect to see your medical team during the week. This may depend on where your office is situated, the doctor's work commitments and preference.

The majority of doctors carry radio pages or bleeps which can be accessed using the telephone or via switchboard. You should familiarise yourself with the protocol for paging different members of your team to pass on messages.

Your work may take you out of the office, or you may be occupied, e.g. with a telephone call when your doctors visit the office. The following tools can assist you in ensuring messages are received and actioned appropriately.

All messages should be clearly and legibly copied into: an A4 message book or diary or onto a white board or pinboard for messages. Alternatively, a hand-written message should be left in the appropriate pigeonhole or tray labelled for a doctor's attention. This may be in the format of a proforma to assist message taking and two examples can be found in Figure 6.1.

You may develop this further so you have a number of different proformas for different types of call. For example:

◆ urgent appointment requests, which require full information to be available to the consultant prior to receipt of the referral letter
◆ domiciliary, home visit, request from GP to a hospital consultant
◆ Home visit from a GP
◆ Ward visit.

Message proformas ensure that a consistent approach is taken and that information can be elicited clearly and concisely from the caller.

| Box 6.3 | The international alphabet | | | | | | |
|---|---|---|---|---|---|---|---|
| A | Alpha | B | Bravo | C | Charlie | D | Delta |
| E | Echo | F | Fox-trot | G | Golf | H | Holland |
| I | India | J | Juliet | K | Kilo | L | Lima |
| M | Mike | N | November | O | Oscar | P | Papa |
| Q | Quebec | R | Romeo | S | Sierra | T | Tango |
| U | Uniform | V | Victor | W | Whisky | X | X-ray |
| Y | Yankee | Z | Zulu | | | | |

(a)

| MESSAGE |
|---|
| DATE |
| TIME |
| TO |
| FROM |
| SURGERY/HOSPITAL |
| TELEPHONE NUMBER/BLEEP |
| |
| PATIENT NAME |
| HOSPITAL/REF NUMBER |
| DATE OF BIRTH |
| ADDRESS |
| |
| TELEPHONE NUMBER |
| |
| MESSAGE<br>RE: _____ |
| |
| OUTCOME/INSTRUCTIONS<br>(as appropriate) |

**Figure 6.1** Examples of message proformas which can be adapted for hospital or general practice use. They ensure a consistent approach is taken and information can be elicited clearly and concisely from the caller.

(b)

| REQUEST FOR A WARD VISIT |
|---|
| DATE/TIME REQUEST |
| TO |
| NAME |
| POSITION |
| TEL NO/BLEEP NO |
| |
| PATIENT NAME |
| HOSPITAL/REF NO |
| CONSULTANT PATIENT UNDER |
| PATIENT ON WARD |
| DATE OF BIRTH |
| ADDRESS (if applicable) |
| |
| ADMISSION DATE |
| PATIENT ADMITTED FOR |
| EXPECTED LENGTH OF STAY/DISCHARGE DATE (if known) |
| HISTORY/CURRENT PROBLEM (including site/extent/time) |
| |

**Figure 6.1** Contd.

# THE TELEPHONE

It is important to remember that when you use a telephone the person to whom you are speaking can only relate to your voice. They will not be able to observe body or facial expressions and you must use your voice to make your points clear. The language you use should be clear and you should avoid the use of jargon. By speaking into the mouthpiece and not across it your voice will not be distorted and you should speak more slowly than normally and pitch your voice slightly lower.

You should familiarise yourself with the telephone system as these are usually programmed to provide some or all of the services shown in Box 6.4.

Some telephones enable you to make calls outside the organisation; they usually require you to dial a key number first, for example a six or a nine, though this facility may be inaccessible before 9.00 a.m. and after 5.00 p.m. Alternatively, you may need to go through switchboard to make an external telephone call. It is your responsibility to listen to what the caller has to say and, if it is necessary to transfer them, to ensure that you are able to tell the switchboard exactly where, or to whom, the caller is to be transferred.

It is important to uphold the corporate image of your organisation when making or receiving telephone calls. You should familiarise yourself with the preferred terminology and style for receiving incoming calls. In a hospital this may involve you giving the name of the department followed by your name, for example, 'Dermatology Department, June Smith speaking' or 'Mr Jones' secretary'; similarly in a general practice, 'Southwark Health Centre' or 'Dr Edward's Practice'. This should be a response to both internal or external telephone calls as internal telephones can be linked to organisations outside your hospital. An informal 'hello' should never be used and you should follow up your introduction with 'how can I help you?' or a similar offer of help.

Try to avoid using negative language, i.e. 'no'. If a doctor or patient asks for an appointment it is better to say, 'I will see what I can do', rather than, 'Sorry, there are no appointments available'. When doctors contact you and ask for patients to be seen urgently, ask them when they would like the appointment and then do your best to accommodate them.

New or existing patients may ask why they have not received an appointment or request to be seen that day. Find out your departmental policy and response to these queries.

Patients are often unaware of the systems and procedures involved. For example, with a new patient referral to a hospital, you might explain to the patient that there is a long waiting time because so many patients have been referred to the service, or by saying, 'I am sorry I cannot help you jump the queue, that would mean putting another patient's appointment back'. Always follow up with a positive statement of action the patient can take. For example, you might say 'If you feel your condition is urgent (or 'as you are feeling unwell', whatever is appropriate) you should make an appointment to see your general practitioner and

| Box 6.4 | Telephone services |
|---------|--------------------|
| Call forward | To forward calls to another extension in your absence |
| Follow me | If you are in another office and wish to have all calls diverted to this extension |
| Ring back | To ring back from a number which is currently busy |
| Save | To save an external number you have just dialled |
| Conference facility | To add one or more parties to your two-way call |
| Pick up group | Ability to take calls at your phone from other telephones within your vicinity and hearing range |
| Page/Bleep | There will be a sequence of numbers you will need to ring to page a doctor, or you may have to go through switchboard |

discuss with him/her'. You may need to explain that only their general practitioner can determine the urgency of their condition and you are unable to act on the request of a patient in this case.

For patients who have been seen in the department or practice previously it may just be the case that you have to point out that 'the next available appointment is for ...' and if they are unhappy then it is best to bring this to the attention of the appropriate member of your medical team.

Confidentiality has to be uppermost when you use the telephone as it is difficult to be sure to whom you are speaking. If in doubt as to the caller's credibility take his/her telephone number and address and other details, obtain the case notes and speak to a member of the medical team before ringing the caller back. It may be necessary, depending on the nature of the call, to ask the caller to send in a written request before any information can be divulged.

Always answer calls promptly, even if you are busy. To avoid sounding abrupt on the telephone, if you are feeling harassed, before lifting the handset pause, take a deep breath and put a smile in your voice. Box 6.5 lists some guidelines for good telephone practice.

## Answerphones

When leaving messages on answerphones be aware that this information will be accessible to those other than the patient whom you are trying to contact and thus raises the issue of confidentiality. Only leave a message if it is vital to do so, or the patient has given prior consent in previous conversations. Keep the message brief and leave the minimum of detail. It is usually best to leave your name and number and ask the person by name to return your call at the earliest opportunity.

In your own office an answerphone should only be used selectively for incoming calls. It is important that you are easily accessible to anyone who needs to get a message to your consultant or a member of your medical team. The constant use of answerphones can be frustrating for callers, especially if the message on the answerphone is out of date or inappropriate.

---

**Box 6.5** Tips and hints for good telephone practice

*Receiving calls*

◆ Answer calls promptly.

◆ Avoid keeping callers waiting – give callers the choice of being rung back if their query requires you to search for information or consult other staff.

◆ Take the caller's name and telephone number in case you should be cut off, and ring back directly if this occurs.

◆ Keep coming back to callers.

◆ Be familiar with staff names and extension numbers for routine requests.

◆ When re-routing calls ensure the called extension wishes to accept the call. If the call cannot be put through or there is no reply, give the caller a choice of ringing back, together with your telephone number or ask if he/she wishes to leave a message.

◆ Do not be over familiar.

◆ If a caller is cut off ring back immediately.

◆ End the call politely.

*Making calls*

◆ Plan what you are going to say and have all the information you may need to refer to at hand and also a list of the points you wish to raise.

◆ Dial the number carefully.

◆ If you dial the wrong number offer an apology.

◆ Introduce yourself by name and organisation.

◆ Give the name of the person you wish to speak to or state the purpose of your call so you can be put through to appropriate person.

◆ Be aware of costs – the distance and length of call.

---

The following guidelines may be helpful when deciding how you are going to utilise an answerphone most effectively.

◆ Aim to use only when you are out of the office.

◆ Avoid using when in the office except for exceptional circumstances, for example, during meetings.

◆ Timely response to messages – take messages off immediately you return to the office, prioritise and ring the caller(s) back immediately, clarify their need and advise that you will get back to them as appropriate.

◆ Update the recorded message regularly, keep it brief, taking into account your organisational protocol, and indicating when you will next be available.

## VISUAL COMMUNICATION

It is important to observe a dress code. Some organisations provide their medical secretaries with a uniform or give them a colour code. If no such guidelines exist you have to consider the impression you wish to give as a representative of your practice or hospital.

**Reflection point**

◆ A well groomed and smart appearance can affect the patient's perspective on the care they are to receive from you and others. Consider how you would expect a member of staff to be dressed should you have to attend for a doctor's appointment. Also be aware of the practical considerations of dress. A medical secretary may need to travel some distance on foot on a daily basis as well as lifting, bending and stretching, for example when moving case notes around the office.

It is also a patient charter standard that all staff should wear an identity badge and it may be a disciplinary offence for staff to be seen without one as this will form part of the security strategy.

Non-verbal signals are as important as what we are saying and how we say it. Here are some areas where you should consider whether the non-verbal signals you are giving can be interpreted positively or negatively by the other person.

*Your:*

◆ posture and positioning
◆ gestures, including body and head movement
◆ facial expressions
◆ eye contact
◆ mirroring of the other person's body language.

**Reflection point**

◆ Think about the positive and negative ways non-verbal signals can be interpreted by the receiver for each of the above.

## WRITTEN COMMUNICATION

### Patient case notes

In addition to the computerised Patient Administrative System, explained fully in Chapter 8 on information technology, your main source of information regarding a patient's care will be found in the patient's medical record or case notes. The primary medical record file should contain the information listed below, and you will make particular reference to the most recent clinic notation and test results as well as patient's personal and demographic data, particularly when copy or audio typewriting correspondence.

A medical record usually includes:

◆ current identification sheet
◆ previous letters (referral and clinic)
◆ copies of discharge summaries following inpatient stays as appropriate
◆ history sheets/clinical notation for each visit
◆ operation and anaesthetic records (hospital records primarily)
◆ diagnostic test results, e.g. chemical pathology, ECG records
◆ X-ray results
◆ pathology results

♦ drug prescription chart
♦ labels with GP and patient data.

It is important that every effort is made to ensure that results and correspondence copies are filed in the case notes promptly. You should make reference to Chapter 12 on medical records and Chapter 16 on the working practice for further details of patient case notes and their organisation.

When patients attend regularly, their case notes may increase and you may find they have a secondary file containing non-current information. This is to ensure that the primary file contains relevant current information only and is easily accessible, thereby reducing the bulk of paperwork handled routinely at clinics. The secondary file may be stored separately from the main filing store and you will only need to obtain this when specifically requested to do so.

It is easy to become complacent and forget that your office contains many confidential documents. Whilst medical records in particular should never be locked away you should ensure that only staff have access to your office in your absence and ensure that confidential information is not left unattended in patient areas.

## WRITTEN CORRESPONDENCE

Typewritten correspondence still forms the primary link between general practice and hospitals. The vital link is established between GPs and hospital departments by the initial referral letter from the GP to a hospital consultant in a specific field of medicine asking the specialist for his/her opinion and appropriate treatment. Once the hospital specialist has accepted the shared care of the patient, a letter following each hospital outpatient visit ensures the GP has current and accurate information available on a patient's progress, their current medication, test results and so on until they are discharged back to the GP's exclusive care.

It is therefore important that any correspondence you produce from audio, hand-written or shorthand dictation can be easily identified to a particular patient and is accurate and complete.

Whilst you may be familiar with the standard organisational format for letters, you will need to familiarise yourself with the format and style of letter used in your department or practice. This may include the use of proformas. You should ensure, however, that every letter contains the following:

The patient's details form the heading of the letter; these must be prominently displayed so that the doctor can easily identify which patient they refer to. You may, for example, choose to use one of these formats. Remember that with the open styles you must leave two spaces between items.

Ralph ARMANDY dob 10.04.35
14 Blackfriars Road, Woolwich, London.
SW1 4TH

*or*

Ralph Armandy dob 10.04.35
14 Blackfriars Road, Woolwich, London.
SW1 4TH

*or*

RALPH ARMANDY dob 10 04 35
14 BLACKFRIARS ROAD WOOLWICH
LONDON SW1 4TH

In addition, you should also include the following:

♦ a reference comprising doctors' initials/your initials/record or case note number if available, e.g. 'SM/sac/MK 12 34 26'
♦ clinic date
♦ date dictated (if not the same as clinic date and this may be optional)
♦ date letter typed
♦ addressee and their address
♦ signatory.

The letter is usually addressed to a doctor.
If it is to a GP you should address the letter as follows:

Dr D Benson
Watling Road Practice
Watling Road West
Milton Keynes
MK12 5MM

If the letter is to a consultant physician you should address the letter as follows:

Dr D Watson
Consultant Gastroenterologist
Milton Hospital
Milton Road
Milton Keynes
MK12 5MM

If it is to a consultant surgeon you should address the letter as follows:

Mr D Watson (or Mrs/Ms/Miss Watson)
Consultant Gynaecologist
Milton Hospital
Milton Road
Milton Keynes
MK12 5MM

For the signatory's name, it is essential to check organisational preferences; for example, your doctors may prefer to have their qualifications listed after their name (e.g. FRCS or MRCP).

It is usual for GPs to put their name only, for example:

Dr D Benson

For a consultant you may put:

Mr D Watson
Consultant Gastroenterologist

See Figure 6.2 and 6.3 for examples of the layout for an outpatient clinic letter.

A copy of the letter should be filed in the appropriate section of the case notes; the most recent letter is usually filed on top of all previous correspondence.

As they form part of the patient's medical case notes, and so that they can be easily referred to, it is important that copies are correct and legible. You must use the spell-check facility on your PC and proof-read correspondence before it is presented for signature to minimise effort and frustration and the inevitable delay when letters have to be corrected, reprinted and presented for signature

once more. In addition, it is helpful to keep a personalised dictionary, entering unfamiliar spelling as you come across them for your own information and for a secretary who might be assisting you with your workload or covering your annual leave.

## Managing the incoming typing workload

The following systems can assist in managing your typing workload effectively.

Your doctors will usually be only too pleased to assist with the preparation of case notes ready for transcription, particularly from audio cassettes, especially if this results in fewer queries or inaccuracies in correspondence waiting for signature and requiring subsequent correction and re-presentation for signature. You will find further reference to audio cassettes in Chapter 13 on the outpatient department.

When the GP or hospital doctor dictates correspondence on patients attending the clinics ask them to:

◆ dictate their name and the clinic date at the start of the audio cassette
◆ keep case notes in an orderly pile, preferably in the order dictated
◆ dictate clearly and precisely.

You should bring any problems in this area to their attention as a great deal of time can be consumed in trying to decipher unclear or indistinct dictation. Remember that the ease of transcription depends partly on the quality of recorded text. If there are problems you should sensitively discuss these with the individual concerned. A mutually beneficial method of working is important if you are going to complete your workload speedily and accurately.

You can assist by taking responsibility for the following points.

◆ Ensure that a supply of batteries and good quality audio tapes are available to the doctors as old batteries and tapes can cause distortion of dictation.
◆ Once an audio cassette has been used it should be sealed in an envelope.

**HOSPITAL HEADING**

Ref:   DW/sac/proform/44 44 21

Date:   10 12 96

Dr D Benson
Watling Road Practice
Watling Road West
Milton Keynes
MK12 5MM

Dear Dr Benson

AL GUPTA dob 21.07.61

9 SEED STREET, CLOVER GATE, MILTON KEYNES MK2 3DT

I regret to inform you that the above patient failed to attend their outpatient clinic appointment on

_____ .

No further appointment will be sent.

Yours sincerely

Mr D Watson
Consultant Gastroenterologist

**Figure 6.2**   Example of a Did Not Attend outpatient clinic letter.

**HOSPITAL HEADING**

Ref:    DW/sac/proform/44 44 21


Date:    10 12 96


Dr D Benson
Watling Road Practice
Watling Road West
Milton Keynes
MK12 5MM

Dear Dr Benson


AL GUPTA dob 21.07.61

9 SEED STREET, CLOVER GATE, MILTON KEYNES MK2 3DT


Your patient attended for _____ surgery on 9th December 1996.

A review appointment has been arranged for _____ .


Yours sincerely




Mr D Watson
Consultant Gastroenterologist

**Figure 6.3**    Example of a letter indicating that surgery has been carried out.

◆ The doctor's name/initials and the clinic date should be written on the envelope as it may get lost or dictated over in error.

◆ Secure the case notes with a rubber band and attach the clinic tape envelope to reduce the risk of notes and tape becoming separated.

◆ Place in chronological order of clinic dates for typing.

When correspondence is printed off for signature it is essential that two copies are made and that one copy is filed in the case notes at the earliest opportunity, ensuring that the case notes are complete and up to date before being passed on for another clinic or to another doctor.

Letters for signature can be kept in pristine condition by placing them in folders labelled appropriately and placed in the doctor's tray or pigeonhole. Check your departmental procedure as some doctors like to be paged when their letters are ready for signature; others may expect you to make them available at the beginning or end of outpatient clinic sessions.

Remember to wipe the cassette clean to avoid confusion with tapes that have old dictation on them but only when you are satisfied that neither you nor the doctor will need to refer to them again.

If there are indistinct words or passages on the tape which you are unable to decipher you should keep the cassette with the case note(s) and clearly mark where the gaps are for the doctor to complete at the earliest opportunity.

Occasionally, case notes have to be taken for other clinics before you have had an opportunity to type the letters. Set up a system whereby whoever removes the case notes leaves you with a patient and GP label from the notes, to be taken together with the other notes and tape waiting to be typed.

In addition, you may provide, for ease and quickness, a label which can be attached to the front of the case notes asking for them to be returned to you so that the copy of the letter to be typed can be filed inside. See Figure 6.4 for an example of a return label which can be stapled to the front of the case notes. Departments are generally familiar with this system and should use internal systems to return the case notes to you and not back to the main store.

---

PLEASE RETURN THESE CASE NOTES

AS SOON AS POSSIBLE TO:

THE DERMATOLOGY DEPARTMENTAL SECRETARY

LEVEL 1, OUTPATIENT BUILDING

EXTENSION 3658

Reason required: (e.g. Dr DW clinic 4.4.96)      date (5.4.96)

THANK YOU

---

**Figure 6.4**   Example of a return label for case notes taken for another clinic or doctor's attention.

Ask doctors to dictate urgent letters if possible on a separate cassette for speedy transcription after clinic as this saves time going through a cassette to find one letter which needs to be sent urgently.

It may be possible within your department to use a number of proforma letters on your personal computer for some groups of patients.

For example, when patients do not attend their hospital appointments it is possible to have a standard letter format (see Fig. 6.2) which has been agreed by the directorate, to be sent to patients. Another example (see Fig. 6.3), might be to confirm that a patient has attended for a surgical procedure in an outpatient clinic.

## Prioritising typing workload

Your working week will to a large extent be determined by your consultants' outpatient and inpatient timetable or GP's surgery sessions. A clinic timetable is therefore a useful piece of information to have displayed on your noticeboard; see Figure 6.5 for an example of a hospital department timetable.

**Reflection point**

Using the information given in Figure 6.5, when would you expect to receive your incoming typing workload?

In this case you may expect an influx of clinic work for typewriting on the Tuesday afternoon, Wednesday afternoon, Thursday morning, Friday afternoon and late Friday or the following Monday morning. The numbers of patients attending each clinic is obviously in direct relation to the number of letters dictated.

| DAY | MORNING | AFTERNOON |
|---|---|---|
| Monday | – | – |
| Tuesday | OUTPATIENT CLINIC<br>Dr Peach, Consultant Physician<br>Dr George, Registrar | – |
| Wednesday | OUTPATIENT CLINIC<br>Dr Fisher, Senior Registrar | OUTPATIENT CLINIC<br>Professor Robert Johns<br>Dr George, Registrar |
| Thursday | – | – |
| Friday | OUTPATIENT CLINIC<br>Professor Robert Johns<br>Dr Fisher, Senior Registrar | OUTPATIENT CLINIC<br>Dr George, Registrar |

**Figure 6.5** Example of general medical outpatient clinic timetable.

The ratio of new to old patients is also important. New patient letters are generally longer than those for follow-up patients because they contain reference to patients' relevant past medical or social history as well as clinical findings.

It is therefore important that you look at your typewriting workload as a continuous cycle of transcription, presentation for signature and dispatch. It is unusual for medical secretaries to have no outstanding clinic typing and some typing should be included as one of your daily priorities. You should also familiarise yourself with your department's policy regarding turnaround of clinic transcription and dispatch of letters. Some hospital departments will stipulate this in the contract for services with the GPs; for example, that the correspondence be dispatched within 5 days of clinic attendance. These times will have been negotiated with GPs and you should do your best to prioritise your workload accordingly and address issues within your control, for example the quality and speed of transcription and organisational skills, as well as taking into account issues outside or partly within your control. These may include poor quality of dictation, delay in dictating or signing letters for dispatch, arrangements for annual leave and sickness cover, all of which can have an impact on the throughput of work.

### Reflection point

◆ What other factors influence the period of time that elapses before correspondence is sent out to GPs and which of these should you be familiar with?

You should familiarise yourself with when your doctors visit your department for signing letters, whether you have to page them when their letters are ready or prepare them for signature during the next outpatient clinic. You will also need to inform new medical staff joining your department of systems already established.

### Hospitals

What are the implications if a member of your medical team delays dictating clinic letters for patients who have attended an outpatient clinic?

◆ Case notes awaiting dictation are static in the department, taking up valuable space and time when searching through for case notes.
◆ Case notes may be taken for other clinics and if the case notes are not returned promptly, or are sent back to the medical records department, in error, a letter may be delayed or missed. This may result in your department or the contracts department being contacted by a GP surgery requesting confirmation of clinic attendance and treatment received, and financial penalties may be incurred.

### General practice

If there are delays in letters being dispatched by general practice then this will result in:

◆ Delays for patients entering the referral system at the hospital including the dispatch of an outpatient appointment. This may result in telephone calls and queries from patients enquiring about their forthcoming appointment.

## INTERNAL/EXTERNAL SYSTEMS TO FACILITATE GOOD COMMUNICATION

It is essential that the staff you work with are also able to find their away around your office, so it is important to label trays and pigeonholes clearly and ensure that files and records are easily accessible.

In addition, it is important to keep up-to-date information available on the different procedures you use as you will be absent at different times throughout the year. This will help minimise the disruption to the daily routine whilst you are away and there will be fewer queries on your return.

# Tracking system for medical case notes and X-rays

It is essential that you have a tracing system for patient case notes entering and leaving your department. Increasingly departments are computerising their systems utilising the Patient Administration System (PAS) and bar coding the case notes for accurate identification and tracking. Alternatively, you may use a manual system, for example by using an A–Z book to draw up hand-written entries, or patient identification labels, as notes enter and leave the office. The most vital information to record is the destination of case notes and the date they leave your office. The majority of case notes are returned to the medical records department for general filing.

You will, however, have requests for notes to be taken to other departments or outpatient clinics and, if the tracer is not updated in the medical records department, the case notes will still be booked to you and considered your responsibility.

In addition, the book can be used for booking case notes to particular doctors' pigeonholes or offices and will save time when looking for case notes. A system is only as good as its users so it is important that medical staff and other staff using your office are made aware of the booking in/out system and that the book is always readily available.

## Diary

You will usually hold the consultant's diary, whether it be computerised or manual. Whichever system you use, it is important that you keep entries up to date, accurate and readily accessible. You will need to clarify times when your consultant sees medical representatives as they may have a regular slot or slots for these visits.

### Notification of cancellation/reduction of clinics

You are usually the first to know when a doctor is going to take annual or study leave. It is advisable to ask your doctors from time to time (perhaps leaving a message to do so in your bring forward file) what their leave arrangements are to be. You may also find it helpful to liaise with the medical staffing department, usually based within the personnel department framework, who usually manage leave requests.

It is essential that information about doctors' leave is passed on as soon as possible, usually in writing, to the appropriate appointments staff so the necessary alterations can be made to the clinic lists. This may necessitate rescheduling of patients already booked into appointments to other clinic dates.

When notification has not been received or there has been insufficient time to contact patients, even by telephone or telemessage, this can result in clinics over running, doctors attending the clinic experiencing a higher than normal workload and patients either having to wait unacceptable times to be seen or being turned away. This situation should be avoided at all costs.

Figure 6.6 shows a proforma which might be utilised instead of a memorandum and illustrates the information required by the appointments staff.

## Bring forward system

You may utilise both computerised and manual systems to highlight work requiring immediate attention. A simple example would be to use a concertina wallet divided into the days of the month, 1 to 31. Correspondence, queries, items to be actioned at a later date can then be placed in the appropriate slot. You can use this system in conjunction with a concertina folder divided into the twelve months of the year, transferring papers and reminders at the beginning of each month.

Any bring forward system must be checked daily and relevant correspondence or messages retrieved and actioned accordingly.

## Computer system

It is imperative to keep back-up disks of work held on computer and you should endeavour to do regular housekeeping, at least once a month, to erase any files that are no longer required.

Build up a glossary facility as you come across names and addresses for each new GP and hospital doctor for quick and easy insertion into correspondence.

HOSPITAL LOGO

### NOTIFICATION OF CANCELLATION AND REDUCTION OF CLINIC

Clinics will only be cancelled/amended when authorisation has been given by the Consultant in whose name the Clinic is held. A minimum of four weeks' notice should be given:

CLINIC LIST IN THE NAME OF: _____

IF JUNIOR DOCTOR, STATE WHICH
CONSULTANT YOU WORK FOR: _____

| DATE | LIST CODE | CANCEL | REDUCE BY | SPECIAL COMMENTS OR REQUESTS e.g. 3 doctors rather than usual 5 |
|------|-----------|--------|-----------|-----------------------------------------------------------------|
|      |           |        |           |                                                                 |

DATE:

CONSULTANT NAME (CAPITALS):

SIGNATURE:

FOR APPOINTMENTS USE ONLY

CLINIC AMENDMENT/CANCELLATION

DATE RECEIVED

AKNOWLEDGEMENT SENT

CHANGE COMPLETED

**Figure 6.6** Notification of cancellation and reduction of clinics proforma.

Set up a macro outline of the format of your correspondence for each member of your medical team, saving you time by not having to repeat the same information for each letter. An example is shown in Figure 6.7 of a skeleton outline of a letter.

Chapter 8, on information technology, looks at computer systems in more detail.

Each time you find a new medical term add it to the spell-check dictionary to make it as comprehensive as possible.

## Reference books

Ensure you have ready access to reference books such as:

◆ medical dictionary
◆ general dictionary
◆ MIMS and/or BNF for checking the spelling of drugs (sometimes obtainable from the pharmacy or your doctors can provide you with a recent copy)
◆ internal and external telephone directories
◆ medical directories.

## Noticeboards

Your noticeboard is a useful tool for quick and easy reference for yourself and colleagues. For a noticeboard to be an effective aid, all information displayed must be current and updated at regular intervals. It is helpful to display:

◆ useful telephone numbers and page/bleep numbers
◆ diagrammatic clinic timetable
◆ diagrammatic doctors' timetables
◆ lists of macros and glossary short forms available on your PC
◆ holiday timetables
◆ calendar
◆ miscellaneous.

## Circulation of information to members of the team

You will be asked to circulate information to members of your team. A proforma can easily be attached to a document with the appropriate action indicated for the receiver; see Figure 6.8.

Similarly, proformas can be used to avoid confusion and requests for photocopying may be aided by the use of a photocopying requisition form; see Figure 6.9.

## Mail

The internal mail system is not generally used for the transportation of patient case notes. Either there will be a delivery service, usually part of the medical records department store, or case notes should be hand delivered.

Hospital patient case notes must never leave the Trust or Health Authority from which they originate, other than in exceptional circumstances. Once a written request for information has been received, and the patient's written consent has also been received, the patient's doctor will indicate whether all or certain sections of the case notes can be copied by you and sent off. The same applies in general practice, unless the case notes have been recalled, for example, for auditing or for dispatch to a patient's new GP.

### Incoming mail

You will need to clarify whether the mail is delivered to your department or you have to collect it from a central point. You can sort it into mail addressed to you, mail for doctors within the department and the consultants' mail. Some consultants prefer you to open their mail, sort and prioritise it. Others open and sort all their mail themselves.

As with some messages, it is important to provide the doctor with as much information as possible to accompany the letter or test result, and this will usually necessitate locating relevant case notes for the patient indicated. If, however, case notes are unobtainable in the first instance this should not delay bringing the letter to the doctor's attention.

Incoming mail for general practice usually includes:

◆ letters from hospital for patients who have attended outpatient clinic visits

---

**HOSPITAL HEADING**

Direct Line:

Fax No:

Ref: DW/sac/

Clinic:          (enter date and then copy)

Typed:          (enter date and then copy)

Dear

                                                        Yours sincerely

                                                        Mr D Watson
                                                        Consultant Gastroenterologist

---

**Figure 6.7**  Outline of a letter which can be set up on computer as a macro or glossary.

◆ discharge summaries for patients who have been discharged from an inpatient stay in hospital
◆ test results.

Incoming mail for a consultant and his team usually includes:

◆ referral letters from general practitioners requesting a specialist opinion
◆ test results from the various laboratories.

Both may receive:

◆ requests for information from solicitors, insurance companies, other hospitals
◆ agenda/minutes of meetings
◆ pharmaceutical literature
◆ medical journals
◆ general correspondence.

## Outgoing mail

Mail will usually have to be sorted into 'internal' mail, which is going to departments or internal organisations, and 'external' mail, which is for the Post Office to deliver.

Mail is usually sent out second class unless you indicate first class on the envelope. Once again, you will need to clarify whether outgoing mail is collected or whether you have to leave it for collection outside the department. Outgoing mail should be dispatched at the earliest opportunity.

There may be an internal transport link system

HOSPITAL LOGO

Date:

To:  _____

____  For your information/circulation

____  Please take appropriate action

____  As requested

____  I should be grateful for your comments

____  Please answer this for me

____  Please read and return

____  For your files

Dr S. Patel

WITH COMPLIMENTS

**Figure 6.8**  Example of compliment slip style action proforma.

between neighbouring hospitals and general practices where post bypasses the Post Office, thus saving postage costs and distribution time and preserving confidentiality.

## Facsimile copies

The fax machine is a relatively cheap way to send information and is very useful when information has to be relayed quickly. It is essential that care is taken in dialling numbers (confidentiality could be easily breached if patient information were transmitted to the wrong destination).

Some safeguards include:

◆ checking with the receiver of the fax where it will be received, for example in an open patient area or office

◆ informing the receiver at the time you send the fax
◆ asking the receiver of the fax to contact you directly it is received
◆ deleting the patient's second name and other personal details which can be subsequently filled in by the receiver.

A top sheet should always accompany the faxed sheets and Figure 6.10 provides one such example.

## E-mail

The use of computer networking to facilitate communication between hospitals and general practice is gradually increasing as more sophisticated hard- and software is being introduced into the health care sector. See Chapter 8, on

## PHOTOCOPYING REQUISITION

Date requested

Department

No. of originals

No. of copies

Print 2 sides

Collated          YES/NO

Other requirements

**Figure 6.9** Photocopying requisition form which can be adapted accordingly to instruct staff on facilities available to them.

information technology, for further information regarding this.

## CONCLUSION

Your role is to process a constant and wide variety of incoming verbal and written data. The dissemi-nation of this information may in turn be verbal or written. Accuracy, timeliness and appropriate disclosure of information is central to the smooth running of your department. You provide the important communication link between the professionals sharing the 'hands on' care of patients. You may often be the first representative of your organisation with whom a patient will come into contact. How you relate to patients and staff is of great importance if patients are to have confidence from the outset in the care they are to receive.

### Exercises

Discuss how you would deal with the following situations.

◆ An elderly patient's daughter telephones you to ask why her mother is attending the clinic as she is very worried about her.

◆ A patient telephones you and asks you to tell him the result of his blood test. He says he was told to ring you for this information.

◆ You receive a call from a friend of a patient who wants to enquire whether the patient is still an inpatient in the hospital.

◆ A solicitor's clerk telephones and gives details of a particular patient whom he says has given permission for her records to be released to him. He asks you to send the case notes to him urgently, as the patient's court appearance is imminent, and to clarify some specific appointment dates on the telephone.

**DEPARTMENT LOGO**

ADDRESS

TELEPHONE NUMBER

FACSIMILE NUMBER

**FAX**

INFORMATION STRICTLY CONFIDENTIAL

TO _____

FROM _____

NUMBER OF PAGES BEING SENT, INCLUDING THIS SHEET _____

IF ANY DIFFICULTIES, PLEASE CONTACT _____

TELEPHONE NUMBER _____ EXTENSION _____

MESSAGE _____

**Figure 6.10** Example of a fax covering sheet.

# 7

# Finance

*Stephanie J Green*

## OBJECTIVES

◆ To enable the reader to appreciate the increasing importance of finance in general practice and the role of specific administrative staff to monitor and manage it

◆ To assist the reader in understanding the sources of finance in general practice

◆ To explain the different demands which private practice will make of the medical secretary

◆ To provide a source of reference material including official publications and journals.

## INTRODUCTION

This chapter is designed to introduce basic financial procedures and to discuss the measures by which income and expenditure are managed in general practice and in private practice. It should be obvious that the finances of a hospital will not be part of a secretary's normal role. However, if this is an area of work which fascinates, there is nothing to stop the secretary undertaking further training to extend experience and ability, in order to fulfil a different role or to find promotion in a different area of administration.

Financial management in medicine has become more complicated over the past few years and the changes in structure generally have made the employment of other professional people a necessity. This does not mean that the medical secretary will have nothing to do with financial affairs, but that whatever the involvement with income and expenditure, it is always important to understand the responsibilities attached to this area of work and the good practice which should be observed at all levels. It is true to say that medical secretaries who work in private practice will probably have more to do with the financial side of their work than a secretary working within the National Health Service.

## GENERAL PRACTICE

In general practice, the financial control of the practice will lie with the practice manager, and in fundholding practices, this may be extended to a fundholding manager, accounts manager or book-keeper, depending on the needs of the practice. Financial work will include the following:

◆ regular checks on NHS claims for work – complete, correct and submitted on time
◆ control of petty cash
◆ administration of invoices and receipts
◆ salaries
◆ insurance
◆ PAYE for staff
◆ maintenance of cheque books and accounts. It is likely that in the future all accounts will be computerised – many are already.

The medical secretary may be involved with some or none of this work, depending upon the nature of the practice. However, there are financial tasks which may well be the medical secretary's responsibility. These are:

◆ Receipt of invoices or payments in the mail – these will need to be recorded in the relevant book and redirected to the practice manager.
◆ Invoicing accurately for work completed, in accordance with the standard fees list, e.g. requests for medico-legal reports. These are usually the responsibility of the medical secretary because of the use of specialist language within the report. A diary system will also be needed to ensure that payment has been received, especially as these reports may be part of lengthy legal debate and payment may therefore be long term.
◆ Invoicing for photocopying of notes requested by solicitors, once patient consent/authority has been given for the use of confidential material. Again, a proper record of this kind of work should be kept and a note of payments made.

Although we have mentioned areas of financial concern specific to the medical secretary, there are some general points that all staff working in general practice will need to remember in order to maintain an efficient system. Today, general practice has to be run like any other business, balancing income against all the usual outgoings and expenditure.

**Reflection point**

◆ Make a list of all the expenses involved with business premises you can think of. Then think of your own general practice or one where you have had work experience and add all the more particularly medical items.

## Income

All general practices are allotted a Practice Allowance Capitation from the NHS via the Local Health Authority. This will vary depending upon a variety of situations such as the number of patients on the doctors' lists, whether it is a rural practice or an inner city practice for which special payments may be made. As well as this, there are a number of common activities known as 'items of service' which must be claimed for if they are to become part of the general practice income. Some examples of items of service are shown in Box 7.1.

**Box 7.1**　Some 'items of service'

◆ Patient registration
◆ Child surveillance
◆ Night visits
◆ Temporary patient care
◆ Contraceptive services
◆ Antenatal care

**Reflection points**

◆ Remember to ask about these claims when you are in a general practice work placement. What does the claim form look like? How is it filled in? Whose responsibility is it?
◆ What else can be claimed for in this way?

Another source of income is from 'targeted' activities. These are items of care which have a special percentage target to be achieved by the practitioners if they are to gain the maximum payment for their work. At the moment claims under this scheme are for:

◆ immunisation of children of 5 years and under.
◆ cervical cytology.

Other sources of income for general practice are:

◆ trainee practitioner scheme
◆ postgraduate education allowance
◆ education of medical students
◆ private patients
◆ insurance medicals
◆ cremation forms
◆ special driving licences and passport forms.

Some GPs take other appointments such as medical responsibility for a local company or for the police as police surgeon.

There are many sources of information, varying from monthly journals to official documents and publications to help staff in general practice. The NHS has its own publication, known as the 'Statement of Fees and Allowances'. You will also hear this referred to as the 'Red Book'. Every doctor and general practice is issued with a copy of this loose-leafed book, which is bound in a red cover – hence its name. It is regularly updated by the department when changes are made to charges, rates of pay or conditions of service. It also contains information on allowances made for premises. It is most important to remember to update the Red Book whenever amendments are issued. A copy should be readily available to staff as a source of reference.

Many general practices are 'networked' to their Local Health Authority to enable them to make direct claims for their work. This may happen automatically when they enter an 'Item of service' onto the computer network.

## PRIVATE PRACTICE

In private practice there is more responsibility demanded of the medical secretary for the mainte-nance of accurate accounts. This will largely fall into three areas:

◆ The maintenance of patient accounts
◆ The maintenance of practice accounts
◆ Banking.

### Patient accounts

Each practice will have a list of set charges appropriate to the work of the practice. This will include the items shown in Box 7.2.

Patient accounts may be kept on a card index or more commonly now may be computerised. The record for each patient will record:

◆ the date of the bill sent for each visit
◆ the date the bill was paid
◆ the date of any reminders sent.

When a patient pays his/her account, a note should be made of the method of settlement, i.e. whether through his/her own account, by cheque,

---

**Box 7.2** Items for which charges are made in private practice

◆ New patients – this is a charge for a first appointment or for a re-referral. As 'history taking' will be involved, these appointments take longer than a normal appointment.

◆ Follow-up visit

◆ Special treatments

◆ Injections

◆ X-ray

◆ Charge for inpatient care, should the patient be admitted to hospital. In this circumstance, the medical secretary must always be ready to take note of the following:

— the number of days in hospital

— any treatment carried out

— any inpatient visits carried out.

These items will be picked up and charged for when the discharge report has been made.

or by an insurance company in that patient's name – this is often the case where patients are subscribers to a private health care plan or are covered in this way through their work.

## Practice accounts

A well kept accounts book will:

◆ assist an accountant in preparing accounts
◆ provide much of the financial information for annual audit
◆ provide necessary information for tax self-assessment.

The accounts book will have separate pages for expenditure and payment-in. It is also useful to keep a separate book for recording cheques written on the account, with all the details noted. Remember, that only the cheque number will appear on the regular bank statement. It is easier to identify cheque details and to trace payments if you have made another more detailed record. All bills and receipts should also be kept as a back-up record.

Each transaction entered into an accounts book should be dated and entered into the relevant column. If the payment has been made by cheque, the cheque number should be entered into that column as well.

Some transactions are made automatically by the bank. These may be identified by particular initials such as:

◆ DD – direct debit
◆ SO – standing order
◆ TR – transfer.

With DD and SO, sums of money are taken out of the account on a predetermined date each month. This is always an arrangement which is made in advance with the full authorisation of the account holder.

TR applies to another arrangement made with the bank and authorised by the account holder. This is not strictly a payment, but a setting aside of money from a current account to a holding account in order to allow for certain bills to be paid on demand on regular occasions. This may be for payments such as income tax. When this demand comes from the Inland Revenue, the secretary must contact the bank and arrange for the correct amount of money to be transferred back to the practice account in order to make sure that there are sufficient funds available to meet the cheque.

**Reflection point**

How long will it take for the bank to complete this transaction? If you do not know – find out!

Figure 7.1 provides an example of a payments page from an accounts book.

## Banking

A special bank account will be held by the practice and with it an accounts book, as a record of all financial transactions undertaken.

As cheques arrive:

◆ record details on the patient's record
◆ enter into the paying-in book
◆ record in cheque record book
◆ bank cheques weekly.

As bills arrive

◆ present the bill and 'made out' cheque to the person authorised to make the payment, and ready for signing and dispatch before the overdue date arrives. (You may find that some practices require two signatories.)
◆ do not present all the bills at once – plan the payment over a sensible amount of time.

Remember that cheques written as payment from the practice must also be recorded with all details of whom they are to be paid to, the date and the cheque number.

| SUNDRIES | | | | | | | | | | |
|---|---|---|---|---|---|---|---|---|---|---|
| | | | | | | | | | | |

PAYMENTS ANALYSIS

| RENT RATES AND INSURANCE | REPAIRS RENEWALS AND MAINTENANCE | SALARIES AND WAGES | PETTY CASH | BANK LEGAL AND ACCOUNTANTS CHARGES | DRESSINGS DRUGS AND INSTRUMENTS | TRANSPORT EXPENSES | | | |
|---|---|---|---|---|---|---|---|---|---|

**Figure 7.1** A payments page.

**Reflection point**

◆ When a bank statement arrives it will only show you a cheque number. How will you trace your payments? What other record should you keep of your payments so that your accounts can be properly checked?

## Petty cash

Petty cash usually refers to transactions which are made by cash payment. This is a system used to account for everyday small payments in most businesses, and staff in general practice and in many other areas of medical administration need to know how this works. If payment is made to the practice for a fee for a service provided, this is a different matter altogether and this should be kept quite separate from the day-to-day petty cash, and should be accounted for properly, with a description in the accounts book and full payment made into the practice account. However, in order to deal with everyday petty cash, a float of money of an agreed amount may be kept to enable small payments to be made for items such as postage stamps. This sum of money is often referred to as 'imprest'. It will often be kept in a petty cash tin with petty cash vouchers and a petty cash book in which to enter the transactions for each month. A petty cash voucher must be issued as an authority to make a purchase, and will be signed by a senior member of staff.

A petty cash book will be divided into columns to describe the expenditure. These headings will vary depending on the character of the practice, but may use such headings as 'post, stationery, office and sundries'. Once the imprest has been decided upon, expenditure will be totalled up regularly on an agreed date (probably monthly) and the sum needed to restore the imprest to its agreed starting amount will be withdrawn from the general account (Fig. 7.2).

## CONCLUSION

From this chapter, the medical secretary should be able to understand some of the complexities of financial management in general practice and appreciate the differences which may be found in private practice.

| IMPREST £ | DATE | DETAILS | VOUCHER NO. | TOTAL £ | POSTAGE | STATIONERY | OFFICE EXP. | OTHER EXP. |
|---|---|---|---|---|---|---|---|---|
| 5.80 | 1 | Balance B/F | | | | | | |
| 44.30 | 1 | Cash Forward | | | | | | |
| | 3 | Stamps | 123 | 15.00 | 15.00 | | | |
| | 4 | Tea/Coffee | 124 | 7.34 | | | 7.34 | |
| | 8 | Taxi | 125 | 6.30 | | | | 6.30 |
| | 10 | Magazines | 126 | 4.30 | | | 4.30 | |
| | 15 | Flowers | 127 | 5.60 | | | | 5.60 |
| | 18 | 2 Electric plugs | 128 | 2.00 | | | 2.00 | |
| | 21 | Rec' Delivery | 129 | 0.55 | 0.55 | | | |
| | 28 | Notebooks | 130 | 1.00 | | 1.00 | | |
| | 30 | Luggage Labels | 131 | 1.50 | | | | 1.50 |
| | | Total Spent | | 43.59 | 15.55 | 1.00 | 13.64 | 13.40 |
| | | Balance in hand | | 6.41 | | | | |
| 50.00 | | | | 50.00 | | | | |
| 6.41 | | Balance B/F | | | | | | |
| 43.59 | | Cash | | | | | | |

**Figure 7.2** A petty cash book page totalled and 'restored'.

**Exercises**

◆ Find out how to write out a cheque accurately.

◆ What is an invoice?

◆ How can you use a credit note?

◆ When you are on work placement, make sure you find out how your practice deals with claims.

◆ Does the practice have a reference source for new staff? Is there one member of staff who is particularly responsible for filling in claim forms? Is this a good or a bad idea?

## FURTHER READING

Harrison J 1996 Secretarial duties, 10th edn. Longman, Harlow

*This book covers the general financial aspects of secretarial duties.*

National Health Service. General Medical Services. Statement of Fees and Allowances. (The 'Red Book'.) NHS Executive

Journals and Periodicals: Medeconomics (published by Haymarket Medical), Pulse (published by Miller Freedman)

# Information technology

**8**

*Phillip Simons*

Before you start reading this chapter, find a bank (or building society current account) statement or a telephone bill (one that has the calls itemised).

## INTRODUCTION

We deal first of all with the role of information in today's NHS and what plans the NHS Management Executive has for information technology (IT) and information.

Then we discuss how you may be affected by IT, first in a hospital setting, then in general practice.

Next we point out the major aspects of confidentiality and security of data wherever you are working.

In the longer term IT brings the prospect of NHS-wide data communications and we deal with this towards the end of the chapter.

Because each institution has different procedures and because there is such diversity of computer equipment we have dealt with topics in a general way, trying to focus on basic principles rather than specific types of computer. We do, however, use some examples taken from actual practice to illustrate the possibilities of IT.

**Reflection point**

This activity will help you appreciate how information appears in different forms. Take a look at either the bank statement or the telephone bill that we asked you to find earlier on.

If you have a bank statement note how each individual transaction is recorded and all the transactions are added up so the final result is a *summary* figure telling you how much money remains in your account. The individual transactions are simply bits of *data* but the summary is *information*. Additionally, the information is sorted into columns of deposits and withdrawals.

If you have an itemised telephone bill you can see how the telephone calls are individually listed but also grouped into local and national calls as well as providing a total amount to pay. Again the computer has collected all the information relating to calls at different times and to different destinations from your telephone and brought them together to make up your telephone bill.

accounts and wants to know who has overdrawn and so that he/she can order action. But the manager doesn't need to see *every* account or *every* transaction, just exceptions and a summary all of which can be created by a computer.

At Headquarters level the management want to know how its branches are performing in comparison with national averages and which are performing poorly and might need closing and the business transferred to another branch. They don't need to know about individual transactions but they need to summarise information created from those transactions.

This shows that at different levels of the bank's management different people need different things from the same information. In the same way different 'layers' of the NHS need different types of information.

In addition, there is a short glossary of computer terms at the end of the chapter.

In these examples a constant factor such as your telephone number or bank account number brings all these different individual bits of data together. In the same way these 'constants' (such as the new NHS number, which we discuss later on) are an important requirement for NHS information systems.

## THE ROLE OF INFORMATION IN THE NHS

### Reflection point

Earlier on we looked at the example of a bank statement and how it provides information for the bank customer. But the tens of thousands of individual transactions for thousands of customers form the basis for a summary for use for managerial purposes. The bank manager is responsible for thousands of customers'

Before you read further you may like to consult Figure 8.1

To run today's NHS a vast amount of information is needed at different levels and for different purposes. The information has to be timely, accurate and relevant to each level of the organisation. This means that the basic information about tens of hundreds of thousands of individual patient encounters with the NHS has to be summarised and codified so that different layers of information can be created for the different levels of authority in the NHS. As the level goes 'up' so the need for individual data diminishes and the need arises to summarise and group the information.

We will describe this going from individual to national level.

## INDIVIDUAL LEVEL

At the individual (and most important) level clinical staff who treat the patient need to have access to individual patient information, to add to that information, and to share that information with other authorised professionals.

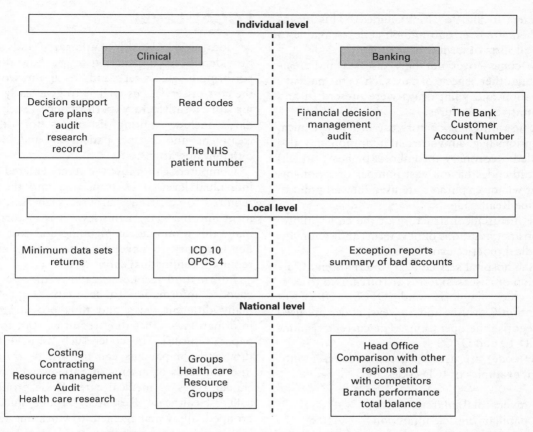

**Figure 8.1** Information requirements at individual, local and national levels in the NHS and in typical banking organisation.

At this individual patient level there is a certain minimum amount of information such as name, age, sex, address and occupation (often called 'demographic' information). In addition, a record is kept of clinical activity associated with that patient. The problem for clinicians is to describe their activity in standardised terms that can be used by computers. In general practice special codes called 'Read' codes are used and are often entered directly into the computer by the doctors.

The Read codes are an agreed dictionary of medical terms that form a kind of 'language of health'. The terms are arranged in a hierarchy so that the appropriate amount of detail can be chosen by the clinician. The example in Box 8.1 shows how it works.

| Box 8.1 | Read codes |
|---|---|
| H | Respiratory system diseases |
| H2 | Pneumonia and influenza |
| H20 | Viral pneumonia |
| H202 | Pneumonia – parainfluenza virus |

The leftmost character defines the broad area, e.g. *Respiratory system diseases*. The more detailed descriptions are covered by characters further to the right. Because each character can be either a number 0–9, or upper case, or lower case, this gives each position 58 possibilities (the characters 'i' and 'o' are excluded). This means that there are over 650 million codes available to cover all sorts of terms.

The codes cover not only diseases and treatment but other aspects of care such as the patient's occupation and what drugs were prescribed and preventative procedures.

Because different doctors use different clinical descriptions (e.g. a myocardial infarction may also be called a coronary thrombosis or heart attack) the Read codes have a vast number of synonyms so that whatever phrases are used they all point to the same Read code.

The hierarchical structure of the codes allows for constant additions of new terms and synonyms as medical practice evolves.

In the hospital service ICD (International Classification of Diseases) terms are often used to categorise the diagnosis and OPCS (Office of Population Censuses and Surveys) codes are used to categorise the operations. The current versions are ICD 10 and OPCS 4.

ICD codes are used to describe diseases only. Typical examples of ICD codes are:

| | |
|---|---|
| Acute myocardial infarction | 410 |
| Acute papillary muscle infarction | 410.8 |

These codes are numeric only and they deal with levels of detail by using decimal points.

OPCS 4 codes describe treatments and operative procedures only. Example of such codes are:

| | |
|---|---|
| Ear operations | D01–28 |
| Drainage of middle ear | D15 |
| Radical mastoidectomy | D101 |
| Simple mastoidectomy | D104 |

These codes are often entered by specialised staff called 'coders' attached to clinical directorates and can be used to describe 'episodes of care', which are the basic units of hospital activity.

The computerisation of diagnoses and treatments facilitates medical audit: the practice of reviewing and comparing how patients with the same type of condition were treated and what the outcomes were.

## LOCAL LEVEL

At local level, Health Authorities and service providers need information to see how they are performing against set standards and to work out the cost of services as well as to give 'early warning' of unsatisfactory performance. Such standards include waiting list times for different treatments and cost per patient day and costs for different operations.

Computers can allow the terms entered at the individual level to be translated into the codes required for different purposes such as management information. At this level it is important to make this grouping for planning and costing but not necessary to have the detail that clinicians require for individual care.

Information technology allows the previously encoded information to be analysed quickly in many different ways and thus provides timely information – rather than requiring staff to fill in paper 'returns'. The codes such as ICD 10 for thousands of patients can in turn be translated into hundreds of groups of patients who require similar types of medical care. These groups are called Healthcare Resource Groups and, thus grouped, allow management to work out costings and compare performance.

Because there is so much information available about the patient and only a certain amount is actually needed for these purposes, Health Authorities use a 'minimum data set' containing only the basic demographic details necessary for their calculations.

## NATIONAL LEVEL

The government has a statutory responsibility to make available information about overall numbers of patients treated nationwide and at what overall cost. This permits planning of new services, reviewing how existing services are going, and deciding what funds to allocate in the future. For example, average waiting times for treatments are an important measure of service level and have significant political implications.

At the same time information at this level can

be used to establish averages and standards, for example the cost per day of treating one patient.

This permits comparisons to be made between health service performance in different parts of the country and to highlight possible problem areas. It also allows international comparisons.

The role of information technology in all this is that it can greatly assist the communication of patient information, safeguard confidentiality and make the aggregation of individual patient records into useful statistical information much more quickly and accurately than before. It is, therefore, possible to take action to remedy unsatisfactory situations whilst the information is still current.

Because computers allow rapid sorting and transmission of information the possibility now exists for accurate information to be available to senior levels in the NHS without delay.

## THE NEW NHS NUMBER

Now we will describe a particular initiative which is crucial for the success of IT in the NHS, the new NHS number.

The new NHS number is a 10-digit number which replaces any previous NHS numbers a patient may have had. In the past there were up to 20 separate types of number, none of which was suitable for computer use. The new number, which is now almost universally used by both hospitals and GPs, is more suitable for computer use. It allows seamless transfer of information between providers and purchasers for invoicing purposes because the number can be checked by the computer; for clinical staff new information such as test results will go directly to the right patient record.

## FOR HOSPITAL-BASED SECRETARIES

Although most medical secretaries use stand-alone computers you may find yourself using a Patient Administration System (PAS) containing the names, ages and addresses of all the patients plus episode history (gives demographic data), including those who are currently staying in the hospital.

The PAS is a very large and powerful *database*. A good example of a database is a telephone directory. Here addresses and telephone numbers are stored in alphabetical order so that, if you know the name and initials, you can find the number.

A computerised database allows far more powerful arrangements of data so that when a logical question is presented to it, it can produce an appropriate output. So, for example, a *computerised* telephone directory would allow you to enter the telephone number and find out the name and address connected with that number.

In most hospitals the PAS is run by a powerful computer which is usually kept in a central secure location and which is connected by cables to a large number of computer terminals around the entire hospital site. This arrangement is called a 'network' and because it normally covers only one site it is typically called a local area network or LAN. The PAS usually covers all the inpatient work of a hospital as well as the outpatient department (see Chapter 13).

As a medical secretary you may have access to a computer terminal connected to the PAS. (You will require a password for this – we discuss this later on in this chapter.) You can extract information from the PAS such as:

1. Details about a patient's age and address, and some basic details about any episodes of care that patient may have had at the hospital, e.g. date and ward of admission; consultant in charge; and the diagnosis. Because this information relates to just one identified person we call it *individual* level.
2. The number of admissions in the past month for a particular consultant. Because this information is calculated from lots of *individual* records we call this *aggregate* information. Your work may involve you in extracting aggregate level information for your consultant or hospital management.

You may also be required to enter information into the PAS such as admission dates and discharge summaries.

### Scenario

At the Midshire Hospital Trust consultant staff add patients to waiting lists whilst they are in the outpatient clinic by entering information directly into the PAS system. They can put a patient on particular waiting lists and designate them as 'urgent', 'routine', etc. The medical secretaries on the orthopaedic unit regularly print out the waiting lists by type of treatment or by surgeon. The list is divided into categories such as 'routine', 'urgent', 'soonest', etc. They can also print out the list by GP and identify which patients are in fundholding practices, and which are extra-contractual referrals.

When you are entering information into a PAS you need to remember that the computer system remembers your identity and has an 'audit trail' and can trace which person entered, or viewed, a particular piece of information.

Most PAS systems allow different levels of access to different grades of staff. For example, non-clinical administrators may be locked out of information such as medical details and test results and you may find that you are not allowed to do certain things. For example, you may find that you are not allowed to modify a patient's NHS number or their diagnosis.

Because the PAS contains personal clinical information belonging to thousands of patients there are stringent security precautions.

### Scenario

At the genitourinary clinic at St David's, a hospital in a large city, the secretaries keep a manual record of telephone enquiries. Each week they transfer the information to a computerised spreadsheet. The spreadsheet creates a graph which shows the range of problems dealt with by the unit (Fig. 8.2).

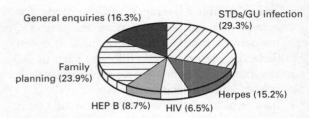

**Figure 8.2** Telephone enquiries to the genitourinary clinic (week beginning 5 February).

You do not have to have access to the PAS to deal with information. For example, you may have a free-standing computer which, besides running word processing for clinical correspondence, has spreadsheet and database programs.

## GENERAL PRACTICE

Already over 80% of practices in the UK have some kind of computer system so you are almost bound to find yourself using a computer in your practice. You will almost certainly find that the new NHS number mentioned above has been implemented for all the patients.

In many practices patient correspondence such as referral letters and reports is done on a free-standing computer or word processor.

However, most of the consulting rooms and the reception desk usually contain computers connected in a 'network'. These computers use programs specially designed for general practice and will handle:

◆ Basic or full patient records with name, age, sex and address.
◆ Records of drugs prescribed for patients. This is useful for printing out repeat prescriptions. Some programs can also warn of dangerous drug interactions.
◆ Recall systems for cervical cytology and children's immunisations. The computer automatically identifies certain patients by sex and age and prints out lists of patients who need certain treatments within a given time period. The computer may also print out standard letters inviting those patients to come for treatment.

◆ Tracking 'item of service' (IOS) payments from the Health Authority. These are payments to the GP for treatments such as maternity care, treatment of temporary residents, night visits and contraceptive care.
◆ Information for medical audit and research purposes. The GP can input special codes to record consultations and treatments for later analysis by the computer. By performing database queries it is possible to compare treatments and outcomes for patients with similar conditions.

### Scenario

In the Anytown practice Dr Green uses her computer at every consultation. She enters the main aspects of the consultation (such as diagnosis, treatment given, drugs used) using special codes called 'Read' codes.

Later on she can perform a database query to search for patients with a condition or group of similar conditions.

For medical audit purposes, she can see the effect of certain drugs on patients with the same condition. Alternatively, if a warning has been issued by the Department of Health for a particular drug Dr Green can get a list of all patients given that drug.

If yours is a fundholding practice the computer system may have programs which keep records of contracts with various health care providers and also track and compare costs between different providers. (At the time of publication the government are considering replacing fundholding with 'locality purchasing'.)

The functions described above are often covered by an 'all in one package' from a specialist computer supplier.

Nearly all practices have a facility called 'GP/HA Links' which combines computers and communications.

The aim of GP/HA Links is to replace paper-based patient registration and IOS transactions previously sent by post with an electronic system. Registrations and item of service details are entered by practice staff and gathered into a computer file for automatic transmission down the telephone line each evening to an electronic 'mailbox' run by a specialist computer company.

To send data down the telephone line a 'modem' is used. A modem takes the digital signal from a PC and modulates it into an analogue signal (sound). The receiving modem will then demodulate this sound signal back into a digital signal at the other end of the line.

The HA computer then dials in to the 'mailbox' and collects the claims. If the claims are accepted a message is sent back to the practice.

Nearly every practice in the country is using GP/HA Links for patient registration and over half are using the system to transmit claims for item of service payments. In addition, the DoH plan to introduce call and recall systems for cervical cytology during the summer of 1998.

If your practice has GP/HA Links you may be involved in entering data. This requires you to observe a certain discipline when keying in information, e.g. not using abbreviations such as 'St' for Street.

The GP/HA Links facility is just the start in a series of initiatives to link up the various parts of the NHS. Plans exist to add hospitals to the network of links and services such as on-line access to waiting lists. We cover this later in the chapter.

## SAFEGUARDING THE PATIENT AND THE DATA

The latest NHS Management Executive's information strategy includes the statement that 'information must be confidential and secure, only available to those who need to know'. This section outlines basic security precautions which you will be required to follow, most of them required by the Data Protection Act 1987.

The Data Protection Act covers NHS authorities. Box 8.2 lists the main provisions.

NHS authorities must:

◆ be registered under the Act

◆ obtain and process personal information fairly and lawfully

◆ hold the information only for the purpose described in the register entry

◆ use information only for those purposes and not disclose for an incompatible purpose

◆ make sure data is adequate, relevant and not excessive for the purpose

◆ keep data accurate and where necessary up to date

◆ hold information for no longer than is necessary for that purpose

◆ provide access to individuals upon request and correct or erase information as appropriate

◆ ensure data is protected by proper security.

Although senior management are responsible for registering your practice or organisation under the Act, everybody has responsibility for compliance with the conditions above.

What this means is that you need to make sure of the following points.

1. Only authorised staff can gain access to the computer system.
2. Accuracy is maintained.
3. Data is not corrupted.
4. Equipment is safeguarded.
5. Back-up copies of the computer data are made frequently.

We now discuss these points in more detail.

## Restricting access to the computer system to authorised staff

This is normally achieved through the use of a password which you will have to enter before you can gain access ('log on') to programs containing confidential data such as a PAS. You need to observe the following precautions.

Do not use your own name, middle name or nickname as your password. Some computers will reject a password consisting only of letters and may insist on you using more than four characters. Ideally you should use a mix of letters and numbers.

Make sure that no-one is looking over your shoulder when you are typing in your password. When you enter your password the computer screen will not display what you have typed but someone could memorise your keystrokes.

Similarly, make sure that no unauthorised people can see the computer screen when you are viewing patient information.

When you have finished using the PAS you must 'log off' the program – each computer has different mechanisms for this. It is vitally important that you do this, even if you leave the room for just a few minutes, otherwise the computer thinks you are still there and will allow someone else to use it. Most computer systems automatically switch themselves off if they detect 2 or 3 minutes of inactivity, but you should not rely on this.

You need to remember that some computer screens go dark automatically to save electricity and to stop the screen from being damaged by 'burn in' – this is not the same as switching off or logging off.

Do not use someone else's password and do not let anyone know or use yours. When you first start work you will probably be issued with a temporary password which you will have to replace almost straight away with one that you think up.

## Ensuring accuracy is maintained

You need to be aware that it is much easier to confuse characters on screen and much harder to detect spelling mistakes. You need to be extremely careful when entering information into databases because the smallest mistake could mean that important test results and communications about a patient are misread or go astray.

Patients have the right to access electronic data held about them under the provisions of the Data Protection Act enacted in 1987 – so be careful what you put in, or are asked to put in – the patient may see it later.

You should also be aware that patients are allowed to see their own paper-based record (see Chapter 12).

## Making sure that information is not corrupted

Computer programs and the data they contain are at risk from corruption or damage from three sources.

### Viruses

Whilst computers can be of great benefit, some destructive people make and distribute computer viruses which cause damage to computer systems.

A virus is a piece of computer code that can attach itself to a program and copy itself when the program is run. This enables the virus to be transmitted to other programs and also from one computer system to another.

The symptoms caused by a computer virus are: messages appear on the screen; data goes wrong; the computer takes longer to load and carry out commands. Viruses can seriously damage your data – which means that vitally important patient information and programs could be destroyed. Networks are particularly at risk because data is being passed rapidly around many computers.

The most common cause of transferring viruses is the use of floppy disks because they can easily be loaded into different computers. What this means for the medical secretary is that floppy disks containing 'shareware' programs or computer games should never be used on your work computer.

Your hospital or practice should have precautions in place against attack by viruses. Viruses can be detected by using a 'scanner' – a specialised piece of software. If you need to use a floppy disk at all, make sure that it is 'write protected' and that you test it with a 'scanner' program before copying data to your computer's hard disk or onto the network.

Viruses are strictly electronic in form and only affect computers but new viruses are being discovered at the rate of about 200 per month, so your 'scanner' software will need constant updating to stay effective.

### Accidental damage

Although modern computers are very reliable they can be physically damaged like any other piece of machinery. So avoid moving the computer when it is in use, and make sure it is placed where no-one can bump into it.

Computers, particularly keyboards, do not like having coffee spilt over them, so do not drink coffee at your desk!

### Electricity supply faults

A lesser known risk to computers is a sudden variation in the electricity supply. These are called 'spikes' or 'surges' and they can cause data to be corrupted. The electricity supply may even break down altogether. This makes it all the more important to follow back-up procedures outlined below. If your computer is on a network there may be a special device for the central computer called an 'uninterruptible power supply' (UPS). The UPS is connected between the computer and the mains supply and acts as a kind of reservoir for electricity, keeping the supply at a constant level. The UPS also provides for a few minutes of battery power in the event of a total mains failure.

## Physical security

Computers and computer components are now a target for criminals. Often entire office blocks of computers are stripped of their valuable memory chips, or simply removed wholesale.

You will need to cooperate with procedures which may include bolting the computers to the desktop or actually locking them away in a secure room every evening.

## Making back-ups

Back-ups are copies of your data to devices that are separate from your computer. At the most simple level, for example, you can copy small amounts of data onto a floppy disk and store it in a drawer in your desk. The result is that if your computer has a virus attack, or is stolen, you can restore the data from the floppy disk.

In practice back-ups are more complicated. Data is constantly changing every hour of every day, so most organisations will make a back-up every day or even every half day. This means that if disaster strikes only half a day's data is lost. Because there is so much data in hospitals and it takes so long to actually copy, special devices such as tapes or optical disks are used.

You may be asked to carry out back-ups and also to make sure that further copies of back-up tapes or disks are kept in a separate location – just in case the ultimate disaster happens and your building is damaged by fire.

None of these measures will work properly if you are working on a stand-alone computer and do not save your work frequently to disk.

The all-important aspect of health and safety at work regarding seating and the VDU are dealt with in Chapters 3 and 17.

## OTHER DEVELOPMENTS IN IT

### Reflection point

You are a secretary in general practice. How would you normally tell everyone that Dr Green has had to take a day off today?

The forthcoming developments in IT in the NHS are in the area of communications. We are going to cover a number of developments here.

### Electronic mail (e-mail)

E-mail is an electronic messaging service where the text that you type into your computer can be sent to other people on the network, either to individuals, or to predetermined groups of staff. Messages are stored in electronic 'mailboxes' within the computer system so that you can pick up your messages from any computer terminal, not just at your own desk.

E-mail can allow people within your practice or hospital to communicate more efficiently because it is transmitted instantly and does not rely on paper systems and postal services. However, it is less intrusive than telephone calls and is thus an ideal way for busy people to keep in touch by dealing with their messages at a time that suits them.

E-mail can work not just within a hospital or practice but around a whole Health District – this wider form of network is called a WAN (wide area network).

### Scenario

In the Whitely village practice the receptionist can use e-mail to pass messages to doctors seeing patients in the surgery without having to interrupt consultations. One of the doctors can send a message to everyone in the practice saying that one of the practice's patients has died.

### Further developments in GP/HA Links – sharing and transmission of patient information

Earlier on you learnt about GP/HA Links and how it is being used to transmit data relating to registrations and claims for payments. Further developments are now in hand which will add important hospital functions to the network so that GPs will be able to receive their patients' pathology and X-ray reports and discharge summaries every day, thus considerably reducing current delays.

The new NHS number mentioned earlier is indispensable for this because it will ensure that this information finds its way to the correct patient record. Similarly, GPs will be able refer patients to hospitals electronically and even book outpatient appointments directly from their own surgeries.

The end result will be more efficient, accurate and rapid communications and a reduction in paperwork and time-consuming transcription of information.

## National database of hospital places

This is in operation in some practices. It allows GPs to find out the range of treatments offered by hospitals around the country plus waiting times and costs. GPs access the database by using a modem attached to their computer. A similar postal system would involve postage and printing costs and would be quickly out of date. But because the electronic database is constantly updated they know that the information is accurate.

## SUMMARY OF KEY ISSUES

◆ Information technology now plays an extremely important part in today's NHS. This has only become possible in recent years with the increasing power and cheapness of computers and their ability to communicate rapidly via telephone lines or specialised cables.

◆ The strategy of the NHS Management Executive is to create a patient record that is accessible wherever a patient is treated. In addition, they want information in the NHS to be person based – so that information about health service performance is generated as a by-product of patient care rather than as an end in itself.

◆ However, all this needs accuracy, otherwise the data will be meaningless and may harm the patient. It also needs confidentiality and this is all the more important because so much medical information can be made available.

◆ It also means that data has to be compatible for it to be shared between computers. This highlights the need to *speak the same language*, hence the development of the new NHS numbers and the investment by the NHS Read codes and Healthcare Resource Groups.

◆ What this means for you, the medical secretary, is that confidentiality and accuracy are vital when working with computers.

## CONCLUSION

Information technology is one of the most powerful developments in today's NHS. However, powerful things can be destructive. For example, if patient information falls into the wrong hands or is lost then the damage can be catastrophic. Data has to be safeguarded against accidental loss or destruction by viruses and you need to be aware of, and cooperate with, the precautions taken by your hospital or practice. Above all you must guard against unauthorised access and use of patient information.

### Exercises

◆ Find out if your hospital or practice has written guidance about data protection.

◆ Find out which clinical coding system your hospital or practice is using.

◆ Dr Brown tells you that he needs to look up a few patients' details but has forgotten his password. He asks you to 'log in' with your password and then allow him to use the computer. How would you respond to his request?

◆ One item of information on the minimum data set is the patient's postcode. What possibilities for medical research do you see for using the computer to sort information using the postcode?

◆ What possibilities can you see for management in using postcode information?

## FURTHER READING

Preece J 1994 The use of computers in general practice. Churchill Livingstone, London

## RESOURCES

For free leaflets and publications on NHS Information Management initiatives, including Read codes and the new NHS number, contact:

Information Point
Information Management Group
NHS Executive Headquarters
c/o Cambridge & Huntingdon Health Commission
Primrose Lane
Huntingdon
Cambs
PE18 6SE

Tel: 01480 415118
Fax: 01480 415160

## KEY TERMS

### Aggregate level information

This is statistical information that relates to groups rather than to individuals. For example, a list of wards with average lengths of stay would be aggregate level, because it is made up of a large number of individual recordings for each patient's length of stay. Another example would be numbers of emergency admissions to different hospitals.

### Audit trail

For computers this is a way of tracing an exact history of when and by whom each new piece of information is entered into the computer system.

### Coder

For management and clinical purposes, details of patients' diagnosis and treatment need to be entered onto a computer so that they can be analysed. Computers cannot handle medical terms because they can be ambiguous (for example MI could mean 'myocardial infarction' or 'mentally ill') or because there is no consistent terminology (for example athlete's foot might be described by a doctor as 'tinea pedis'). So diagnoses have to be converted into unambiguous identifiers. Coders are members of health staff whose job is to enter the correct clinical codes (such as ICD, OPCS and Read codes) to cover each patient's encounter with the hospital or health unit.

### Data Protection Act

The purpose of this Act is to protect the rights of individuals about whom data is obtained, stored, processed or supplied. They may find out information about themselves, challenge it if appropriate and claim compensation in certain circumstances. Data users, such as Health Authorities, must be open about their use of data and follow sound and proper practices.

### Database

An organised collection of information rather like a card index or telephone directory except that the computer's database is far more sophisticated and powerful.

### Demographic information

This is information that refers to basic domestic details (e.g. name, sex, age, address, occupation) about a person rather than detailed clinical information.

### Episode of care

This is now the basic statistical unit of clinical care in hospitals and was one of the recommendations of the Körner report on ·health service information. The episode of care usually begins when a patient is transferred to the care of a new consultant. This allows statistics to be recorded in a uniform and accurate way.

### Extra-contractual referrals (ECR)

Health Authorities arrange contracts for the care of patients in their catchment area, as do many GPs who are fundholders. An extra-contractual referral occurs when they need to refer a patient to a hospital or health facility where a contractual arrangement does not already exist. This may occur when specialised treatment is required or where there is an urgent admission.

### Floppy disks

These are disks covered in a magnetic coating which permits recording of electronic data. Most floppy disks are about 3.5 inches in diameter and are protected by an almost rigid square plastic case, so the term 'floppy' is somewhat misleading. A typical floppy disk can store the equivalent of about 400 A4 pages of single-spaced text. Because they are portable they can be used to transfer data and programs between computers.

### GP/HA Links

This is a system for allowing electronic transmission of information between general practices and Health Authorities. This will speed up patient registration and de-registering procedures and claims for item of service payments, besides reducing clerical effort.

### ICD (International Classification of Diseases)

These classifications (published by the World Health Organization) are used to code each patient's diagnosis, normally on discharge. Because they are standard throughout the world they can be used for comparisons of health problems between different countries. The current version is ICD 10.

### Individual level information

Information which can be related to individuals' individual entities. A good example of individual level information is a telephone directory because each record (i.e. a name, an address and a telephone number) is about an individual.

### IOS (item of service)

This occurs only in general practice. It refers to services and treatments which fall outside the definition of 'General Medical Services' and for which the GP can claim a payment.

### LAN (local area network)

A network is a number of computers connected together and sharing information. A *local* network means that all the computers are in the same building or on the same site. So, for example, a computer system on a large hospital site encompassing many buildings would be called a LAN.

### Log in (also sometimes called log on)

The process whereby an individual keys in details about his/her identity into a computer system so that he/she can interact with that computer system. This process will often include entering a password known only to that individual.

### Log off (also sometimes called log out)

The process whereby a user of a computer system tells the system that he/she is ceasing to use it. It is

important to log off when leaving the computer, even for a few minutes.

### Mailboxes

A mailbox is a kind of electronic pigeonhole where people can send you electronic messages. Your mailbox must have an 'address' unique to you such as your name or initials. Usually you will need to enter a password into the computer to read the messages in your mailbox.

### Minimum data set

This refers to the basic information about a patient that is necessary for contractual procedures in the NHS. It consists of a range of basic demographic information about the patient, details of the service provider, the consultant to whom the patient was referred, the referring clinician, the ward details, GP name, GP's correspondence address, GP's code. There are different minimum data sets for different encounters with the NHS, e.g. outpatient visits and emergency treatments.

### Network

A number of computers connected together (usually by special cable) and sharing information.

### NHS number

A new number which will uniquely identify each user of NHS services. This number will apply wherever the user is in the UK and whichever branch of the NHS they use. This will enable important clinical and demographic information to be available to authorised staff throughout the UK. Unlike previous numbering systems, which had 22 different formats, the NHS number will be designed for use with computers.

### OPCS (Office of Population Censuses and Surveys)

This refers to classifications of surgical procedures (e.g. procedures that require the services of a surgeon and an anaesthetist) carried out on patients. The current version is OPCS 4.

### PAS (Patient Administration System)

These are networked computer systems that make patient information available to authorised staff at numerous terminals around a hospital. This speeds up the creating and interchange of clinical and statistical information.

### Read codes
A set of codes for accurately describing a wide range of clinically relevant information and used mostly in primary care. The codes were designed from the start to be used by computers and were created by a practising GP, Dr James Read. The latest version (version 3) of the Read codes allows for sophisticated analysis by computers.

### Scanner
A device (similar in function to a modern photo-copier) for converting the information in paper-based documents and images into digital form. They can then be stored, manipulated and trans-mitted by a computer.

### Shareware
Computer software that users can make use of for a trial period to see if they like it before electing to pay for a full licence to use the software. These programs may contain viruses and should not be used on NHS computers without the authority of senior staff.

### Spikes
A sudden momentary increase or variation in the mains supply voltage which can occur from time to time without warning. The data in computers can be lost or corrupted by these sudden variations in the normal electricity supply voltage.

### Surges
Surges are similar to spikes (see above) but because they are of much longer duration and the energy concerned is greater, they are more liable to cause permanent damage to both the data and the computer and its associated equipment.

### Uninterruptible power supply (UPS)
Computers rely on electrical power to process information. If the mains supply to a computer fails, or changes suddenly (see 'Surges' and 'Spikes' above), a computer will lose vital data in its electronic memory. The UPS is a device which ensures continuity of supply of power to the com-puter. Generally, it is the central computers or 'file-servers' in a health building that are connected to a UPS because they store vital data.

### Virus
A virus is a self-replicating computer program that can cause loss of data and seriously harm com-puter systems. They are created by individuals with malicious intent and can be passed on by fail-ure to use correct computer procedures. The most common cause of virus 'infection' is the use of floppy disks containing unauthorised software such as computer games on NHS computers.

### WAN (wide area network)
These are networks that connect computers on more than one site and over a large area. For example, a network that connects several health centres and hospitals is a WAN.

### Write protected
This refers to information in a computer file, drive, or floppy disk. It means that you cannot amend the information already existing by, for example, copying or saving new files. The protection can be achieved by physical means (such as sliding a small plastic catch on a floppy disk) or by software.

# 9

# The use of the word processor in medicine

*Phillip Simons*

## OBJECTIVES

◆ To explain what you can achieve with your word processor other than churning out plain correspondence

◆ To explain how to set about enhancing your documents with your word processor

◆ To introduce you to some 'desktop publishing' terms

◆ To warn you about the pitfalls you may encounter with enhanced word processing.

## INTRODUCTION

You may already be familiar with the term 'desktop publishing'. We will use a different term in this chapter because we will be concentrating on what you can do with a conventional word processing package.

For the purpose of this chapter we concentrate on what you achieve using 'WordPerfect version 5.1' for DOS or 'Word for Windows version 6' rather than dedicated desktop publishing packages.

Instead of desktop publishing we will use the terms 'enhanced word processing' and 'enhanced documents' because we aim to show you the sorts of results you can achieve without having to use a specialised desktop publishing package. Moreover we will be concentrating on things that you can achieve with a few hours of practice, assuming you are already familiar with basic word processing features. Now and then we will use a few desktop publishing terms which we explain.

Firstly we will discuss briefly why there is a need for enhanced word processing in today's NHS, with the aid of some examples which we will refer to throughout the chapter.

Then we go into details of how to set about creating your own enhanced documents and introduce you to some simple steps that will help you achieve a good result.

Finally we give some brief 'health warnings' about getting carried away with it all and we outline some pitfalls to watch out for and give you some hints and thoughts about the cost and time implications of using word processing.

Throughout the chapter there are examples of

enhanced word processing including good (and not so good!) features which we ask you to examine closely.

We begin by asking why the medical secretary should bother with enhanced word processing.

# WHY ENHANCED WORD PROCESSING?

## Computers have got a lot better

In recent years the cost of computers has dropped considerably yet their speed and capacity has increased enormously. This means that modern computers are able to handle sophisticated graphical displays that help you organise your document's appearance on the screen. You are no longer limited to alphabetical characters but can include graphics and can see how your document will look on the printed page before you actually print it.

This means that if your word processor is running under 'Windows' you will probably be able to see your page layout as you type – this is called WYSIWYG (What You See Is What You Get). A similar Print Preview feature is also available in WordPerfect for DOS but it is separate from the typing screen.

## Printers have got a lot better

In the last few years printers have come down in price. Nowadays a decent laser printer can now be purchased for around £350. Another sort of printer known as an 'inkjet' printer can be bought for about £200. This means that good quality text and graphics can be produced from your desktop computer.

## Software is easier to use

Software publishers now take a lot of trouble to ensure that their programs and their manuals are more 'user-friendly' than they used to be. This means that you don't need a degree in computer science to use their advanced features.

## There is more need to communicate

In today's NHS there are more demands for clear communication and transfer of information between the service and patients, and within the service itself. There are, therefore, numerous possibilities in this area for using enhanced word processing, some of which are listed below.

For general practices to communicate with their patients:

◆ the practice leaflet
◆ the annual practice report
◆ patient group newsletters
◆ posters (Fig. 9.1).

For hospitals to communicate with their patients:

◆ patient awareness of hospital services, particularly as new services are constantly being created or modified which are different from 'traditional' patterns of care; e.g. a 'drop in' psychology clinic
◆ patient information before admission for outpatient procedures such as day surgery or X-ray (Fig. 9.2)
◆ outpatient information, e.g. information about a genitourinary clinic (Fig. 9.3)
◆ patient questionnaires (Fig. 9.4).

For managerial purposes *within* the NHS:

◆ timetables, schedules and duty rosters (Fig. 9.5)
◆ project planning (Fig. 9.6)
◆ form design
◆ management reports
◆ staff newsletters (Figs 9.7 and 9.8)
◆ temporary signposts and labels.

### Reflection point

◆ What are the advantages of enhanced word processing and how will it affect the medical secretary?

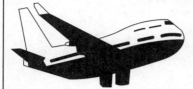
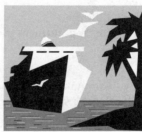

DRS QUINN CAMERON FEGAN
SWIFT & HOLLEY

Where are you going this year?

If it's hot and sunny it's probably got bugs you never heard of.

We can provide vaccination against many of the nastier infections.

To discuss your travel vaccination needs come and see one of the practice nurses.

*Vaccination is cheap insurance*

**Figure 9.1**   A general practice poster.

## Benefits of enhanced word processing

1. *Interesting layouts*. Your word processing program can make your documents more dynamic by allowing you to produce text in columns, import graphs, etc., depending on the purpose of the document (Fig. 9.7).

2. *Different type styles*. You are no longer confined to 'Courier' fonts with modern word processors. Instead you have access to a range of interesting and stylish typefaces (assuming your printer can support them).

3. *Savings in time and money*. On layout costs for simple documents, and for short runs of certain documents such as clinic timetables or labels for temporary purposes.

4. *Greater control over the process*. Unlike sending rough drafts to a printer and getting back something that doesn't *quite* do what you wanted, you can experiment with different layouts and designs and go through several versions until you are satisfied with the outcome.

## How it can affect the medical secretary

◆ It means that you can become more involved in the managerial and public relations side of your work and can broaden your computer skills.
◆ It also means having to allocate more of your time trying out the more advanced features of your word processing program.

**Reflection point**

◆ Look at the questionnaire in Figure 9.4. Note the use of WordPerfect 'graphics boxes' of different sizes. These can be copied and pasted from place to place. Can you think of other applications for this, e.g. creating forms?

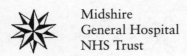 Midshire
General Hospital
NHS Trust

**Department of Clinical Radiology**
Midshire General Hospital
Midtown
Midshire **MD1 1XY**

 0123 456 789

Date: **5th February 1998**

Dear Mr Smith

● An appointment has been made for you to attend for a **Sialagram** at the X-ray department, West Wing, Midshire General Hospital (see enclosed map) on –

**Wednesday 5th March at 2.30 pm.**
If you are unable to keep this appointment please write enclosing this letter telling us the times you are unable to attend.

● **What is a Sialagram?**
A Sialagram is an X-ray examination of the salivary glands in your mouth. A small amount of dye is introduced into the duct of the salivary glands using a small flexible tube.

● **What happens during the examination?**
   ○ Before the examination actually begins we will take some preliminary X-rays of your mouth.

   ○ The examination itself will be performed by a Radiologist (a doctor who specialises in diagnosis using X-rays). The doctor will pass a small tube into the salivary gland duct inside your mouth.

   ○ When the tube is in the duct the doctor will pass some dye through it into the glands. This is not painful but you may feel some mild discomfort if the gland is full – at this point the tube will be removed and more X-ray films will be taken.

   ○ You will then be given a small amount of lemon juice and some further X-rays will be taken. (The lemon juice makes the glands contract and causes them to empty.)

● It is very important that you keep perfectly still during the examination.

● If you have any worries or questions please feel free to contact the department (Direct line 345-789).

Yours sincerely

Eric Pode
Superintendent Radiographer

**Figure 9.2**   An appointments letter.

The newly built Midtown clinic offers a range of services specifically for your sexual well-being. All these services are free and confidential.

The following services are provided:

- Information and advice on sexual health

- Screening for sexually transmitted diseases

- Counselling

- Psychological assessment and treatment

- Cervical smears

- Colposcopy

- HIV testing, counselling and care

- Hepatitis B testing

This service is an **open access service**. This means that you do not have to be referred by your GP.

We suggest that you make an appointment. You will usually take about 2 hours to complete your visit to the clinic.

No information will be released (not even to your GP) unless you give your consent.

*How do I make an appointment?*

You can make an appointment either in person or on the telephone at any time during clinic open hours.

| Monday | 9.00–5.30 |
| Tuesday | 9.00–5.30 |
| Wednesday | 2.30–7.30 |
| Thursday | 10.00–5.30 |
| Friday | 9.00–4.00 |

*What will happen when I visit the clinic?*

This will depend on why you have come to the clinic. However, you will always receive an initial examination by the doctor. If you need a test or treatment this will be arranged and may be carried out by nurses. Health advisors will be available to discuss ways of promoting good sexual health. Clinical psychologists are available if you need more specialised counselling.

*How will my visit to the clinic be followed up?*

You may have a problem that requires you to visit the clinic again. In some cases results of tests can be given to you by telephone.

*Where is the clinic?*

The clinic is in Broadway Road, just to the left of the main Midtown Hospital site.

*How do I get to the clinic?*

The clinic is easy to get to by public transport. Bus numbers 23, 11 and 49 all stop outside the hospital.

Please see the map overleaf.

**Figure 9.3** A leaflet for a sexual health clinic.

**NEEDS QUESTIONNAIRE – MIDTOWN SEXUAL HEALTH CLINIC**

Please give the following information about yourself and tick the relevant box:

1)    **Age**

2)    **Sex**   Female          Male

3)    **What is the postcode or area where you live?**

4)    **Occupation**                                              (if unemployed please say so)

5)    **How did you hear about this clinic?**

GP          Friends          Hospital

Partner          Magazine          Leaflet          Yellow Pages

**Figure 9.4**   A questionnaire. These are WordPerfect 'graphic boxes' with no content, anchor type 'character', vertical position 'centre', a variety of sizes set. These boxes can be copied and pasted from position to position. The font has been changed to proportional to give a more polished appearance.

Junior House Officers' Rotation

| Dr\Month: | Feb | March | April | May | June |
|-----------|-----|-------|-------|-----|------|
| Smith | Medical | Medical | Surgical | Surgical | Elective |
| Brown | Surgical | Surgical | Elective | Medical | Medical |
| Green | Ortho | Ortho | Medical | Elective | Surgical |
| Gray | a\leave | Medical | Ortho | Ortho | Elective |

Note: Changeovers take place on the first Monday of the month.

**Figure 9.5** A duty roster.

Project Plan for Clinic Move

| Weeks before move: | 8 | 7 | 6 | 5 | 4 | 3 | 2 | 1 | Responsible |
|--------------------|---|---|---|---|---|---|---|---|-------------|
| Activity\Week beginning | 1st Mar | 8th Mar | 15th Mar | etc | | | | | |
| Agree layout | | | | | | | | | Dr Green, Mrs White |
| Warn patients | | | | | | | | | Mr Black |
| Arrange transport | | | | | | | | | etc |
| Packing | | | | | | | | | |
| Temp closure | | | | | | | | | |

**Figure 9.6** A project plan.

# Surgical Unit Update

| Volume 1 Issue 9 | March 1998 |
| --- | --- |

WAITING TIMES DOWN

## We've met our Target!

**We are pleased to announce that our waiting lists are below 12 months for all categories within our directorate. The graph opposite shows the progress that has been made in the last year.**

'This shows that our improvement in services to the public is being maintained' said Eric Brogan, the Unit's Clinical Director, as he toured the wards congratulating key staff.

He continued 'We want to aim for a target of 6 months maximum wait over the next 2 years. This will be a priority for the management team to plan for.'

The reduction in waiting times was achieved by sweeping changes to the way resources are used. The operating theatre maintenance sessions were moved to evenings and weekends to free up an additional 4 sessions. In addition a dedicated theatre was used for emergencies only. This meant that routine surgical lists were no longer disrupted, resulting in less cancelled operations.

Further initiatives being planned include the conversion of two wards into a combined day surgery and 5-day unit. This will allow for the increase in short-stays for many operations.

**Figure 9.7** A page from a newsletter.

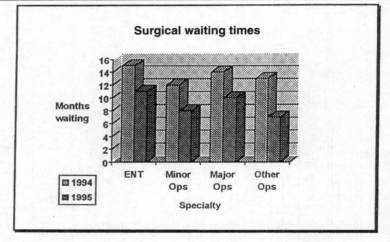

## Confidentiality

Last Thursday a page from a patient's medical record was found left inside the photocopier on Level 4. **This represents a serious breach** of our basic responsibility towards patients – that of confidentiality. We ask **all** staff to be on their guard against leaving confidential documents lying around where they can be seen by non-medical or non-hospital staff.

## Visit by Chairman

Next week the Surgical Unit will be visited by Sir Eric Pode, the Chairman of the Midshire Hospitals Trust.

As well as seeing the work of the existing Day Surgery Unit Sir Eric will be talking to staff and patients on all the wards.

His visit will take place on Wednesday afternoon between 2 and 4.30 pm.

## Inside This Issue

| | |
| --- | --- |
| 2 | The New NHS number |
| 2 | New Day Surgery Sessions |
| 3 | 5-day wards: a patient's view |
| 4 | New House Officer appointment |
| 4 | Eric Jones retires |

# Surgical Unit Update

## Volume 1 Issue 9 — March 1998

## We've met our Target!

**W**e are pleased to announce that our waiting lists are below 12 months for all categories within our directorate. The graph opposite shows the progress that has been made in the last year.

'This shows that our improvement in services to the public is being maintained' said Eric Brogan, the Unit's Clinical Director, as he toured the wards congratulating key staff.

He continued 'We want to aim for a target of 6 months maximum wait over the next 2 years. This will be a priority for the management team to plan for.'

*The reduction in waiting times was achieved by sweeping changes to the way resources are used. The operating theatre maintenance sessions were moved to evenings and weekends to free up an additional 4 sessions. In addition a dedicated theatre was used for emergencies only. This meant that routine surgical lists were no longer disrupted, resulting in less cancelled operations.*

Further initiatives being planned include the conversion of two wards into a combined day surgery and 5-day unit. This will allow for the increase in short-stays for many operations.

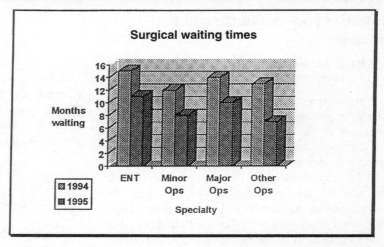

### Confidentiality

LAST THURSDAY A PAGE FROM A PATIENT'S MEDICAL RECORD WAS FOUND LEFT INSIDE THE PHOTOCOPIER ON LEVEL 4. THIS REPRESENTS A SERIOUS BREACH OF OUR BASIC RESPONSIBILITY TOWARDS PATIENTS – THAT OF CONFIDENTIALITY. ALL STAFF MUST BE ON THEIR GUARD AGAINST LEAVING CONFIDENTIAL DOCUMENTS LYING AROUND WHERE THEY CAN BE SEEN BY NON-MEDICAL OR NON-HOSPITAL STAFF.

### Visit by Chairman

Next week the Surgical Unit will be visited by Sir Eric Pode, the Chairman of the Midshire Hospitals Trust.

As well as seeing the work of the existing Day Surgery Unit Sir Eric will be talking to staff and patients on all the wards.

His visit will take place on Wednesday afternoon between 2 and 4.30 pm. and he will be accompanied by Mrs White plus a representative of the Midtown Observer. On his visit Sir Eric will be taking particular interest in our latest developments in

## Inside This Issue

**Figure 9.8**    A different version of the page shown in Figure 9.7.

## HOW TO GET STARTED

A very important point for you to remember is the aspect of design. Before you rush into detailed work on a document, there are some aspects you need to consider.

### Consider your audience and the message

◆ What is the document for?
◆ How is the reader going to use it?

For example, a work of fiction doesn't need an elaborate design because the reader becomes absorbed in the narrative. But sometimes when you are trying to convey a lot of factual information the reader may find it boring, even though it may be important that the reader understands and acts on this information; for example, the instructions in an admission letter will usually be very important, and so a layout that draws the reader's attention to the significant points is desirable.

Another example is where you provide information in a newsletter (Fig. 9.7). Here the user can assimilate information in short bursts so an active layout is necessary.

Considering the audience will guide you in which layout to select.

### Consider the layout

Your document doesn't *have* to be plain A4. You could fold it in two. Or you can fold it in three (a gatefold), but remember that the inside fold has to be a bit smaller (about 4 mm or 1/8 inch) than the other two leaves. Of course, folding means a lot more work in finally producing the document.

Will your document be double sided? This may be so if you adopt the gatefold layout described above. This may cause problems if your laser printer won't accept previously used paper which may be brittle after passing through the laser once. You can get around this if you have a photocopier that can do double-sided copying. In addition, you need to beware of text 'showing through' onto the other side.

### Reflection point

◆ Figure 9.3 shows one side of a gatefold leaflet. This was produced using WordPerfect with columns and text boxes. Can you think of some other applications for this kind of layout?

White space is important. It is not good enough to create a plain slab of text filling the whole page. White space is needed to define important text such as headings and to make the page more attractive to the eye.

### Reflection point

◆ Look at the poster (Fig. 9.1) and consider how the generous use of white space emphasises the opening question and the subsequent short paragraphs.

If your text is in columns you may need to decide about lines between the columns. It is probably best to have lines between different articles and white space *within* an article.

### Reflection point

◆ Look at Figure 9.8. Does the use of lines between the columns assist the layout?

It doesn't have to be difficult working with columns. For example, the basic newsletter layouts in Figures 9.7 and 9.8 were created in 2 minutes in 'Word for Windows' using the 'Wizard' facility. If you don't like working in columns you get around this by making up individual narrow pages and then pasting them together for photocopying in columns.

Don't make the lines too long. The eye reads in *groups* of characters, so anything longer than about 60–65 characters (approximately 10 words to the line) is uncomfortable to read. Moreover, the eye gets tired and it has further back to travel to the beginning of the next line, which it has to struggle to locate.

Avoid full justification. It may look fine on official correspondence but within the columns of a newsletter it can make 'rivers' of white and can look rather ponderous. An example of this is in the third text box in Figure 9.3. Use left justified text but consider using your word processor's hyphenation facility so that words get split up. This fills up the line space more.

Don't make margins too narrow for your printer. Some printers such as laser printers have to have a 0.2 inch margin all around the page and some printers need a 1 inch margin at the top. If the document is going to go into a plastic folder you need to allow extra margin space on the left for the binding. This space is often called the *gutter*.

Remember for documents intended for patients that your readers may have poor eyesight or may be colour blind. Don't expect patients to be able to read text in grey panels, for example.

## Consider how you will group the information

Paragraphs organise information into groups and give the eye time to pause besides providing a reference point to return to. They also break up 'forbidding' slabs of text.

Different types of information can go in different parts of a document, as you can see in the example of the genitourinary clinic (Fig. 9.3) where different boxes are used for this purpose.

Consider the use of the tables facility to do layouts. The examples in Figures 9.5 and 9.6 were created using the WordPerfect Table feature.

**Reflection point**

◆ Look at Figures 9.5 and 9.6 and think of some other management purposes that the 'Table' feature could be used for, e.g. room allocations, clinic timetable blanks.

## Consider what paper you will use and any features

Most laser paper is not very thick and may look flimsy for some types of document. However, thicker paper may not be accepted by your printer so it best to check first before ordering expensive paper.

If you decide to use a paper colour other than white try to choose a pastel colour – they are much easier to read from than a dark colour.

## Choose your fonts – and what is a font anyway?

With modern programs, particularly those running under 'Windows', you have a choice of interesting and creative fonts.

A *font* is a design for a set of characters. Figure 9.8 shows a number of different fonts, albeit too many on the one page!

Fonts can exist in different *point sizes*. A point in 1/72 of an inch. So if you select a point size of 12, each character will take up about one sixth of an inch – we say *about* because in fact the point size is *not* based on the size of the character. Instead it is based on the block that the characters would be mounted on if it were an actual printer's character. What this means is that different fonts in the same point size may take up different amounts of line. To avoid space problems it is a good idea to print out a sample sheet with different fonts in the same point size.

Usual point sizes you will work in will be 10 or 12, with 14, 18 or 24 being used for headings.

Beware of using too many fonts in the same document even though you may have lots of fonts at your disposal. The result (Fig. 9.8) will look like a case of 'fontitis'! Instead, use a maximum of two fonts per document and use different point sizes for the more important paragraphs and headings. For example, a heading can be two point sizes bigger than the body of the text and the text for a quotation could be two point sizes smaller.

### Reflection point

◆ Compare the two versions of the same newsletter in Figures 9.7 and 9.8. Do you think the extra number of fonts in Figure 9.8 makes it any easier to read?

Also, do not be tempted into using very small font sizes. This can lead to lines that are too long.

Fonts can be 'serif' and 'sans serif'. Serifed fonts have finishing strokes at the end and look more elegant. Research suggests that serifed fonts are easier to read because they give the eye more 'clues' about the characters. So use a 'serifed' font for the body of your text and reserve the sans serif fonts for titles, footnotes and introductory paragraphs.

When choosing fonts you have to consider if they will photocopy well – some fonts copy particularly badly when in italics.

Avoid using a lot of capital letters (see Figure 9.8, second column). They are fine for titles or headlines or OCCASIONAL emphasis but not for whole sentences or paragraphs.

Also you should avoid long amounts of text in italics (see Figure 9.8, column 1). Italics work best *in contrast* with plain text.

Blobs (●) can be tempting and useful for making a list of 'bulleted' points, but if you use them, make sure they are all the same size.

White on black text can be powerful for titles and short bursts of text but make sure your printer can support it. The next best thing is bold black on grey (Fig. 9.5).

## Consider graphics

You don't need to go overboard on graphics. Just one or two icons or drawings can balance the text, emphasise points and invite the reader in (see Fig. 9.1). You can use clip art provided with the program or maybe your hospital or practice has its logo obtainable as a computer file. For example, Figure 9.2 uses a 'logo' in its header which could be printed from the computer rather than on pre-printed paper. It also uses a simple telephone graphic to liven up the page.

Although we have mentioned that you can make use of clip art libraries, you should not overdo the artwork so that it looks too fussy and overwhelms the text.

Figures 9.7 and 9.8 show the use of a graph generated in another program and imported into the text.

If you want to include a photograph you can always use a blank image box in your document and then paste the photo in it before photocopying.

If you do use a photo or an image don't forget to give it a caption – but don't tell the readers what is obvious from the picture; e.g. *not* 'Building work in progress on the West Wing' but 'West Wing – £4 million budget'.

Beware of breaching copyright with graphics. Most clip art is free if you are only producing a small quantity of the document and are not selling it. However, photographs and cartoons that you copy from books and magazines will require permission from the copyright holder. Beware too of location maps which may originate from Ordnance Survey, who are very strict about copyright nowadays.

## Consider your writing style

You need to modify your style according to your audience and the document.

◆ In newsletters you will find it difficult to write headlines – use of present tense seems strange but past tense is stranger!
◆ Remember that for patient information your writing needs to be clear and active and reassuring for the patient. See Figure 9.2,

where the information the patient needs to know is clearly structured.

◆ 'Publishing' text calls for extra care and it will be worth checking your wording on a willing volunteer to check that the message has been understood. You also need to make sure that your text is correct clinically.

## Get some feedback

Try a rough sketch layout first and if you are not sure about how different fonts and shaded panels appear, create a page with examples of different shade intensities and font and line sizes for you to refer to and get reactions to.

It is always a good idea to get feedback on your ideas and your work before printing or copying (Box 9.1).

## A WORD OF WARNING

Although software is a lot easier to use these days, you still need time and training to learn some of the advanced skills. Above all do not be tempted to imitate the layouts of daily newspapers or magazines – it takes highly skilled layout experts to create these. Instead try to detect what aspects of their designs seem to work and think about copying just one or two of them. It's easy to go 'over the top' and forget that the purpose of presentation is to enhance the content and not to distract from it.

If you want best quality layout and paper then you have to consider using a commercial printer.

---

**Box 9.1**   Getting feedback

◆ Try reading your text out loud. This is a good way of revealing 'nonsense writing', which can arise if you cut and paste text carelessly.

◆ Get reactions to your layout from colleagues.

◆ If the document is meant for the public, try it out on a willing volunteer patient or friend to make sure that every instruction is understood.

---

Here you can use your word processing skills to prepare rough layouts for discussion amongst your colleagues so that less time is spent by the printer in expensive layout work.

Consider the time cost of producing multiple copies.

---

**Reflection points**

◆ If your laser printer can print 4 pages per minute how long would it take to print 1000 copies? And how many reloads of paper would you have to do if the paper tray only holds 50 sheets of paper?

◆ Consider also the *cost* of producing copies. For example, if the cost of a toner cartridge for a laser printer is £50 and it lasts for 2500 copies what would be the cost (excluding paper) of laser printing 1000 copies? How does that compare with photocopying costs (nominal cost of 3p per copy)?

---

Local photocopying costs can be reasonable for short runs but above a certain number it might be cheaper to get a commercial printer to print it from 'camera ready' artwork supplied by you from your laser printer. The saving here is in the pre-printing stage.

Take the trouble to make back-ups at frequent intervals of documents you are working on. You may spend hours on layouts only to lose them if your disk gets corrupted or someone accidentally overwrites the file. It's a good idea to save your work under different version numbers (e.g. 'newslet1.doc; newslet2.doc, etc.) so that you can always return to a previous version if you are not happy with your latest version.

Also, you should make the most of your work by saving settings, blank 'templates', etc., so that they can be reused later. (A good example is the gatefold leaflet in Figure 9.3.) Alternatively, you could use the 'styles' facility to store and reproduce your work.

attention. Needless to say, attention will have been paid to the planning of all areas and surfaces, so floorings and coverings should all be hard wearing and easy to clean. In some instances such as spillage it will be necessary to be able to clean a surface with bleach. (See Chapter 17.)

The typical environment that patients will encounter, whether in hospital or general practice, should have a variety of different areas, including a welcoming and comfortable waiting area, an office which is well planned for its purpose and close to the reception area and treatment and consulting rooms. Although all will have different characteristics none should be intimidating to the patient and attention should be given to details such as blinds or screens to allow privacy, a mixture of lighting – bright and directable in clinical areas, softer and warmer in counselling or waiting areas, and toys for children, which should be washable and relatively quiet. Even the way in which furniture is arranged should be considered, with chairs placed to the side of a desk, rather than in front, as this is considered to be less confrontational and intimidating to patients. The safe exit of staff in cases of aggression also needs to be considered, so obstructions within clinical areas should be avoided.

**Reflection point**

◆ Think of two areas in a doctor's surgery you have visited either as a patient or on work placement. What impression did you take away with you and why? What might you like to change or improve and how would you try to achieve it?

## THE CLINICAL ENVIRONMENT

Although nurses will mainly be responsible for the work carried out in the treatment rooms, we all need some understanding of what is safe and acceptable in such important areas. These princi-

ples are relevant to both general practice and hospital work.

Ideally a treatment area should have:

◆ enough space to allow treatment or minor surgery to take place
◆ space for consultation and paperwork
◆ a preparation area
◆ storage areas.

It is usual for a screened couch to be provided along with the necessary linen in any consulting area. Adequate lighting to enable examination to take place must also be easily available; this can be of the flexible variety and may be wall mounted or on a movable base. Some form of desk or writing surface must also be provided and with it, storage facilities for a variety of forms and other paperwork. Trolleys may also be used during clinical procedures so adequate space needs to be allowed for them.

As far as preparation goes, this will depend upon the variety and extent of procedures that are to be carried out. However, it is considered best practice to separate used and therefore dirty instruments and equipment from clean areas or sterilised equipment. In the hospital context this can be readily achieved and in many general practices this is the accepted mode of practice, especially where minor surgery is a regular occurrence or a developing feature. We have mentioned the need for adequate storage in the treatment room. This will generally fall into three areas:

◆ lotions
◆ dry goods
◆ vaccines.

**Lotions.** These should be stored separately from any other goods and adequate stock control should ensure that they are always within their shelf-life.

**Dry goods.** These tend to fall into either clinical or non-clinical categories and so might usefully be kept in separate cupboards or storage areas. Some examples are given in Box 10.1.

**Vaccines.** A selection of vaccines used in treatment which will require refrigeration. There should be a regulating gauge inside the refrigerator to enable correct storage to take place; this is

**Box 10.1    Dry goods**

◆ Stationery

◆ Forms

◆ Paper couch roll

◆ Non-sterile gloves and household gloves

◆ Disposable protective aprons – plastic

◆ Sterile packs and dressings – these need to be kept in a dry area and a check kept on expiry dates

◆ Syringes and needles – a full supply of all sizes

◆ Specimen and blood bottles – a variety of different bottles will need to be stocked – these are often colour coded

◆ Suturing material – this will depend on the extent of work undertaken

◆ Examination equipment – this will obviously vary from hospital to general practice and specific items are listed later in this chapter

◆ Surgical instruments – checks should regularly be made on the state of repair and working order of instruments. Cleaning, preparation and sterilisation of these articles is usually a nursing task, but there may be occasions when other staff need to stand in when there is a crisis. In these cases, relevant health and safety recommendations must be adhered to and great care taken that the job is done thoroughly and efficiently

especially important for vaccines. Again, expiry dates should be checked regularly and the refrigerator should be lockable.

It goes without saying that any piece of equipment used in the treatment area must be cared for efficiently, whether it is a piece of electrical machinery such as an ECG machine, a specific surgical instrument, or only a pupil torch. Many of these instruments and machines are extremely expensive and regular maintenance is of utmost importance, both to keep them in efficient working order and to prolong their working life wherever possible.

Some machines require specialist overhaul and correct storage and many will require special parts or spares, which will also need to be stored carefully and replaced when necessary to ensure that a full stock is always available. Do not forget that this includes the ordinary bulbs and batteries, which are essential to so many pieces of equipment and so easily overlooked.

**Reflection point**

◆ How might you ensure that equipment is properly looked after?

## CLINICAL PROCEDURES

Although all clinical procedures will generally be carried out by professionally trained staff whether nursing or medical, it is useful for the medical secretary to understand the principles by which they work and the practicalities that are involved, including some of the pieces of equipment which are used. This section of the chapter will look at:

◆ the sterilisation of instruments and equipment by autoclave

◆ maintenance of the sterile field and aseptic technique

◆ commonly used clinical equipment.

### Sterilisation by autoclave

Autoclaves are special pieces of equipment in which instruments are sterilised. They will vary in size depending on where they are to be used. Hospitals may have a whole department devoted to the safe care and sterilisation of surgical equipment, called the CSSD (Central Sterile Supply Department); they use several very large autoclaves. Doctors and dentists may use smaller 'table-top' versions, but all must meet British Standard specifications. However large or small they are, they all work on the same principle of steam

## Treatment

Some of these instruments listed in Box 10.3 will be used daily; others will only be used for special procedures.

There is an increasing tendency to use 'single use' instruments in general practice and in some outpatient departments. These are usually made of plastic and should be disposed of after one use. Instruments which are likely to fall into this category are basic forceps.

A variety of prepacked disposable sterile blades and sutures should also be available.

It may be considered necessary to keep a small supply of oxygen available in a cylinder and many general practices have a supply of nebulisers available for cases of severe asthma.

Conversion charts are also useful.

Emergency equipment is also necessary in order

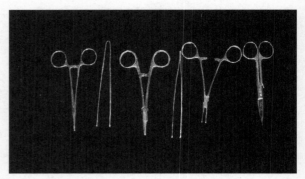

**Figure 10.3** Instruments used for insertion and removal of sutures.

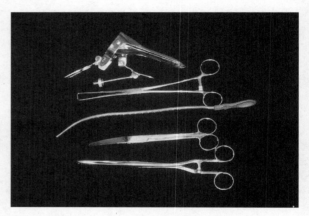

**Figure 10.4** Instruments used for intrauterine contraceptive device (IUCD) insertion. From the top: Cusco's speculum, volsellum forceps, uterine sound, scissors, sponge holder.

to resuscitate patients who have collapsed, perhaps due to anaphylaxis. The items listed in Box 10.4 should be readily available and preferably kept together ready for such an event.

| **Box 10.3** Instruments used in treatment |
| --- |

Aural syringe – with interchangeable ear pieces of different sizes. Some are now electrically operated

Scissors – a variety of size and type

Diathermy/cautery

Tooth dissecting forceps ⎫
Spencer–Wells forceps    ⎬ These instruments are all used in minor surgery or for suturing (Fig. 10.3) with other items, e.g. scissors
Bard–Parker knife handles
Sponge holders ⎭

Uterine sound ⎫ These are used for IUD insertion with other items (Fig. 10.4), e.g. Cusco's speculum and scissor
Volsellum forceps ⎭

Skin hooks

Curetting spoons

Probes

Clip removers and stitch cutters

| **Box 10.4** Emergency equipment |
| --- |

Airways – adult and paediatric – Brooks design

Laryngoscope

Endotracheal tubes

Giving sets

Various drugs to be given by injection, such as hydrocortisone and adrenaline

Syringes and needles

In some general practices it is the policy for each member of staff to have responsibility for a particular consulting room. This will include overall monitoring of basic cleaning and the restocking of forms and equipment and may include the clearing of used instruments at the end of a surgery. The treatment room will be the responsibility of the practice nurse. In the hospital environment this will also be undertaken by nursing and auxiliary staff.

**Reflection point**

◆ Do you know where the resuscitation equipment is kept in any of the places you have been to on work experience?

## CONCLUSION

When you have finished studying this chapter, you should have a better idea about the responsibilities held by other members of the team with regard to clinical activity. You should understand more about some of the procedures being carried out, and feel more prepared to be involved should the need arise.

**Exercise**

Try planning a waiting, reception and office areas to allow patients and staff to benefit from a well thought through environment. Consider patient and staff needs. Consider how you would protect confidentiality.

## FURTHER READING

Medical secretaries and students who wish to further their understanding of the clinical environment in either hospital or general practice may like to take advantage of many books written for nursing education. You may find the following useful:

Clarke M 1991 Practical nursing, 14th edn. Baillière Tindall, London.

Jeffree P (ed) 1990 The practice nurse. Chapman and Hall, London.

Hampson GD 1994 Practice nurse handbook, 3rd edn. Blackwell Scientific Publications, Oxford.

The reader should also remember that many professional magazines and journals will have relevant and interesting articles, which may be a useful source of information. These include:

*Pulse*
*The AMSPAR Magazine.*

# Personnel

*Jayne Pearce*

**11**

## OBJECTIVES

◆ To identify principal health care staff groups and their roles

◆ To illustrate liaison between these groups and the medical secretary

◆ To highlight the importance of effective communication and teamwork.

## INTRODUCTION

In any health service, whether public or private, community or hospital based, the care delivered will be reliant on many diverse teams of staff cooperating effectively to provide a high standard and efficient level of care. As a medical secretary, you will be an essential component of the delivery team. In a general practice environment you will be a member of the primary health care team (PHCT – also referred to as primary care team), providing a key point of contact for the other team members (see Chapter 16 – The Working Practice). You will also be required to liaise with a wide range of other external organisations and individuals. In the secondary care environment, a variety of teams will exist and be called upon at different times to deliver a service to each individual patient. You will form part of the support structure which allows the medical and nursing care to be effectively delivered. You will also be a key liaison point for members of the individual patient's PHCT. Through this chapter we will aim to demonstrate the range of personnel who are involved in patient care and support, and the way in which primary and secondary care teams are linked to form an extended team to ensure the patient's needs are fully met. Members of the PHCT are fully described in Chapter 16, so only brief reference will be made to individual functions in this chapter. It is worthwhile noting that the NHS spends more on staffing resources than on any other category of expenditure.

matters can wait until the consultant is freely available. If there is ever any doubt as to the urgency of a situation, the medical secretary should always demonstrate caution and contact the consultant immediately, unless prior experience dictates otherwise.

## Administration and clerical staff

A very large group of staff come under the general heading of administration and clerical. Medical secretaries are included within this group, along with medical receptionists, ward clerks and medical records clerks. Medical receptionists will be found working on the reception desk of an outpatient clinic and will be responsible for logging patients' arrival to the clinic and for making follow-up clinic or investigation appointments. They will also be involved in ensuring that the medical records are sent through to the clinic area in the correct order. Ward clerks, sometimes referred to as ward coordinators or administrators, will be based within a ward working with the nursing staff to ensure patients' records, results and X-rays are available and in order. They will often be involved with making follow-up and discharge arrangements for the patients and for liaison with the admissions office on a daily basis. Medical record clerks or assistants are usually based within the central medical records library and will work as part of a team under the supervision of a medical records officer or manager. Medical records clerks play a vital role by ensuring the correct recording and filing of all patient-related documentation. They will prepare and check clinic lists and retrieve notes for clinics, search for and file results, collate the records with X-rays and other tests, arrange follow-up appointments and generally assist the medical records officer in the smooth running of the department. Much time is spent searching for and filing case notes, usually housed in huge filing areas operating a numerical system. Each patient is allocated an individual registration number and set of notes at their first attendance at a hospital, which are then kept and used for every future visit or admission. The role of the medical records department is further explored in Chapters 5 and 12. Medical

records clerks will also undertake general repair and maintenance of the records folders as they pass through the system. Clerks may also be required to staff the clinic reception desk as part of their normal job description.

Other medical administration staff will be found working in specialised areas such as the admissions office, appointments office, transport office, radiology department, clinical coding and medical audit. Whilst all require basic office skills, each will develop specialised knowledge and skills in their own particular area of responsibility and may have the opportunity to achieve formal qualifications such as the Clinical Coding Certificate offered by the Institute of Health Record Information and Management.

### Reflection point

◆ The list below contains many different departments within a hospital. What members of staff would be in each?

| | |
|---|---|
| Speech and language | Rehabilitation |
| General outpatients | Oral surgery and orthodontics |
| Diagnostic imaging | Audiology |
| Blood tests and pathology samples | Restaurant |
| Chapel | Boardroom |
| Dietician | Antenatal clinic |
| Social services department | |

## Professions allied to medicine

There are a large number of specialist staff who are referred to as PAMs (professions allied to medicine).

◆ *Physiotherapists or physical therapists:* assisting in rehabilitation and providing advice on appropriate exercise for those with orthopaedic conditions, general injuries, sports injuries, those recovering from surgical procedures or medical conditions, and the elderly.

◆ *Occupational therapists*: working with those who are permanently or temporarily mentally or physically disabled to enable them to cope with everyday tasks and to learn new skills.

◆ *Speech and language therapists*: providing treatment for all types of speech and communication problems afflicting the hearing impaired, trauma patients, the disabled, children and adults with speech impediments and those learning to speak following major surgery to the larynx or oesophagus, and those recovering from strokes or other medical conditions.

◆ *Dieticians*: providing individual dietary advice for patients suffering from specific food allergies, obesity, swallowing problems, malnutrition, kidney disease and other medical conditions. They also provide information on healthy eating, and safe alcohol consumption, in general.

◆ *Chiropodists*: provide expert advice on the care of feet, which may be particularly important to diabetics, the elderly and those with circulatory problems. They also undertake gait assessments and other related tasks.

◆ *Pharmacists*: responsible for dispensing drugs via the pharmacy in all hospitals, for both outpatients and inpatients. They will also provide drug information. Each pharmacy will be managed by a senior pharmacist.

◆ *Social workers*: responsible for coordinating the needs of patients who are to be discharged, either to their own home or to another environment, such as a hospice.

◆ *Radiographers*: working with the team of radiologists providing a range of radiological investigations.

All PAMs undergo specific professional training and will gain recognised qualifications before being able to practise. Their professional status will be governed by their own professional body, e.g. the College of Speech and Language Therapists.

## Technicians

This term covers a range of specialist staff, some of whom are described in Box 11.3.

---

**Box 11.3** Technicians

◆ EEG technician: undertakes the electroencephalograph test

◆ ECG technician: undertakes the electrocardiogram test

◆ ODA: operating department assistant (also known as ODP – operating department practitioner) – working in operating theatres mainly with anaesthetists

◆ Audiology technicians: undertake a range of hearing tests

◆ Laboratory technicians: assisting pathologists with processing of test samples

◆ Phlebotomists: on call within the hospital for taking blood for testing

---

## Management

We have already outlined the Trust Board and senior executives but these individuals will be supported by a team of middle and first line managers, administrators and secretaries to ensure the management of the organisation as a whole is well maintained and cost-effective.

## Human resources

The human resources department (HRD) is also commonly referred to as personnel. There will normally be a senior personnel officer or manager who will be supported by a team including a deputy personnel officer, a personnel secretary and clerical staff. The work of the HRD will include staff recruitment, interviews, appraisals, health and safety training, liaison with trade union representatives and all general staffing issues. They will also be instrumental in ensuring that staff receive adequate contracts of employment and copies of

If Mrs Andrews' discharge from the ward is postponed, who needs to know?

Once you have deliberated this question, you should see that there are many individuals who may need to be updated on the current situation. The patient's consultant or his/her medical secretary must be informed. The transport officer needs to be told so that if official transport has been arranged, this can be cancelled. The patient's relatives will need to be contacted as soon as possible. The admissions department will need to know that the bed is not being vacated as expected, as they may have ·to cancel the admission of another patient to prevent a wasted journey. The patient may also have an assigned social worker who will also need to be kept informed. It may also be necessary to advise the patient's GP by telephone that the patient is not being discharged home, particularly if a home visit had already been organised. It is possible that the medical secretary may be required to undertake some or all of these communications.

## CONCLUSION

In this chapter we have examined a number of staffing groups to be found within a health care environment outlining the who, where and why in some instances. It is important to note that staff from all these groups may be found working within both primary and secondary care. Each member of staff has an important function in the delivery of health care services, whether they are involved in direct patient care or in a supporting role. As a recipient of health care, as we all will be at some point in our lives, we will rely on the efforts and expertise of an extensive network of professionals and support staff who will work together to ensure an acceptable level, and quality, of care.

As a medical secretary you have a duty to familiarise yourself with the staff and services available within your place of work. Ensure that you obtain a copy of the in-house directory detailing the names, departments and contact telephone numbers for all staff. Get to know your line manager and ensure you are aware of the terms of your job description. Nurture good working relationships with all other staff. You should also ensure that your colleagues are aware of who you are, how you can be contacted and what the full extent of your role is. Your aim should be always to make a worthwhile contribution to the service received by the patients. In this way you will help to create an environment conducive to effective communication and promote your own value as a member of the team.

### Exercises

◆ Find out what other specialist nursing qualifications are available by further reading and contacting recognised nursing bodies and associations.

◆ Through further reading and group discussion, make a list of professional bodies responsible for the training and conduct of PAMs in the UK.

◆ On your work placement or at your place of employment, find out who is responsible for training and development within the organisation. What development opportunities do they offer which might be useful for medical secretaries? Do they actively promote the attainment of professional qualifications?

## FURTHER READING

Irvine D, Irvine S 1996 The practice of quality. Radcliffe Medical Press, Oxford

Pringle M (ed) 1993 Change and teamwork in primary care. BMJ Publishing, London

# Medical records

*Grizelda Moules*

**12**

## OBJECTIVES

This chapter aims:

◆ To examine some important aspects of patient notes including the ownership of hospital records, length of time that they should be kept and means of accessing them

◆ To explain the different methods of compilation and storage of medical records in the hospital environment

◆ To highlight the importance of confidentiality and accuracy in all record-keeping activities

◆ To outline the most important forms used in hospital

◆ To explain the way in which contracts for outpatients and extra-contractual referrals are made

◆ To describe the role of audit and the part you need to play to ensure accurate information is recorded, with particular reference to research purposes

◆ To show how you may need to oversee the needs of other secretarial staff or assistants.

## INTRODUCTION

This chapter focuses primarily on medical records in the hospital environment, but also covers the important documentary links between hospital and GPs. One of its key themes will be the importance of confidentiality and accuracy in all record-keeping activities.

## PATIENTS' NOTES

### Ownership of records

Any records that are in writing are made up of the following two elements:

◆ the physical paper on which the words are written; and
◆ the information contained in them.

Within the NHS, the records belong physically to the NHS Trust or hospital (or the Family Health Services Authority (FHSA) for GP records) and ultimately to the Secretary of State.

The records of *private patients* belong to the health professional with whom they have a contract.

This ownership is unusual in law in that the 'owner' has a custodial responsibility, but is unable to sell or dispose of records. It is also an obligation that the 'owner' has to provide patients with access to them under the Access to Health Records Act 1990. All those who are aged 16 and over have the right to see any of their case notes which were created since November 1991. This is described later in the chapter.

There is a *duty of confidence* whereby the contents should not be disclosed to unauthorised

*Be aware* of the possibility that patients may have difficulty with reading and writing. A possible way of them avoiding saying this directly can be that they have 'forgotten their glasses'. They may also have difficulty in hearing or in understanding English, so be sensitive to these needs. Many hospitals are able to provide interpreters or people who can assist with sign language when needed. The GP should alert the hospital if he or she knows of these needs, but is not always aware of them.

*Remember to update information.* It is important to update any changes in patients' details. These may include changes of name, title, address, phone number and GP and/or GP address. It is quite possible that just one detail may change at a time and this can mean that data is lost from the hospital record or that it is misfiled or never reaches the correct GP. From the clinical side it is also important that medical staff are updated and informed of any changes in medication. Inaccuracies in medication are potentially very serious.

## Protocol for registration of patients

A protocol needs to be agreed for patient registration and several steps need to be followed. This is covered in Chapter 13 on the outpatient department. Ideally all details should be supplied on the (Blue) GP referral form (HMR 3) or on a plain paper referral and it is very important when working in general practice to ensure all details are given. If you are working in general practice, you can find a reference to a hospital number at the beginning of either a letter from a clinic or sometimes from a laboratory test result. Make sure these relate to the hospital to which the patient is being referred.

In the medical records department, firstly the referral letter needs to be approved. Providing that the patient has not previously been registered at the hospital, a pre-registration hospital number will be allocated and a hospital record file prepared. The allocation of a number is usually made on a computer and the method must ensure that the specific number is unique to that patient, so that even if several clerks access the computer simultaneously, the number allocation is controlled. Patients will be sent a questionnaire to complete and to bring with them when they attend for their first appointment.

The PAS computer database should be able to identify a set of hospital records from the details given. It is important to check that these relate to the right patient, particularly when several people may have the same name. In cases where details may have changed, such as GP and address, a note should be made and attached to the records or recorded on screen so that clinic reception staff can check that these are the right notes.

Normally patients will be allocated a hospital number on their first attendance at a hospital and this number may be specific to that hospital, or may be used within a specified group of hospitals. This is a particular case where GP staff can help tremendously. In whichever situation you are working you need to try and quote the current hospital number accurately and draw attention to any changes of name, address or GP. It is also worth identifying any different hospital numbers which may have been used previously at the same hospital, so that all details on that patient can be amalgamated.

### Reflection point

◆ How could you try to ensure all the data on a patient is *kept* up to date?

*Possible ideas*: Incorporation of reminder notices in the waiting room or at reception desk.

## Protocols and checklists for reception/nursing staff

It is advisable to compare previous letters from the GP to see if they include different addresses or other information. Such changes of data need to be checked with the patient to see what is accurate, e.g. they may have been staying at a temporary address.

The patient may be encouraged to bring a current repeat prescription card or even the bottles of medicine themselves for a first attendance or when changes in either dosage or medications are made.

### Pocket guide for junior doctors

This idea may help to encourage junior medical staff to help to maintain a good quality of patient record. The Welsh Medical Records Forum has designed a pocket guide in the form of a card. The importance of the medical records is emphasised and the doctor's responsibility towards them is outlined. The advice includes the points listed in Box 12.1.

---

### Reflection points

◆ Do you think this guide is a good idea? Why/why not?

◆ What points would you suggest adding or changing to this list?

◆ Which other categories of staff do you think could benefit from such an aide-memoire?

---

### Box 12.1 Patient record guidelines for junior doctors

◆ The case notes must not be removed from the hospital.

◆ The patient must be identified on all documents.

◆ All entries must be written legibly, in black ink, dated and signed.

◆ Consent forms must be completed and signed.

◆ Test results must be signed when seen.

◆ Discharge letters must be timely, neat and accurate.

◆ Senior staff need to check coding of diagnosis and procedures.

### Compiler records

A record should be kept of who compiles this information. Data entered on computer during or after a hospital consultation *should be automatically attributable to the health professional who entered it*. This would normally be part of a computer audit trail and for this as well as other reasons, it is important that staff do not borrow or use other people's password identifiers.

In the case of manual records, initials may be used, but these should be readily decipherable and there should be a means of identifying them back to their originator.

## Access to notes

### Patient access to their medical records

The Access to Health Records Act 1990 allowed all people over the age of 16 to see their own case notes created since November 1991. This is unless a clinical case is made for access being denied. Access to any records created before that date is at the discretion of the physician involved.

Following the Data Protection Act of 1984, patients have a right of access to any information held about them on computer. Applications have to be made in writing to the holder of the record and the application must be processed within 40 days. Applications for access are usually dealt with by medical records staff. Record holders who supply information are entitled to charge a fee and may also charge for copying and postage.

### How it works in practice

A patient who wishes to have access to his or her notes may be asked to complete a request form. This form will ask for the person's identification details and will require the person's signature. In the case of a person under 18 a responsible adult needs to certify that the child understands the nature of the application. The young person will need to sign an authorisation of release of any personal health records relating to him or her.

The application will then go to the consultant concerned and if approved the notes will be prepared.

Reasons why details *may not have to be released* include:

◆ if the information identifies a third party
◆ if legal issues are being considered by solicitors
◆ if the information is thought to be potentially mentally damaging
◆ if the information was recorded prior to the Data Protection Act of 1 November 1991.

Patients may also request to see their records during a consultation. It is recommended that when a patient is accessing notes, someone who has the appropriate expertise and ability should be present to 'explain' where necessary.

This situation may change with patient-held smart cards or patient-held notes. Currently maternity patients often keep a set of obstetric notes with them which are passed back to a health care professional a few weeks after the baby's birth. Similar records for child care may be held parentally to encourage partnership of care between parents and health care professionals.

## CLASSIFICATION FOR FILING

### The contents of the medical record files

*On the outer cover* of the record, the name of the hospital is printed. In addition, the patient's name is written, usually with the surname first and the hospital number in a position so that it is prominent when filing. It is also helpful to put a patient identification sticker on the outside, so that should two patients with the same name be attending the same clinic, they can be more readily differentiated.

*Inside* the medical record envelope there should be the following items.

**Patient information sheet.** This should include the patient minimum data set and additional information, which is also often kept on computer.

It should be possible to print this out and to attach it at the front of the records. It is a good idea for it to be glued inside the front cover so it is easily accessible to anyone reading the records and a recognised place for data to be updated. There

should be plenty of room for changes of detail, such as address or GP, particularly in areas of a fluctuating population. It is very important to keep the records up to date.

Other details which should be included here are:

◆ telephone number
◆ details of religion
◆ next of kin
◆ details of known allergies or hypersensitivities.

**Reflection point**

◆ What other details should or could be included here?

**The patient questionnaire.** This may have provided a source of useful information and could be included in the record and used to complete data held on the computer. Another questionnaire may be used to ask for details of medical history. If it covers general information, it may be included at the front, perhaps on a colour of paper which can be easily identified. Other questionnaires may be included in a departmental section (see 'Specialty coding', below).

**Stickers.** These should give basic patient details (name, address, GP, date of birth, etc.) and should be included in the notes. It may well be your job to ensure that they contain current information (and relate to the right patient). If they have run out or need updating a note could be put on the front of the records before they are returned to the medical records department.

**History sheets.** These should be included here, if not already within the departmental sections (see 'Specialty coding', below). They should be headed with patient details or a sticker.

The question as to how the history sheets are stored varies. In some cases these are chronological, from the top downwards (like a book), in others the most current (and most relevant notes) are kept at the top. The latter method is often used in general practice for history cards. The sheets may be held together with treasury tags or with a flexible plastic device which clips into place and hold the notes tightly, but is sometimes difficult to open and close.

**X-ray reports.** These are often stored at the back of the notes on a set of single pages and are attached by a sticky strip. Some hospitals report that they stop sticking after a while and can fall off. Some recommendations include glue, others suggest staples

**Pathology laboratory results.** These are stored in a similar way to X-ray results, but are particularly likely to accumulate with some patients. They may need to be culled from time to time and an agreed protocol for this needs to be in place. It may be your job to alert the doctor to the situation that the notes are getting full or that information is at risk of being lost. It may be that a summary of results is required at some stage, and in some cases computer-held results can provide a summary printout easily. A graphical representation may also be provided to show a pattern over time, perhaps of levels of hormone in relation to the use of a particular drug. The order in which these sections are arranged can vary between hospitals.

**Nursing records.** While a patient is an in-patient, records will be kept of the nursing care and this is incorporated in the notes in a separate section.

**Specialty coding.** This can be a very effective way of distinguishing the notes of different departments. Each department is assigned a different colour for a dividing folder, e.g. dermatology notes may be kept within a green folder and orthopaedics within a red one. The name of the department and consultant are then stamped on the front of this section and if a particular questionnaire relating to that treatment has been completed it can be included at the beginning of that section.

*History sheets* should also be stamped with the department and consultant's name and headed with the patient's details (on label where possible). This can save time when the consultant or other doctors wish to see the patient's progress with a particular condition, without necessitating them wading through a perhaps considerable amount of notes relating to other complaints.

A possible drawback of dividing the case notes by department is that this method does not allow the notes to be totally chronological of all that relates to the patient in hospital and consultations in other departments may shed light on what could be an interrelated condition. A particular effort may need to be made to look at other notes or question the patient about other illnesses for which they are being seen. From a medical secretary's point of view, it does facilitate the location and maintenance of the notes relating to a particular department within the patient's records.

Whatever the method used for filing within the record, it is important that this is consistent, so that everyone knows where to look for the information they need.

It may also be necessary for you to let the medical records department know if the notes have become badly torn or are just too big to be kept together effectively. In some cases notes need to consist of more than one volume. If it is not possible for clinical or other reasons to cull the notes further, they may be stored and clearly labelled as a series of volumes and stored in an area known as 'Fat notes'.

## Filing of medical records

Within a medical records department records awaiting filing should be stored in the order in which they will be filed to enable rapid access should they be required. Records should not be kept in cupboards or on shelves where they would be difficult to locate when needed should an emergency situation arise. It is also important that this applies in your own office.

### DOB index

A method of cross referring back to other details such as date of birth, name and address is essential to check that a hospital number has not previously been allocated and to enable records to be located when the hospital number is not specified or not known. This had previously been in the form of a series of cards filed in order of date of birth, then alphabetically by surname. This method is sometimes still used, particularly in small hospitals.

## Systems of filing

Medical records in general practice are usually filed alphabetically, but in a hospital, where large numbers of records are held and there can be many patients with the same name, numerical filing systems are preferred.

Hospital numbers are allocated chronologically. The number is often of six figures. In some hospitals, usually smaller ones, straight numerical filing may be used. This has the advantage of being easy to understand, but may result in misfiling through transposition of numbers; for example, a record with the number 324558 may be filed as 325458.

One of the main drawbacks of this method of filing is that the part of the filing area which has most activity and needs to be available to the most staff at once is that of the newest records, which in this case would have the highest numbers and would be filed next to each other.

To prevent such bottlenecks of use occurring, other filing methods have been introduced.

**Terminal digit filing system.** The terminal digit system is a popular method of filing health records in hospitals. It relies on locating records by use of the patient's hospital number. A record number of various lengths can be used but often six-figure numbers are used. A six-figure number can be divided into three pairs of two numbers, which may be written with a space between each pair.

The terminal digit filing system is easy to operate and efficient in the use of space in the records department but does require some training. The last two digits of the record number are termed the 'primary digits', the middle two are the 'secondary digits' and the first two (on the left of the number) are the 'tertiary digits'. For example, with the number *67 80 54*:

*67* are *tertiary* digits, *80* are *secondary* digits and *54* are *primary* digits.

In the terminal digit file there are 100 primary sections from 00 to 99. Each individual record is filed in straight numerical order according to its *tertiary digits*.

When filing a record, you would look at the primary digits first (remembering that these are the

last two, on the right of the number). On finding the section for those primary digits, you need to look at the secondary digits next. On finding that part, the record should be filed in straight numerical order according to the terminal digits, i.e. the first two numbers.

Examples of file numbers arranged this way are given in Box 12.2.

Should an odd number such as a five, seven or nine figure number be used, the middle group of numbers are regarded as a group on their own, with pairs on either side. This may happen, for example, if the files are more numerous or if the number is the same as another number used by the patient, e.g. NHS number or Social Security. An example using a nine-digit number is given in Box 12.3.

**Use of colour.** The spine and cover of medical records can be of different colours. These colours can be used to indicate the *year* of first attendance at a hospital. In this case records which precede a certain date can be clearly identified and selected

---

**Box 12.2** Numbers arranged by terminal digit filing system

| | |
|---|---|
| 56 87 90 | 98 99 41 |
| 57 87 90 | 99 99 41 |
| 58 87 90 | 00 00 42 |
| 59 87 90 | 01 00 42 |
| 60 87 90 | 02 00 42 |

---

**Box 12.3** Terminal digit filing using a nine-digit number

For the number 571–02–64–39, the group could be divided as follows:

| 57102 | 64 | 39 |
|---|---|---|
| Tertiary digits | Secondary digits | Primary digits |

The tertiary digits would then be filed sequentially. So the next ones would be: 57103 64 39, 57104 64 39, etc.

for possible culling or retention in a different form such as microfiche.

**Colour coding.** Colour coding of the notes may be done to aid filing and identify particular notes. For example, a coloured strip of adhesive tape may be added to the spine of notes to identify a particular part of the hospital number. Alternatively, a hard plastic divider may be used which projects from the edge of the notes and can be readily seen when the notes are filed. Misfiled notes can then be easily spotted, as ones with a colour which does not match the others is more readily noticeable than an incorrect number.

**Classification by geography.** In a hospital which contains the records of other, peripheral hospitals; the records which relate to other hospitals may have a different coloured outer cover or other features to identify them, such as a different design or a form colouring or tagging on the spine. The numbering system may start with a letter to indicate which hospital they belong to. By keeping these notes separately, they can be more readily accessed for clinics at the peripheral hospitals.

You need to ensure that on returning clinic bags or other groups of records, records from these hospitals are kept separate from those of the main or other hospitals. On requesting records from the medical records department, it is helpful to medical records staff if you group together requests for records from a particular hospital. You may also need to use a separate booking-out book or a separate section of the general booking-out book to identify these records.

Be especially careful when a patient who normally attends an outlying hospital needs to come in for investigations or for an operation in another or in the main hospital. Multiple sets of case notes may come to light. In this case clear reference to the other notes needs to be made on the outside of each set. For future records, the consultant needs to be informed to ensure relevant documentation is included in both while not duplicating information unnecessarily.

# MICROFILMING

Microfilming is a photographic method which is used to reduce the size of the records stored. The size of the reduction can vary. If the original is reduced to 1/24 of the original size, the reduction rate is 24 to 1 and described as 24×. This is the usual rate for reduction of medical records and can result in a 95% saving in storage space.

It may be necessary to agree a criterion for deciding which medical records should be microfilmed and whether all or only part of the contents should be included. The equipment necessary to microfilm can be quite expensive. Several hospitals are now employing or looking towards more sophisticated methods of storage which involve more advanced information technology methods such as optical disk.

For microfilming to be carried out, it is necessary to have a range of equipment including cameras. In addition, to assist with the selection and inspection of the images by providing an enlarged view, it will be necessary to insert the microfilm into jackets. Special equipment called 'lay up equipment' is used to provide microfiche masters. Duplication equipment will provide the microform.

In order to see the microfilmed records, it is necessary to have special machines, called readers, which act as projectors, as well as reader-printers. It is also possible to use computerised microfilm indexes by using CAR (computer assisted retrieval). This may be worth considering when the rate of retrieval or reference is high.

The technique of filming the record is not difficult to learn, but an alternative may be for a hospital to contract out the filming part of the process. This may be done on a fixed rate per exposure. The confidentiality of these records must be ensured. The resulting films need to be checked before the original paper versions are destroyed.

It is not always easy to read microfilmed notes and they can be of poor quality if derived from sources that have used carbon copies, darkened paper or have been torn or crumpled. Records need to be prepared by ensuring that the patient's name and number are included, that they are in chronological order and that any staples are removed. Each page is then photographed and presented in chronological order on a small card.

It is important that microfilmed notes are stored

in appropriate conditions and are clearly labelled and catalogued.

# FORMS

## Hospital referral form (blue PRL 1) or referral letter written on computer

When a GP refers a patient to be seen at a hospital this can be done either on a blue referral form, or on plain paper. The information needed on the referral letter will include the clinical reasons for the referral, but may also include information such as drug sensitivities or allergies. You may find that a method needs to be agreed with the consultant so that this information can be recorded in a suitably prominent position. Other information will form the basis of the patient data set which can then be included in the PAS (Patient Administration System) and is used for preliminary patient identification. Where GP/Hospital Links are in place, this can be done electronically (see Chapter 8).

## GP request forms

GPs may request the hospital to carry out pathology laboratory reports on a variety of specimens or may request X-rays or other investigations to take place. Often this is carried out electronically through GP/Hospital Links. It is important that data kept on the patient is up to date.

The cost implications of requests depend on the contract the GP has with the department.

Possible types of contract are shown in Box 12.4.

---

**Box 12.4    Types of GP contract**

◆ *Cost to case contract*: each case is costed and billed separately

◆ *Block contract*: to be paid no matter how much activity takes place

◆ *Trigger contract*: up to a certain amount is agreed to be paid for and beyond that trigger, new agreements need to be made

---

## Investigation request forms

Unfortunately it is often the case that the doctor's handwriting is not totally clear, so as a medical secretary working in general practice or in hospital you can help ensure the right patient's details relate to the right sample and that the result of the investigation returns to the doctor who requested it.

The consequences of accurate results being sent to the wrong doctor who has a patient by the same name could be disastrous and it has not been unknown to happen. Scrupulous care needs to be taken here.

Labels kept in patients' case notes can be useful, but ensure that a separate label has been used for each piece of the form. This sometimes needs three labels per investigation. A method of assisting the results to return appropriately is to prerecord details such as department code on sample requests.

If you are helping to prepare for a clinic where all the patients are likely to have the same samples taken, e.g. particular blood tests or cervical cytology, the appropriate forms and labels can be prepared and labelled for each patient. The use of clear, legible writing, usually in capitals, makes everyone's work easier.

Where a particular doctor has exclusive use of a consultation room, many forms can be prepared by ensuring the doctor's code and practice or department code are already written on request forms. This can also be done with sample bottles and containers. It may be that someone else can help with this and that a medical receptionist or nurse or ward clerk may be involved. The result is more efficient collection of data. Samples can otherwise easily be sent to a different doctor who has similar initials and never reach its true destination, which means that both the doctor's patient's and laboratory technician's time is wasted plus that of others, including yourself, who try in vain to locate the missing information.

Another benefit is that there is a better use of doctors' time by minimising their clerical work, which will allow them more time in consultation with the patient.

It is very important that each sample is checked before sending it off.

An input of a little extra time initially can achieve good results.

## Form MED 10 – inpatient certificate

This can be used by a patient who is currently attending or who has attended hospital as an inpatient. It needs to be completed and signed by an authorised member of the hospital staff. This form can be used to support a claim for statutory sick pay or to continue a claim for state benefits. To start a claim for state benefit, patients need to use form SC1 (Rev) if self-employed, unemployed or non-employed, or Form SSP1 (E) or SSP1 (T) if they are an employer.

## Private patients

In the case of private patients who have undergone treatment whether as an outpatient or inpatient, the appropriate forms from their insurance companies will need to be completed, if applicable. The consultant may need to refer to the patient's notes for completion of these forms and it may be necessary to hold them back for this purpose.

## Registration of birth

Following the birth of a baby in hospital an orange notification form is sent to the local Register Office. In the case of a birth being in the community, the midwife will send a similar form to the Register Office. The parent should register the birth within 6 weeks and will be given a birth certificate. The parent will also be given a pink registration form which should be given to the GP on registering the baby there, and not included in the baby book as some parents do.

## Death certificate

This will be issued if the death occurs in hospital. It is very important to record full details, including telephone number of next of kin so that they may be notified promptly should a death occur. It may also be of particular importance if the person who died had offered to be an organ donor as decisions may need to be made within a short space of time.

Following a death, if a *coroner* is involved the coroner will send Part A of a form to the Register Office. If a post-mortem occurs, the coroner will send Part B to the Register Office. The next of kin is advised to go to the Register Office to register the death.

When a body is to be *cremated* one doctor needs to sign Medical papers Part B. This can be either the deceased's registered GP or hospital doctor. Form C is completed by another doctor, either a hospital doctor or one who is from a different practice. Each doctor must see the body and they must not be related to each other.

## Contracts

Contracts need to be agreed by the consultant following a patient being referred by a GP. Where patients are in hospitals which are not of Trust status, Local Authority contracts apply. For non-fundholding GPs, fundholding comes from the Local Authority. (Refer to Chapter 13 on the outpatient department.)

## Extra-contractual referral

When an extra-contractual referral has been made, an *ECR Outpatient Appointment Authorisation Request Form* is prepared by the accrual officer of the hospital Trust and sent to the relevant GP for its completion and return. Details of the approved contract doctor or other approved person will be added and their account code, authorisation number and signature given.

If the patient needs to be admitted for an investigation or an operation or treatment, an *ECR Waiting/Booking List Authorisation Request Form* is prepared. Following discharge, the form is completed, with dates of admission and discharge and codes such as OPCS/ICD 10 codes given. (See Chapter 8 for further details.)

In the case of emergency treatment, *ECR Notification of Emergency Inpatient Treatment Form* will be issued and completed following treatment. In the case of a road traffic accident, insurance companies will be involved in the payment of treatment.

## Road traffic accidents

When a road traffic accident (RTA) has occurred, the hospital can request reimbursement of emergency treatment costs. The fee is payable by those using the vehicle at the time of the accident and liability for payment is unconnected with any question of responsibility or liability for the accident itself. Usually these costs can be met by the relevant insurance company, but can be settled by the individuals themselves. This is covered under the Road Traffic Act 1995 Section 158. Records of patients involved in RTAs are sometimes filed separately and may have separate numbers. It is important to note when emergency treatment has related to an RTA.

## Form PU1 – notification of tertiary extra-contractual referral

Tertiary referrals are from consultants in hospitals which are outside the area of the hospital to which the patient is being referred, e.g. a consultant in Devon may request a referral for their patient to a hospital in London.

This is completed by a referring consultant to the purchasing authority or fundholder. Each set of forms is numbered and is written on self-duplicating NCR (no carbon required paper). The form is completed by the receiving provider unit. The top copy is white and sent to the purchasing authority or GP fundholder. The second sheet is pink and is sent to the receiving unit and retained by them. The third copy is blue and is sent to either the purchasing authority or the GP fundholder. This last copy gives more detailed information regarding the estimated costs of the procedure.

## GP/hospital/consultant links

Although usually a letter will be sent in paper form between the GP and hospital, another method is now in use. Requests for referral may now be sent electronically direct to the hospital, where GP/Hospital Links are in place. The letter to the GP following an outpatient appointment or following inpatient treatment can also be sent electronically which, in addition to similar transfer of pathology laboratory data, can speed up considerably the process of information transfer as a whole.

# AUDIT

Audit should be an ongoing process. The purpose of audit may be to monitor and review current performance. It may be connected with research into new methods or new drugs or equipment. It may also be to assess either quantitatively or qualitatively certain aspects in greater depth than had previously been carried out. Related to audit is the clinical coding, which can be used to identify cases of particular interest.

Some forms of audit may be carried out from data already collected and available *electronically*. This can assist analysis of the data from a point at source.

In order to carry out a particular audit, ways of collecting the data efficiently should be considered at the outset and electronic methods will often provide the best solution if a suitable method can be found. For retrospective studies where such data is not easily accessible, the patient's notes may need to be accessed.

As a secretary, you may need to request particular notes from the records department for audit purposes. It may be important also to retain particular notes of patients involved in an audit study, particularly if it is part of a clinical trial. These notes should be stored in a specific area and a list of them kept up to date and visible. This can prevent the need for someone to go through all the notes in their search for one particular set.

It may also be important to ensure any rotating junior medical staff have been able to complete their part of the study before they may move on to another department or leave the hospital. It is important that a method of monitoring audit notes is maintained, so that the data can be collected as soon as appropriate and so that the records can be released back to the medical records department as soon as possible.

## Research

On occasion, audit may be carried out for specific reasons into particular areas. For example, an orthopaedic surgeon may wish to study the effectiveness of different surgical procedures, for research purposes. Another research study could be into the incidence of postoperative infection and consideration of which form of treatment for a specific infection is most effective. Or it may be a study of the efficiency of different forms of prostheses in different categories of patients – how soon do different prostheses need to be replaced and why. In addition, and of increasing importance nowadays, many current forms of audit attempt to discover what are the quality of life benefits and the cost implications of different treatments.

## Links to medical records officers

A typical line of accountability can be seen in Figure 12.1.

# ACCOUNTABILITY

An established line of responsibility and accountability should be decided so that each member of staff knows to whom they are accountable. In addition, they should be aware of whose work they should be overseeing and monitoring.

The job description of individual members of the medical records department may vary considerably. The medical records assistants may be responsible for working in the medical records department and may stay there while outpatient clinics take place. In other situations the role may involve reception of patients during the clinic. Sometimes staff are based in the clinic most of the time and only visit the medical records department to pull (locate and take) records for use during the clinic.

Each member of staff should have a job description, but it is important to remember that this needs to be updated. Any changes in their role need to be agreed and made clear. When new members of staff begin work, they should be able to clarify any areas about which they are unsure of their role. Such areas may come to light particularly during the first week, but other areas may not be encountered until later on. By providing a method of checking that the nature of the work is explained fully and clearly, problems may be avoided in the future.

# TRAINING

Staff in a medical records department often receive only one day's general induction training. In

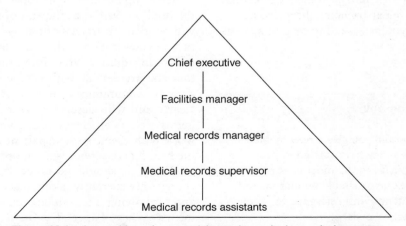

**Figure 12.1**  A typical line of accountability in the medical records department.

addition, some training may be given on PAS systems. It is important that thorough plans should be made for both induction and ongoing training of staff so that they are fully aware of what their jobs entail and of the importance of working to a high standard. This may involve an investment of time and money and extra staff need to be available to cover for those involved in training.

Needs analysis of the training needs of staff in the department should be made and a plan of training objectives set out. Ongoing monitoring and reassessing of training needs should be made and evaluation of training sessions made, so that staff are kept up to date of changes which may affect them or the work of other related departments.

When training of other staff in the hospital or Trust is being considered it is important for them to be aware of the work of the medical records department so that there is an overall appreciation of how each other's work interrelates, particularly with regard to the resulting effect on the availability of notes. These staff may include nurses, doctors, ward clerks as well as others working outside the department.

There is a particular need to consider the training needs of staff who may be devolved to clinical directorates. This is because following devolution, they may not be included in training courses which had previously been provided centrally.

*Temporary staff*, if untrained, may be unused to the medical environment and may be in particular need of guidance. It may be important to ensure that they have a particular person to whom they can refer, if they are experiencing difficulties.

It may be that you are asked to help new members of staff in this way.

### Reflection point

◆ What advice would you give a new member of staff? Imagine they have started in your department. What are the most important points and what areas should be emphasised in their job outlines with reference to hospital medical records?

You may be involved in preparing job descriptions or notes on how the work is done. As well as including information on how a record should be kept of where the notes are and how they should be filed, it is important to remember to include guidance on the importance of records being accurate and on the nature of confidentiality. By doing this, you can help others become aware of how the records should be kept.

## CONCLUSION

As a result of working through this chapter you will now:

◆ be aware of the issues concerning ownership of and the length of time that health records should be kept, and know of the means of accessing health records
◆ be aware of the different methods of compilation and storage of health records in the hospital environment
◆ have an outline of the most important forms used in hospital
◆ be able to update information concerning service agreements for patient care
◆ be able to describe the role of Audit and identify how and why it is important to record information accurately
◆ be able to describe how you may need to oversee the needs of other staff.

Most importantly it is hoped that throughout the book as well as at the end of this chapter you will build an awareness of the significance of accuracy in your work and the importance of confidentiality. In addition, it is important to remember that you are dealing with people who may not be able to communicate their needs and feelings clearly and who deserve respect and understanding as well as efficiency in the way in which you work with them, so that patient care throughout the health care service is at an optimum.

Finally, it should be noted that a number of changes are currently taking place within the NHS and, following the publication of the Government's White Paper *The new NHS. Modern. Dependable*, further change is likely (see Chapter

2). Contracts are now service agreements, usually in the form of 3–5 year rolling agreements, Primary Care Trusts are likely to replace GP fundholding after 1999 and the new Patients' Charter may alter patterns of work at various levels of health care.

## ACKNOWLEDGEMENTS

Bristol Royal Infirmary Trust, Royal United Hospital Trust, Bath.

### Exercises

◆ Find out how your local hospital stores its medical records; which system is it using now? Are they happy with the way it works? And do they have any plans to change the system in the future?

◆ Monitor the access to records procedures which are currently used. Are they working well? Are records already being kept on computer? Record access both by patients and by other bodies?

◆ Work in a small group of three to four colleagues or other students. Each choose 5 six-digit numbers. All write down the complete list of numbers and as a group decide how these would be filed by terminal digit filing.

◆ Visit your local reference library and ask to view newspaper articles which are kept on microfilm. What do you think are the advantages and disadvantages of this method?

◆ Ask a laboratory technician if all samples are clearly, legibly and appropriately labelled! What suggestions can you make to help ensure a high level of accuracy?

## FURTHER READING

Audit Commission 1995 Setting the records straight. A study of hospital medical records. HMSO, London.

Department of Health 1995 National Health Service Charges to overseas visitors. Patient's guide. Annex 6, Appendix 2, January. DOH, London.

Department of Health 1994 Being heard. The report of a review committee on NHS complaints procedures. DO16/BH/2M HSSH JO6 3055, June. DOH, London.

General Medical Council 1995 Duties of a doctor. GMC, London.

Hauffman EK Health information management, 10th edn. American Health Information Management Association, Physician Record, Illinois.

Markwell D 1995 Computerised patient records in general practice – guidelines for good practice. Produced for NHS Executive Performance Management Directorate Clinical Information Consultancy 24.03.95.

NHS Executive 1995 Guidance on the revised operation of notification arrangements for tertiary extra contractual referrals. HSG(95)20, March.

Primary Health Care Specialist Group of the British Computer Society 1996 Proceedings of Annual Conference, Downing College, Cambridge.

# 13 Outpatient department

*Sara Ladyman*

## OBJECTIVES

◆ To describe the systems and procedures that take place in an outpatient department, including those requiring a secretarial input, with examples of a new patient referral system, the use of PAS, preparation and administration before, during and after an outpatient clinic and correspondence

◆ To outline other aspects which require special consideration, in particular procedures for urgent referrals, for patients who fail to attend appointments, tertiary referrals, overseas visitors, hospital transport, domiciliary and ward visits

◆ To highlight throughout the chapter the interdependence of procedures and staff responsibilities and the repercussions when there is a breakdown in communication

◆ To consider throughout the chapter the non-routine and the irregularities that may occur which may involve secretarial input to resolve.

## INTRODUCTION

This section is concerned with the administration of outpatient clinics in a hospital. You may find it helpful to obtain a copy of the national Patient's Charter and a copy of the patient charter standards for your local hospital or a department within it.

## OUTPATIENT CLINICS

The majority of consultants will share a purpose-designed outpatient clinic area within the hospital staffed by outpatient nurses and reception staff. Clinics will be held at set times. Other consultants may have access to their own outpatient clinic area, where specialist equipment has to be accessed, for example in the radiotherapy department.

Referrals to hospital may come from a variety of sources and not necessarily from GPs. They may include:

◆ self-referral (for example to a genitourinary medicine clinic)
◆ consultant, following emergency admission
◆ consultant, following domiciliary visit
◆ accident and emergency referral
◆ GP referral.

Not all clinics have an appointments system. For example, genitourinary clinics may have walk-in clinics. Some departments will keep their own confidential patient records, which may never leave their department, for example psychiatry and genitourinary medicine.

Some clinics are for patients requiring specific treatments, for example surgery to be carried out as a minor operation. This may include some ophthalmology and dermatology procedures. You should always be aware that there may be a manual appointment system running parallel to that on the Patient Administration System (PAS) for these types of clinics and you should familiarise yourself with the necessary procedures.

# NEW PATIENT REFERRAL SYSTEMS AND PROCEDURES

The majority of new patient referrals are received from general practitioners (GPs), seeking specialist advice and consultation or a specific procedure for their patients. We will look at different sources of referral later in the chapter.

You will need to familiarise yourself with the computerised PAS at the earliest opportunity as it is integral to your day-to-day activity. (See Box 13.1.)

---

**Box 13.1** The computerised Patient Administration System (PAS)

A PAS will usually include:

| | |
|---|---|
| Patient Master Index (PMI) | Personal and demographic data on all patients who have attended hospital |
| Modules linked to PMI | Provide management and record keeping functions |
| Modules include: | Outpatient Module |
| | Waiting List Module |
| | Accident and Emergency Module |

In addition, the system may also be linked to pathology and imaging departments, thereby providing access to patient results by medical and nursing staff.

More specifically, the Outpatient Module of PAS provides for the effective management of outpatient clinics. Outpatient Module functions may include:

- maintaining a 'diary' of past and forthcoming clinics, identifying patients booked on to specific clinics and their attendance times
- production of a variety of letters, reports and statistical analyses
- clinic rules specifying the frequency of the clinic, duration, number and type of appointments available
- screen transactions to enable you to answer queries and to make, cancel or change appointments
- lists of patients booked on to specific clinics that can be printed to:
  — assist patient services departments in collecting the patient case notes required for a clinic
  — assist medical, nursing and reception staff with clinic management
  — gather statistics for Department of Health requirements to collect patient charter standard data such as patient waiting times in clinic.

You may use PAS, Outpatient or Inpatient Modules to:

- answer general queries
- register patients
- generate patient identity labels, front sheets, case note labels
- generate new and follow-up appointment letters or cancellation letters (e.g. due to a death)
- amend patient details
- make transactions on patient records, e.g. add attendances, make appointments
- cancel clinics and reschedule appointments
- print statistics and reports
- produce outpatient clinic prints
- add waiting list episodes, print waiting lists and so forth.

Different staff groups will have password access to different parts of the system, according to their role. The way in which a hospital's PAS system actually operates will not be described as they differ so much between individual hospitals.

A new patient referral indicates that a patient is being referred for a particular ailment to a particular consultant and will start a new patient care episode. This is irrespective of the patient having any episodes of care running concurrently with other consultants or having been referred to the same consultant, treated and discharged back to the GP in the past.

Figure 13.1 outlines the procedure for processing both new and old outpatient referrals.

The GP referral letter is sent to the hospital. It may go directly to the consultant or to a centralised appointments department. See the sample referral letter in Figure 13.2.

It is incumbent upon whoever receives the letter first, the appointments desk or medical secretary, to date stamp its receipt and to enter the patient identifying details onto the PAS Referral Module at the earliest opportunity.

### Reflection point

◆ Why is this so important?

The reasons why it is important that the letter is date stamped upon its receipt and details entered on to the computerised PAS are that these actions:

◆ commence an audit trail for the accurate tracking of the patient through the new patient referral system to provide evidence that the hospital is meeting its contractual specifications and obligations
◆ facilitate gathering of statistics for national and local patient charter and quality standards on waiting times for first outpatient appointment times
◆ enable verification and appropriate changes to be made to patient details, for example GP, patient name or address changes

◆ enable patient's date of birth, sex, address, postcode, marital status and registered/referring GP/practice and consultant, which are key to contract validation, to be analysed. By entering the date of birth into the Patient Master Index (PMI) on the PAS Referral Module, and then making a further check using their name, it is possible to discover whether the patient is new to the hospital. If among the selection of patients shown it is apparent they have already been allocated a hospital number, there should be a corresponding set of patient case notes in existence.

### Reflection point

◆ If a patient has been seen at the hospital previously what are the variables which may have changed and require verification and subsequent changes to the Patient Master Index and any case notes in existence?

The changes which may have occurred since a previous visit to the hospital include:

◆ name
◆ address – including postcode
◆ referring GP
◆ the existence of duplicate registrations and case notes for a patient where similar details have resulted in separate registrations, requiring amalgamation.

At this point we should mention that if the referring GP is not a fundholder and there is not an existing contract between the hospital consultant and GP's Health Authority to provide this service then this patient is an extra-contractual referral.

Agreement has to be sought before an appointment is sent to the patient that the Health Authority is willing to pay the extra-contractual fee for this patient to be seen and the contract department usually administer this procedure.

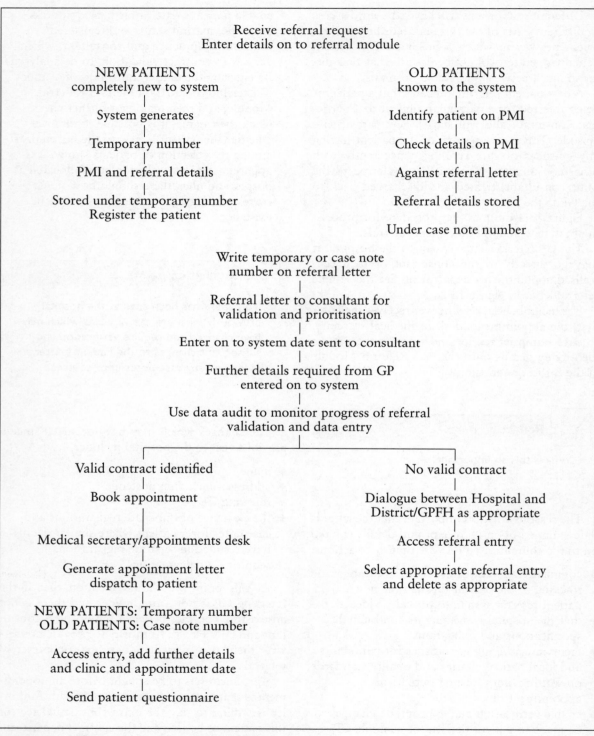

**Figure 13.1** Procedure for processing outpatient referrals.

Water Mead Practice,
1 Meadow Walk,
Buckingham
MK18 2HP
Tel 01280 854329
Fax 01280 833441

Dr. R. Mott
——

Dr. M. Sread
——

Dr. L. Khan

—— February ——

Contract I.D.

Practice Code

Mr. A. McAllister,
Consultant Urologist,
General Hospital NHS Trust,
Forest Lane,
Milton Keynes MK13 2DF

Dear Mr. McAllister,

**Mrs. Anne BAYLISS dob 14.04.**          **NHS No:**
    **Hospital No:**
**6a Water Mead Gardens, Buckingham MK14 6HP**
**Tel 356212**

Thank you for seeing this lady in your Out-patient Clinic. She has no past history of note apart from bronchitis in childhood. She attended recently with a two-week history of severe pain in the left loin. At that time she had cystitis and I prescribed antibiotics for a urine infection. She returned to the surgery today still complaining of pain in the left loin and she says she still has pain on passing water. I would be grateful if you could see her as soon as possible as I feel she requires further investigation.

Yours sincerely,

Dr. R. Mott

**Figure 13.2**  Sample referral letter.

The GP code is necessary to identify if the GP is a GP fundholder. The patient's postcode is used to identify the Health Authority of resident.

A valid contract has to be identified before an appointment can be given. If this information is omitted or requires clarification there may be a delay to the patient being seen.

A temporary hospital number (pre-registration number) may be allocated to the patient who has never been seen at the hospital before which will alter to a permanent hospital number once the patient has attended a first appointment. The pre-registration or existing hospital number must be written on the referral letter.

The referral letter must then be passed to the consultant, or nominated doctor, for validation and prioritisation. By marking the letter for an urgent (e.g. 0–2 weeks), soon (e.g. 2–4 weeks) or routine (next available) appointment, the consultant validates and accepts the GP referral. All consultants will have their own appointment criteria and may have specific new patient appointment slots for urgent or soon referrals. Each clinic will have a reference code on the PAS and appointments are made in the outpatient module.

**Reflection point**

◆ Although the word 'routine' is used, there is nothing routine about an appointment, for example, to attend a breast clinic. We should therefore be continually aware that each appointment will highlight for patients their own particular concerns about a disease, and possibly their own life process.

In addition to new patients having their appointments prioritised clinically, it is important to remember that new patient clinic appointment slots are generally allocated a longer time with the doctor than a patient returning for a second or further visit.

**Reflection point**

◆ Why is it important to ensure the new patient is given a new patient appointment slot and not a follow-up patient slot in error?

The reasons it is important a new patient is allocated a new patient clinic slot and not a follow-up clinic slot are:

◆ to allow sufficient time for history gathering, patient examination, tests to be carried out and for further tests to be organised
◆ it may be policy for the consultant or nominated deputy to see all new patients, whereas follow-up clinic slots may be allocated to other members of the medical team.

Once the referral letter is validated by the Appointments Module and the consultant, the appointment must be booked and a computer-generated letter may be produced by the PAS and dispatched to the patient. Part of this letter may constitute a patient questionnaire to gather further patient data to be entered on the PAS. This data, known as the minimum data set, is a Department of Health requirement, but data may also be collected to ensure the hospital is responding to the needs of its local population and thus is used for statistical purposes. Analyse the information provided and information requested in the example proforma letter and patient questionnaire shown in Figure 13.3.

The clinic code, date and time of appointment should be recorded on the referral letter and the letter filed in the case notes so that it is subsequently available for the clinic visit. Alternatively, for new patients for whom no case notes exist, it may be your responsibility or that of the appointments staff to keep the referral letters in a bring forward system ready for the new patient clinic preparation, to be married up with the patient questionnaire sent to the patient with their appointment time, and subsequently returned. Whenever possible, the whereabouts of the referral letter should be indicated on the PAS and it should be readily accessible should staff be absent. Note that the practice in some hospitals is to make up a set of new patient case notes, file the referral letter inside and then file within the medical records department library until they require pulling for clinic preparation.

The procedures and systems associated with the running of a busy outpatient clinic quickly become routine. It is important for you to remember that all calls and enquiries regarding appointments should be vetted before any information is given about clinic attendance. Even the disclosure that a patient is on the PAS is confidential and every care should be taken to validate callers and the reasons for information requested and given.

## CLINIC PREPARATION FOR NEW PATIENTS

Medical secretaries, appointments desk staff or clinic reception staff may be involved in preparing case notes for new patient clinics. The principles remain the same and Figure 13.4 outlines the procedure that takes place.

It is possible to print a list of patients booked in to attend the new patient clinic from the PAS Outpatient Module and this may be done 3–5 days prior to the new patient clinic being held (Fig. 13.5).

Outpatient clinics can be organised in a variety of formats, some with a mixture of new patient appointments and those for patients returning for follow-up appointments, and the consultant may have different clinics for different conditions. It is important for you to familiarise yourself with the types of appointment available to patients seen in the department.

**Reflection point**

◆ What are the ramifications of the referral letter being unavailable for the clinic attendance?

If the referral letter is not available for the clinic attendance the consultant may not agree to see the patient until the referral letter providing clinical information about the patient is available. Obtaining a fax copy or taking dictation over the telephone may cause delays in the smooth running of the outpatient clinic and unnecessary distress for the patient kept waiting. This can adversely affect the local and national patient charter waiting time statistics collected for patients attending clinic.

## PROCEDURE FOR NEW PATIENT CLINIC

In the new patient clinic the patient will be clinically examined and this may result in:

◆ diagnostic tests being performed or ordered
◆ an admission to hospital for surgery, or being placed on the waiting list
◆ an appointment with another specialist
◆ a further follow-up appointment to return to the clinic.

The appointment date and time will usually be given to patients before they leave. You may be required to make or change a follow-up appointment and this can be done on the PAS with a standard letter generated. The patient may, however, be discharged back to the GP's care, thereby ending this particular patient care episode.

It is usually the clinic receptionist who attends and 'sits' the outpatient clinic. We will look at the receptionist's role before concentrating on that of the medical secretary. See Figure 13.6 for procedures relating to the outpatient clinic.

During an outpatient clinic patients will have various tests carried out. Samples will either be taken by the nursing or medical staff and the appropriate documentation completed on the request forms, or the patient will be sent to the appropriate department. Box 13.2 indicates the different departments the patient may be required to attend prior to, during or after an outpatient clinic attendance.

General Hospital NHS Trust,
Forest Lane,
Milton Keynes MK13 2DF
Appointments: 01908 465887/547986

6a Water Mead Gardens,
Buckingham
MK14 6HP

DATE
HOSPITAL NUMBER

—— February ——
NP (Pre-registration No. ZA334466)

Dear Mrs. Bayliss,

An appointment has been made for you to attend MR. McALLISTER'S NEW
PATIENT CLINIC, C6, on — FEBRUARY —.

Please report to Registration Desk TWO on the FOURTH FLOOR OUTPATIENT
CLINIC at 2.00 P.M. If you have been handed a referral letter by your doctor please
bring it with you. We hope that this date and time is convenient for you. If you
cannot come please let us know as soon as you can.

If you have not been to this Hospital before, or if the details printed are wrong, please
fill in the Patient Questionnaire and send it to us now. If you have any query
regarding this appointment, please have your hospital number (if you have one) or
this letter available for reference.

Yours sincerely,


June Davies
Appointments Manager

(Enc. Schematic Map of Hospital with public transport services indicated)

**Figure 13.3** Example of proforma appointment letter and patient questionnaire.

**PATIENT QUESTIONNAIRE**

Hospital Number     NP (Pre-registration No. ZA334466)

Surname     Title

First Names

Date of Birth     Sex

Civil State     Single     Divorced

     Married     Separated

     Widowed     Other

Current Address

Postcode

Telephone (home)

Telephone (work)

Name of GP (own doctor)

Address

NHS Number     Have you lived in United Kingdom for past 12 months YES/NO

Surname at Birth

Other surnames

Town and Country of Birth

Religion

Ethnic origin (This is needed because people of different ethnic origins may have specific health needs. Please tick the box which best describes your history, values and culture.)

Occupation

Industry or Name of School

Occupation of Spouse

Industry

Name of Next of Kin

Relationship

Address

Telephone

CLINIC     APPOINTMENT     DATE     TIME

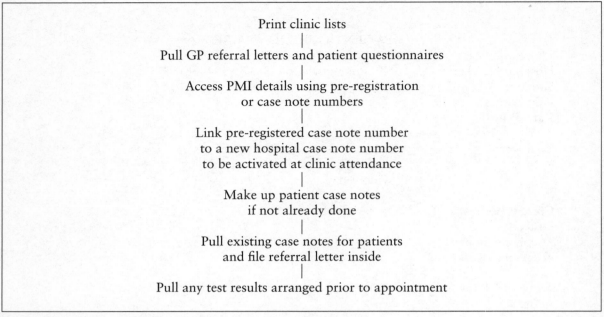

**Figure 13.4**  Procedure for processing new patient outpatient clinics.

NEW PATIENT PULLING LIST

CLINIC Mr. A. McAllister          SPECIALTY          Urology Clinic Code C6    DATE

PULLED          —.02.—CLINIC DATE —02—

| TIME | NO. | NAME/ADDRESS | DOB HOSPITAL NO. | GP LETTER | PREVIOUS X-RAYS | |
|------|-----|--------------|------------------|-----------|-----------------|---|
| | | ROUTINE/SOON/URGENT | | | | |
| 2.00 | ZA334466 | BAYLISS Anne | 14.04.- | L | N | R |
| | | 6a Water Mead Gdns Buckingham | | | | |
| 2.15 | | HUGHES Keith | 12.10.-GH386432 | L | N | R |
| | | 39 Brown Rd Buckingham | | | | |
| 2.30 | ZA498723 | PIPER June | 06.09.- | L | N | R |
| | | 12 Westcroft Lne Gawcott | 05.07.- | | | |
| 2.45 | | PATEL Myra | 31.03.-GH279432 | L | Y | S |
| | | 6 Bierton Road, Bishopstoke | | | | |
| 3.00 | ZA857322 | JONES Peter | 27.01.-    Bringing letter  N | | S | |
| 3.15 | | LAMBERT Clare | GH328954 CANCELLED APPT. | | | |
| 3.30 | URGENT SLOT | | | | | |
| 3.45 | URGENT SLOT | | | | | |

**Figure 13.5**  New patient pulling list.

---

(a) Immediately prior to and during an outpatient clinic

---

Copies of referral letters obtained
as applicable
|
Copies of clinic list printed from PAS and distributed to consultation rooms.
Cancellations and late bookings may need to be added manually
|
Patient reports to reception desk
|
Receptionist confirms patient arrival on PAS. Checks PMI data with patient
|
Referral details transferred to case note number system
and new patient number confirmed
|
Endorse details on printed clinic list

---

(b) At the end of and following the outpatient clinic

---

Identify patient
|
Enter attendance details on to PAS outpatient attendance module
from the attendance form (completed by doctor)
|
**PATIENT ATTENDED**
|
Temporary number deleted.
Allocated a hospital number
(if not already allocated one)
|
Add outcome details to outpatient module
i.e.
follow-up appointment
booked/or not booked
or patient discharged back to GP's care
(decided by clinician)

---

**PATIENT DID NOT ATTEND (DNA)**
|
Referral details remain on temporary number
|
New appointment booked/or not booked
(decided by clinician dependent on locally agreed procedure)

---

**Figure 13.6** Outpatient clinic procedures.

**Box 13.2** Departments a patient may be required to attend prior to, during or after an outpatient clinic attendance

### Imaging department

All clinical specialties have access to imaging services, with the majority of outpatients being examined on demand. Where appointments are required for special examinations, the waiting time may be as little as a week.

Equipment may include:

- magnetic resonance imaging machines
- CT (computed tomography) scanners
- Ultrasound equipment.

### Haematology department

In addition to clinical advice and interpretation of results, the range of investigations available may include: full blood count, ESR (erythrocyte sedimentation rate), blood film and differential, monospot, sickle cell screening test, serum B12, red folate, platelet function studies, blood grouping and antibody screens. Routine specimens are processed during weekday office hours and Saturday. The department will be computerised and reports may be available on PAS VDUs within minutes of completion.

### Chemical pathology

The department will offer a comprehensive range of services. The range of tests will include urea and electrolytes (U&Es) and liver function tests (LFTs).

### Histopathology

A full range of histopathological and cytological services will be available, including:

- routine histological processing and diagnosis from frozen sections – immunocytochemistry
- electron microscopy
- routine cervical smear diagnosis
- non-gynaecological cytology and fine needle aspirates.

### Microbiology

A range of diagnostic services will be available, including:

- bacteriology, virology, parasitology, mycology
- public health and environmental microbiology.

It will also be closely involved with all aspects of infection control and will work closely with the infection control nursing officers.

Routine specimens are processed during weekday office hours and reports can be accessed on PAS VDUs.

### Nuclear medicine

Investigations carried out routinely may include:

- the study of organ function
- evaluation of ischaemic heart disease
- the detection of cancer and its spread
- differential diagnosis and assessment of dementia
- the monitoring of renal function, transplant
- diagnosis of acute bleeding
- screening of infection and inflammation
- acute embolic lung disease.

The majority of services are available on an outpatient basis, most requiring only a single visit to the department. Radionuclide therapy is carried out for benign and malignant thyroid diseases.

*Physiotherapy*    See Chapter 11 on personnel.

**Reflection point**

- What are the ramifications if the request form accompanying a specimen or a request form accompanying the patient is incorrectly completed. How can this be avoided?

You are not usually expected to be present in the clinic area but should be readily available whilst the clinic is in session.

Finding the times when your consultant and the medical staff are available to deal with queries, sign correspondence, check incoming results and mail may include time before the clinic commences or immediately after the clinic finishes. It is important to be prepared beforehand.

Doctors usually dictate their correspondence using handheld dictaphones, although shorthand is still used in some clinics, and it may be your responsibility to ensure there are sufficient dictaphones, audio cassettes and replacement batteries available for the outpatient clinic session.

If you have access to an additional handset this could be designated for urgent letters to save time finding this text somewhere on a tape.

Dictated audio cassettes in particular can be easily misplaced. Encourage medical staff to place the audio cassette in a window envelope and seal it, writing the doctor's name and the date of the clinic on the outside and securing it to the dictated clinic notes with an elastic band.

## PROCEDURE AT THE END OF AN OUTPATIENT CLINIC

You should familiarise yourself with the system used at the end of the clinic for ensuring the patient case notes and dictaphones, etc., are taken to your office.

The consultant and members of the medical team are responsible for ensuring the GP is kept informed of their findings and this is usually in the form of a letter and may include a preliminary diagnosis, prognosis and drugs or other treatments prescribed for the patient.

GPs require written confirmation of all outpatient attendance to fulfil their auditing obligations. Regular checks will take place by the purchaser that billing is accurate. This includes checking that letters stating when the patient has attended the hospital are found in the GP patient notes, indicating that the patient is currently in a consultant patient care episode or has been discharged back to the GP's care. Purchasers contact the contracts department at regular intervals and the contracts department will contact consultants to discover the reasons why a particular letter has not been received by the GP and get the matter rectified.

Whilst the referral system is rooted in medical ethics and etiquette, the production of prompt written feedback to the GP will form part of the contract specification and is a patient charter standard. Failure to comply may result in contract penalties being imposed by the purchaser. Make reference to a copy of the Patient's Charter, and a copy of a contract specification if available.

When the clinic finishes, responsibility for the case notes and accompanying dictated audio cassettes transfers from the clinic staff to the medical secretary.

The case notes will have been traced out to the clinic. It is in the medical secretary's interests to have a system for recording case notes subsequently found in the office. This usually takes the form of a 'booking in/out book' which may involve using patient labels or handwriting the patient's name, hospital number and date case notes were received from the clinic, with a space for the date and destination of case notes once the case notes are no longer required. Bar code tracking systems linked to the PAS may also become available.

A booking in/out system of case notes to the office is only as good as the user. Ensure that all medical staff and staff using the office are familiar with the system in place and that it is easily accessible. Whilst it may appear laborious, tracing notes can pay dividends when a past entry in the book can be referred to, rather than searching through all the case notes in your own and adjoining doctors' offices.

The pattern of your working week will be governed by the number and type of outpatient, inpatient and, if your consultant is a surgeon, operating sessions he/she is contracted to provide to the hospital. It is therefore a good idea to familiarise yourself with your consultant's timetable at the earliest opportunity to assist you in prioritising your main weekly activities and then to fit the other duties expected of you around these.

**Reflection point**

◆ You have been away for 3 days. What are the implications if the outpatient clinic typing falls behind?

# OUTPATIENT CLINIC LETTERS

Letters dictated for patients attending their first clinic visit may be longer than those for patients re-attending as follow-up patients because the consultant will include the history of the patient's condition. Therefore the number of letters to be transcribed for a new patient clinic may be fewer but may take as long, if not longer, than a follow-up patient clinic where many more patients have been seen.

You usually transcribe outpatient correspondence in chronological order, using the clinic date as a guide. You will be required to follow the departmental house style for correspondence. You should ensure each letter contains the information shown in Box 13.3.

You should ensure that information, including patient details, extracted from the case notes is the most current for each letter typed. The doctor will have made handwritten notes about the patient in the case notes and these, together with test result

forms, previous correspondence and clinic entries, provide an invaluable aid to accurate transcription from audio cassette. You should make a habit of spell-checking and proof-reading all correspondence as part of the process of preparation for signature. Doctors may only visit the department at a certain time during the week so an opportunity is lost to dispatch the letter promptly to the GP if alterations have to be made and the letter has to await signature once more.

A copy of the dictated letter must always be filed in the case notes and this should be amended with any changes a doctor may make when he/she comes to sign the top copy. Each department will have its own policy regarding additional copies of correspondence on disk or on file.

**Reflection point**

You should book the case notes back to the medical records department in the booking in/out book as soon as they are no longer required.

Why is this a good policy to adopt?

It is a good policy to book case notes back to the medical records department at the earliest opportunity because:

◆ the medical records department is the first port of call for anyone trying to access case notes quickly and easily
◆ there is a direct correlation between the number of case notes you hold in your office and the number of queries and interruptions you will receive from staff searching for them, ultimately increasing your workload
◆ there is generally limited space available to store case notes
◆ when case notes are needed outside working hours, for example in the accident and emergency department, this necessitates searches being made in offices which may be some distance from the department where they are required.

---

**Box 13.3** Details required in an outpatient clinic letter

◆ A reference, including the doctor's and typist's initials and the patient's case note number
◆ Clinic date and the date transcribed by secretary
◆ The name and address of the referrer
◆ The name, date of birth and address of the patient
◆ The name and designation of the doctor dictating the letter

**Reflection point**

◆ What are the legitimate reasons for case notes staying in the office?

**Reflection point**

A clinic receptionist telephones you to ask for a set of case notes required for a clinic in 2 days. You need them to type a clinic letter. How will you resolve this situation?

Legitimate reasons for case notes being in your office include:

◆ awaiting transcription of outstanding correspondence
◆ a doctor's specific request, for example research patients
◆ awaiting test results and for the doctor to respond to these
◆ a query to be resolved
◆ arranging an admission
◆ patients for whom a return visit is imminent.

Therefore, once the letters have been typed, case notes should be booked back to the medical records department. These case notes are usually collected at regular intervals throughout the week from the secretary's office.

## FOLLOW-UP OUTPATIENT CLINIC APPOINTMENTS

The medical records staff or the clinic receptionist will generally prepare the follow-up outpatient clinics, although this may be the responsibility of a medical secretary.

The medical secretary's relationship with the receptionist or medical records staff preparing case notes for future clinics is of paramount importance. It requires cooperation and under-standing to accommodate the different needs of the individuals involved, i.e. when a patient's case notes are needed by you to resolve a query or type a letter and get the copy in the case notes, but are equally needed by the receptionist to complete preparation of case notes ready for a forth-coming clinic with the same or a different consultant.

## THE FOLLOW-UP OUTPATIENT CLINIC

Figure 13.7 outlines the procedures for a follow-up clinic.

The patient will attend a follow-up outpatient clinic:

◆ to receive test results following their initial visit to the new patient clinic
◆ to have further investigative procedures, for example admission to hospital, added to the waiting list for admission for surgery or requested to come back to the clinic at a later date for reassessment of the initial problem
◆ to receive a diagnosis post-surgery
◆ to have surgical wounds examined, dressed or sutures removed
◆ for routine 3-, 6-, 9-monthly or annual check-up
◆ to have a check-up and then be discharged back to the GP's care, thereby ending this particular patient care episode.

Occasionally patients may turn up to a follow-up clinic without an appointment. You should familiarise yourself with the consultant's policy regarding this occurrence and the procedure for obtaining case notes, test results, etc., should it be agreed to see the patient. It may be that each case has to be taken on its own merit; for example, a patient may arrive as a result of an administrative error on the part of the hospital and have travelled some distance to get there.

As with the new clinic appointment, there will be a clinic receptionist in attendance and he or she will be responsible for updating the PAS Outpa-tient Module as explained previously. You may

A clinic list for the follow-up clinic
will be generated from PAS
(similar to the new patient list, Figure 13.4)

|

An initial search for case notes will be made
in the medical records department

|

Tracer cards for case notes not in medical records
will form a vital clue as to the case note
whereabouts
as will the PAS

|

Medical secretaries will be contacted for
case notes booked out to them
Case notes to be released as soon as possible

|

Case notes are prepared for the doctor,
i.e. all outstanding test results, X-rays, etc. are entered into case notes
so the doctor has all information to hand for return clinic visit

**Figure 13.7**  Procedure for a follow-up clinic.

wish to refer to the ENT attendance form, in Figure 13.8, to identify the possible outcomes for the patient who has attended the follow-up clinic.

A clinic may overrun for a number of reasons: staff arriving late, absent doctors for whom the necessary clinic changes have not been made, overriding the number of appointment slots for that clinic, time spent locating missing case notes or results before patients can be seen.

The implications of an outpatient clinic overrunning include:

◆ Ambulance transport arrangements disrupted
◆ Overcrowding of clinic areas
◆ Escalation of stress levels
◆ Clinics held after this clinic are delayed or disrupted
◆ Patients and staff leave later, perhaps in darkness, especially in winter months
◆ other patient and staff commitments are affected, e.g. those caring for others.

**Reflection points**

◆ What are the implications of an outpatient clinic overrunning?

◆ Who will be affected and how?

◆ Make reference to your copy of the Patient's Charter guidelines. What does this say about outpatient waiting times?

**Reflection point**

What steps can you take to assist the clinic run to schedule, in particular with regard to doctors' planned leave arrangements, the appointment system, availability of case notes, etc.?

---

<u>ENT ATTENDANCE FORM</u>

Time Patient arrived in Clinic
Time seen by Nursing Staff
Time seen by Doctor
Time of leaving Clinic

| Diagnosis | 1 | Code: |
| | 2 | Code: |

Procedures

| TICK | | TICK |
| --- | --- | --- |
| None | | Microtymp |
| Antral washout/suction clearance | | Biopsies of ulcers |
| Reduction of fracture | | Removal of salivary calculus |
| Cautery of nasal septum | | Audioscope |
| Aural polypectomy | | Nasal polypectomy |
| Myringotomy/grommets insert | | Drainage of abscess |

Endoscopy of nose or larynx                    Other

| Outcome | TICK | Further appointments |
| --- | --- | --- |
| DNA | | 1    C    D/W/M/next routine |
| Cancelled by patient | | 2    C    D/W/M/next routine |
| Discharge | | 3    C    D/W/M/next routine |
| Cross Referral | | |
| W/L Minor Operation | | X-rays required    Yes/No |
| W/L Day Case | | Pathology Reports    Yes/No |
| W/L Inpatient | | Audiology    Yes/No |
| Other | | |

PATIENT TRANSPORT REQUIRED          YES/NO        Authorised
Medical
            Signatory

**Figure 13.8**   An example of an attendance form which the receptionist or medical records staff will then transfer to the PAS.

Keeping patients and staff informed of waiting time delays empowers the patient and doctors who can then, within limits, make decisions based on the information to hand. For example, a patient may choose to cancel and rebook an appointment rather than wait if outside commitments cannot be altered.

The consultant and his/her medical team will once more dictate a clinic letter to be sent to the GP to update them on the patient's care. It is the medical secretary's responsibility to prioritise and type the follow-up clinic letters, preparing them for signature and despatch. Once the case notes have been finished with, they should once again be booked back to the medical records department until they are required again.

Patients, for the most part, are unaware of the complexity of outpatient clinic procedures and systems and you should use your discretion to explain to patients the reason for delays or breakdowns in system whilst offering them a positive solution to the problem within departmental guidelines.

## ADDITIONAL INFORMATION REGARDING OUTPATIENT CLINICS

You should familiarise yourself with the departmental policy and procedure regarding the following points.

### Urgent referrals

These may be in letter form or by telephone from GPs or other sources of referral, for example the accident and emergency department. If an urgent appointment is given for an imminent clinic you should ensure that:

◆ Permission is sought from the consultant, or nominated deputy, if policy to do so.
◆ The referral letter will be available for the clinic – this may either be given to the patient to bring, a copy faxed through by GP and only sent through the mail if time allows.
◆ The appointment is made on the PAS.

◆ A request is made for a case note number and folder to be generated or for existing case notes to be found by the medical records department at the earliest opportunity if the clinic list has already been printed and clinic preparation completed.
◆ Clinic reception, nursing and medical staff are made aware that the patient is attending on a particular day in the clinic, particularly as the patient's name and appointment time may not be printed on the clinic listings because they are a late booking on the PAS.

### Patients who fail to attend their outpatient clinic appointments

The GP will need to be informed of all patients who fail to attend their clinic appointment. They do not usually need to know when a patient has cancelled and re-booked an appointment. There is usually a standard proforma letter, either stored on the word processor or a photocopied proforma letter, completed by hand, which should indicate whether or not the patient has been discharged back to the GP's care. See Chapter 6 on communication for an example of this.

### Tertiary referrals

The referral must be from one named consultant in an NHS provider unit to another named consultant in an NHS provider unit; this may be within the same hospital or to another hospital. A standard form has to be completed in order for the purchaser's approval to be sought. The tertiary referral validation is usually managed by the contracts department.

### Outpatient overseas visitors

The patient questionnaire (Fig. 13.3), should identify patients who have not lived in the United Kingdom for the last 12 months. Should this come to a medical secretary's attention then the appropriate manager should be informed, probably within the patient services department, as a decision has to be made as to whether they are 'liable to pay' for treatment given or whether there are reciprocal agreements with their country of origin. The patient will need to attend a 'Stage II interview' with a nominated member of staff who has had the appropriate training.

## Transport

As a rule, transport for new patients has to be booked by the GP as he/she is responsible for paying for it. Once the patient has attended a first clinic appointment the clinic doctor will decide whether hospital transport will be required for future clinic attendances and the appropriate form (Fig. 13.9) will need to be completed each time the patient attends and authorisation entered on the PAS. You must familiarise yourself with the hospital procedure for booking hospital transport in order to avoid missed appointments or unnecessary delays.

There is usually a manual system running parallel to any entries made on the PAS. The transport office will therefore need to be notified in writing if a transport patient cancels or changes an appointment. This is particularly important if you are notified of a patient's death, to avoid transport arriving at the relative's home and causing distress to relatives.

## Domiciliary visits

A GP may write or telephone to ask if the consultant will visit the patient at home if he or she is too ill to attend an outpatient clinic. Familiarise yourself with departmental procedures regarding this. Your consultant will be able to claim a fee for a domiciliary visit agreed by a GP.

## Ward visit

You may receive a request for a ward visit from a hospital consultant or a member of his or her team. It is important to take down all details regarding the patient and pass this on to the consultant at the earliest opportunity.

---

TRANSPORT REQUEST

TRANSPORT REQUIRED
Patient walking unaided
Carrying chair, can sit in ambulance
Full stretcher case
Is escort medically necessary?

DATE OF JOURNEY
TIME OF APPOINTMENT
APPROX LENGTH OF STAY
NATURE OF ILLNESS

WILL PATIENT WEAR
OUTDOOR CLOTHES?

HOSPITAL NUMBER:

SURNAME:
FIRST NAMES:

DATE OF BIRTH:
CONSULTANT:          WARD:

TO BE TAKEN FROM:
TO BE TAKEN TO:
This is to certify that because of his/her medical or physical condition this patient is unable to travel by any forms of public conveyance.

SIGNATURE OF MEDICAL OFFICER

DATE:

**Figure 13.9** A transport request form.

## CONCLUSION

In this chapter we have looked at the practical administrative issues in running an outpatient department by demonstrating the variety of tasks required to do so and the importance of effective communication between all staff groups involved. Emphasis should be placed on staff adhering to systems and procedures as this is essential when we consider the volume of outpatient clinics and appointments being processed in a hospital. It is important for you as a medical secretary to have an overview of the whole system to enable you to resolve queries, or to refer patients to the appropriate department or staff member, as you are often the first point of contact for patients and staff involved in patient care.

### Exercises

◆ A woman telephones and asks why she has not received an appointment yet to see your consultant. What procedure will you follow to resolve this query and what information do you need from the patient to do this efficiently?

◆ A man telephones and says that his new patient appointment is for 3 months' time and he wants to see the consultant now. What procedure will you follow to resolve this query and what information do you need from the patient to do this efficiently?

◆ A GP telephones and asks you to make an urgent appointment for a patient to be seen in the next available clinic. What procedure will you follow to resolve this query efficiently? Consider the information you need and whom you need to inform in order to resolve this matter satisfactorily.

# 14

# Admissions and discharges

*Sara Ladyman*

## OBJECTIVES

◆ To explain the differences between routine, urgent and emergency admissions

◆ To examine an example of an inpatient management system which utilises PAS, including monitoring bed availability

◆ To outline discharge procedures, including the communication with the referring doctors and community

◆ To outline other aspects that require special consideration, including day surgery, intensive therapy unit, when a patient dies, clinical audit and the accident and emergency department

◆ To consider throughout the chapter the non-routine and the irregularities that may occur which may involve secretarial input to resolve.

## INTRODUCTION

This chapter is concerned with the administration of inpatient episodes of care. You may find it helpful to obtain a copy of the national Patient's Charter and a copy of the patient charter standards for your local hospital, or a department within it.

Consultant physicians and surgeons are allocated a number of beds on specific wards for the admission of their patients, giving patients access to specialist medical and nursing inpatient care. Once a specialty has filled its allocation of beds, routine admissions are not usually allowed until some patients have been discharged.

Consultant surgeons will also be allocated specific theatre times during the week when they can perform operations on patients who require surgical intervention as part of their inpatient care; for example, they may be given a half-day operating session each week. It is important to utilise all resources effectively, especially when we consider the specialist medical and nursing care and the involvement of other staff required during an inpatient stay.

For the purposes of this chapter we will assume that the following duties are carried out by the admissions department. However, you should note that you may be required to deal with some or all of the procedures for admitting patients.

There is usually a bed manager who will be supported by senior nurses and the duty medical team. A team of doctors in a department may also be referred to as a 'firm' of doctors. Each medical team, or firm, will nominate a duty medical/surgical registrar who is responsible for allocating empty beds. Each medical team will also take it in turn to be 'on take'. This means they take on extra responsibility for a set number of days for the overall allocation of beds in the hospital. This is particularly relevant in arranging emergency admissions to beds which could be made available or not currently in use by different medical teams.

A patient's admission to hospital may be routine, urgent or emergency and different procedures will apply for each and these will be outlined in the chapter. The computerised waiting list system, described in Chapter 13 and referred to as PAS (Patient Administration System), facilitates the operational admission and discharge procedures by the use of an Inpatient Module. This allows staff to register, add waiting list episodes, admit, transfer, discharge and amend inpatient details, generate letters and labels, print reports and statistics.

## ADMISSION FROM A WAITING LIST

Admission to hospital may result from an outpatient clinic episode when a patient may be given a 'booked date', that is, a specific date for admission agreed by the medical team and based on information made available from the current bed occupancy. Alternatively they may be placed on a waiting list and become what is commonly referred to as a *routine elective admission*. In this instance the patient's admission is non-urgent and he or she will be selected for admission from the waiting list at a point in the future.

To be placed on a waiting list it is essential that a 'To Come In' request form (TCI form) is completed fully and accurately (Fig. 14.1) by a member of the medical team and for this information to be transferred accurately on to the PAS by the relevant staff.

When a TCI form is received, a check is made that there is an existing contract for this patient's care episode. Otherwise the patient will be treated as an extra-contractual referral (ECR) and permission to treat sought by the contract validation unit from the GP fundholder or Health Authority. This department liaises with GP fundholders and District Health Authorities to autho-

rise admissions for patients for whom no contract exists. A patient's episode of care will usually include costs associated with outpatient and inpatient treatment required. It is usual for a minimum of 2 weeks' notice to be given for patients to be admitted from waiting lists to enable the administrative tasks, including notification and confirmation from patients that they are available, to be carried out. Copies of the TCI forms are generally kept by the admissions department or medical secretary.

A printout of the waiting list is used by a nominated member of the medical team in your department to plan forthcoming admissions and it may be your responsibility to ensure that this is available in your department on a regular basis. A short notice list may also be kept for patients who have specified they can be admitted should cancellations or spaces become available. This enables flexibility for the medical team and ensures that valuable resources are fully utilised.

Whether it be the admissions department or yourself, a procedure similar to the one outlined below will be followed. This cycle is ongoing, week to week. An example of an admission procedure is outlined in Figure 14.2. One month prior to an admission date the the procedures shown in Figure 14.2 will occur.

Each medical team will have their own selection criteria for taking patients off the waiting list for admission. This will include medical factors, such as investigations and treatments to be provided, or the type and length of operations to be carried out to fit available operating time, as well as bed availability. Patients may not therefore be selected on a purely sequential basis. Likewise it is the doctor, not the admissions staff or yourself, who decides which short notice patients are to come in. The letter may include instructions, such as advice on no food or drink intake 12 hours prior to admission. (See Fig. 14.3, for an example of an admission letter.)

Similarly, whilst a standard letter is sent to each patient who has not confirmed their admission date, informing them they will be seen in an outpatient clinic or referring them back to their GP, the decision to send these is a medical decision and letters should be signed by a doctor.

## ECR & Elective Admission Request Form

Please complete all information in BLOCK CAPITALS and TICK BOXES as appropriate

Hospital No. _____

Address _____

Surname _____

Forename/s _____

POSTCODE

DOB [ ][ ][ ]

D.H.A. _____

Sex [ ] Male [ ] Female

Tel No: Work_____ Home _____

Referring Practitioner:

Registered GP (only required for patients not registered on PAS):

[ ] Reg GP | [ ] Other GP | [ ] Consultant | [ ] Dentist | [ ] A & E | [ ] Other

(Name & address only required if referral is not by Registered GP)
Name _____

Name _____

Address _____

Address _____

POSTCODE: _____

POSTCODE: _____

Consultant _____

Intended/Estimated
No of Episodes        Proposed Date

Specialty/Sub Specialty Code [ ]      New Patient [ ]      Inpatient

Day Case

Price Band [ ]      Follow-up Patient [ ]

Provisional Diagnosis _____

Intended Procedure _____

Admin Category:      NHS [ ]      Private [ ]      Amenity [ ]  .      Overseas Visitor Status [ ]

### Admission Details

Date Decision to Admit _____

Waiting List [ ]

### Admission Type

Booked [ ]

Priority Type
Routine [ ]      Emergency [ ]

Planned [ ]

Deferred [ ]

Urgent [ ]      Soon [ ]

Deferral Reason _____

Patient Available at Short Notice [ ] Yes [ ] No

Proposed TCI Date _____

Patient Informed [ ] Yes [ ] No

Letter of Confirmation [ ] Yes [ ] No

Admission Time _____

Nil By Mouth from: Date _____ Time _____ am/pm

Ward _____

Operation Date [ ][ ][ ]

Transport Required      None [ ]      Walking [ ]      Chair [ ]
                        Stretcher [ ]   Escort Req [ ]

Dates to Avoid (Annual Leave, etc.) _____

Investigations to be Arranged Prior to Admission: _____

On Admission: _____

Comments on Admission (Medical, etc.): _____

Name of Doctor Completing:
(Please Print)

Date of Completion _____

Computer Input By (Initials) _____      Date _____

For CVU Use
Approved: [ ] Yes [ ] No

Agreement No._____

Signed _____      Date _____

**Figure 14.1**   A 'To Come In' (TCI) request form.

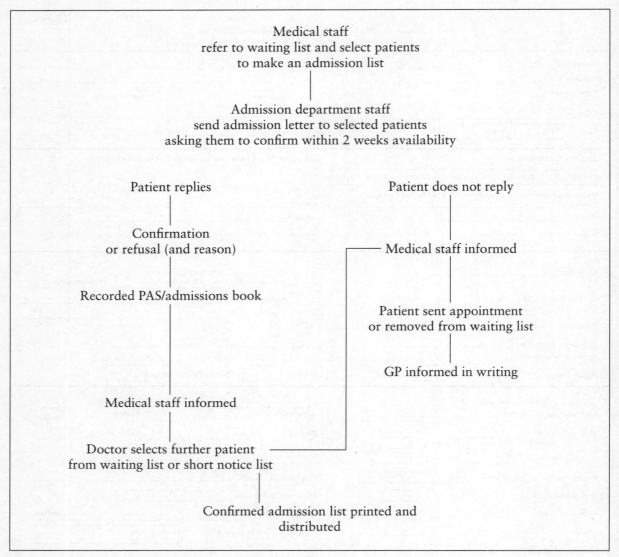

**Figure 14.2** An admission procedure.

A patient telephones to ask you if he needs to follow any special instructions prior to admission. How would you deal with this query?

All patients who have been on a waiting list for a year will be automatically validated, to ensure that admission is still required by the patient and their registration details are still correct. Up-to-date patient details are essential for this to be effective. Currently the patient charter standard (laid down by the Department of Health) requires

Dear

We have provisionally booked a bed for you in
................................................... Ward on ....................................... under
the care of ..................................................

On receipt of this letter please telephone the above number to confirm
or refuse this booking. Failure to do so may result in the cancellation of
the booking.

Please telephone this office between 10.00 a.m. and 11.00 a.m. on the
day you are due to come in to check there is a bed available for you as
we occasionally have to cancel a planned admission.

Please report to the Front Hall Reception Desk at          p.m. where you
will be directed to your ward.

We enclose a handbook 'Coming into Hospital' with information on
what to bring and routine in the ward. We trust this will be helpful to
you.

Yours sincerely,

Admissions Officer

**Figure 14.3** Example of an admission letter.

statistics to be collected; for example, for the number of cancelled operations and whether cancelled operations are then carried out within the recommended 30 days of the original date, as well as the percentage of admissions carried out within 3 and 12 months of being placed on a waiting list. The comparative performance of hospitals is published annually and measures these and other areas and compares with the English average. Waiting list validation procedures may also be agreed in the contract for services between the purchaser and provider.

The medical secretary assists with this by checking that personal and demographic details are completed accurately and comprehensively on the TCI form, that PAS and case notes are updated with information received, that forms are forwarded on correctly and that patients are actually placed on the waiting list. (See Figs 14.4 and 14.5 for examples of PAS computer-generated letters to assist in validating waiting lists.)

## URGENT ADMISSIONS

As well as providing waiting list management information the admissions department will be responsible for communicating any telephone and written enquiries and cancellations as appropriate. For example, in the case of urgent admissions (as opposed to emergency admissions), it is important that admissions staff are informed whether the patient has already been advised of an admission date by you or the outpatient clinic staff. When patients have not been informed of their admission date, admissions staff will contact the patient, by telephone if possible, and update the PAS waiting list system immediately once confirmation is made. An existing TCI form will also need to be updated and the ECR team and contract validation unit notified if there is no existing contract so that agreement for payment can be sought from the patient's Health Authority.

## EMERGENCY ADMISSIONS

This usually refers to a same-day admission and where the patient requires to be admitted immediately from the accident and emergency (A&E) department, an outpatient clinic, through a GP or from another hospital. The referring doctor should contact the admissions staff with the patient's name, sex, age, diagnosis and specialty. The admissions staff are responsible for finding a bed, agreeing this with the duty medical registrar or duty surgical registrar (i.e. a member of the medical staff with responsibility for admissions on that particular day) who will then contact the GP (if relevant) to bring the patient in.

## DAILY INFORMATION ON BED AVAILABILITY

The admissions staff are also responsible for collecting information on bed availability to assist in bed management and monitoring. This information is provided by the 'bed state'. The bed state is a continuous record of the status of each bed in the hospital and this is held and updated on the PAS. The status of each bed is defined in four ways (Box 14.1).

The admissions staff will operate a number of different systems to ensure that timely and accurate information is gathered on bed occupancy.

### Manual bed state list

Nursing staff complete a bed state form for their ward(s) and will notify admissions immediately a bed becomes empty and when a discharge has been decided upon. These are collected daily by admissions staff. The PAS system is then updated and patient listings printed off for use by reception staff, for example in the evenings.

### Telephone collections

Admissions staff will telephone at set times during the day to check the bed state for inaccuracies, caused by discharges and deaths. (See Fig. 14.6, for an example of a manual bed state form.)

In an acute bed shortage the bed manager, supported by the 'take' firm, will contact all firms and

---

**Box 14.1    The bed state**

◆ Occupied: a bed which currently has a patient in it

◆ Booked: a bed which has a patient coming into it in the next 24 hours

◆ Available: a bed which does not have a patient booked in the next 24 hours

◆ Reserved: a bed which has a patient coming back into it within 48 hours, not a planned admission but perhaps an urgent planned admission

5th May

Dr. B.E. Smith (GP),
10 Blackhorse Road,
Bakers Town
BT22 7QD


Dear Dr. Smith,

| | |
|---|---|
| RE | KEITH DAVIDSON |
| DOB | 10.12.49 |
| | |
| ADDRESS | 14 White Cross, Bakers Town |
| POSTCODE | BT21 8SK |
| | |
| HOSPITAL NUMBER | 243675 |
| | |
| OPERATION | FASCIECTOMY |

Resulting from recent validation of my Waiting List, the patient detailed above has been contacted and has expressed a wish to be removed from my Waiting List. After studying the patient's case I have decided to remove this patient from my List.

If you know of any reason why this patient should be reinstated, please do not hesitate to contact me.

Yours sincerely,



Mr. J. Daniels
Consultant in Plastic Surgery

**Figure 14.4** Example of a PAS-generated letter to a GP to assist in validating a waiting list.

ask that patients are discharged or moved to create beds for the 'take' firm. There will be a clinical referee to help resolve difficulties. The Emergency Bed Service and Ambulance Service must also be notified of these decisions.

The Emergency Bed Service provides a central information service for GPs and hospital doctors on the availability of beds in other hospitals.

# BED MANAGEMENT AND MONITORING INFORMATION

There will be a Bed Allocation Committee who will be concerned mainly with retrospective monitoring of bed management and to assist in planning services, statistics generated from the PAS, including hospital initiated cancellations and

HOSPITAL NUMBER      243675

4th May 19

Mr. K. Davidson,
14 White Cross, Bakers Town
BT21 8SK

Dear Mr. Davidson,


As requested recently you have now been removed from Mr. Daniel's Waiting List. Should you wish to be reinstated please make an appointment to see your GP who has been informed of your decision.


Yours sincerely,



**Waiting List Officer**

**Figure 14.5**   Another example of a PAS-generated letter.

patients remaining in A&E for 24 hours or more (i.e. patients who should be moved to an appropriate ward within 48 hours of admission, before routine cases are admitted).

Regrettably, some patients' admission dates have to be cancelled, sometimes on the day of admission, and this can cause a great deal of distress and inconvenience for patients. This may be due to emergency admissions, delays in discharges or the closure of beds due to infection. For example, in recent years MRSA (methicillin resistant *Staphyloccocus aureus*) has emerged as a major infection control problem. It is an organism spread relatively easily from person to person and difficult to eradicate. It can cause infections, ranging from minor wound infections to more serious ones.

**Reflection point**

In what ways can a medical secretary assist with minimising the stress caused by a potentially traumatic cancellation of a patient's admission date?

Once the admission list of patients has been confirmed a computer-generated admissions list from the PAS is given to the admissions department or medical records staff responsible for locating the patients' case notes before their admission. The case note folder will need various sheets added, including an inpatient history sheet, consent forms,

**BEDSTATE** AT 8 a.m.

WARD ___  DATE ___

| Bed No. | Hospital No. | Name | Consultant | PATIENTS – IN | | | PATIENTS – OUT | | | | |
|---|---|---|---|---|---|---|---|---|---|---|---|
| | | | | DATE of Admission/Transfer | FROM | DATE Return to Ward | DATE of Discharge/Transfer | TO | DATE of Death | DATE Home on Leave | For Discharge or Transfer Today |
| 1 | FW0000 | DAVIES CLAIRE NHS | PB | 12.3.90 | OAS | | | | | | |
| 2 | FW0000 | DAVIES CLAIRE NHS | PB | 12.3.90 | W/LIST | | | | | | |
| 3 | FW0000 | DAVIES CLAIRE NHS | PB | 12.3.90 | CLINIC | | | | | | |
| 4 | | | | | | | | | | | |
| 5 | | | | | | | | | | | |
| FX | | | | | | | | | | | |

**Figure 14.6** A manual bed state form.

various charts and patient care documentation for completion by the nurses. X-rays and outstanding results will also have to be located and filed in the case notes to enable doctors and nurses to complete the initial interview and assessment of the patient satisfactorily upon their arrival on the ward. You may be contacted regarding case notes and results in your possession and these should be released at the earliest opportunity.

The admissions list is also circulated to other departments, including the ward, the chaplains and the medical social worker, so that they can make their arrangements accordingly.

The case notes will usually be held by the reception desk responsible for receiving and admitting patients. Once the patient arrives on the ward inpatient care commences and the case notes will be made available for the medical and nursing staff on the ward. The PAS will be updated. The majority of wards have a full- or part-time administrative assistant, sometimes known as a ward clerk or ward assistant. The ward clerk's duties include maintaining the case notes, for example ensuring results are filed, sorting incoming mail and receiving visitors to the ward. They may also have responsibility for updating the PAS, assisting with the bed state and liaising with other hospital departments.

## THE OPERATING LIST

If you work for a consultant surgeon your medical team may ask you to type up the operating list and distribute it accordingly. It is usually handwritten by the house officer and will include each patient's name, age, hospital number, ward, operation details, type of anaesthetic required (general or local) and blood group, and will be typed in the order the patients will be operated upon. You may liaise with the theatres and anaesthetics departmental secretaries, who coordinate all the operating lists for the various specialisms. This information in turn will be circulated, for example, to the central sterile supplies department (CSSD), who provide sterile instruments and equipment for investigative, diagnostic and therapeutic treatments for invasive medical procedures

for inpatient and outpatient care, and the haematology department for blood matching and so on.

## Confidentiality

You may receive a telephone call asking which ward a patient is on – perhaps to send a card or flowers. Anyone with a knowledge of the wards and the types of operations or treatments given in a hospital may deduce the reasons, rightly or wrongly, for a patient being on a particular ward even without you specifying this. For example, Ward 10 may be for the care of patients who are HIV positive and have associated illnesses. Care should be taken when giving this information to callers and a check made beforehand that the patient is happy for this to be done. The PAS may have a facility for recording a patient's wishes.

## DAY SURGERY UNIT

The unit will usually provide facilities for adult patients and children who can safely be admitted for surgical, therapeutic, diagnostic or endoscopic procedures and sent home on the same day. Specialties using a day surgery facility may include general surgery (e.g. inguinal hernia repair), ophthalmology (e.g. cataract extraction), orthopaedic surgery (e.g. arthroscopy), ear, nose and throat (ENT) surgery, urology and plastic surgery. They will have their own operating theatres and team of staff. There may be overnight hostel accommodation available for patients when travelling time would otherwise make it difficult for them to attend for treatment. You will need to familiarise yourself with the procedures involved for admitting patients from your department for day surgery, including the use of proformas, and the production of discharge summaries may be your responsibility or that of the medical secretary within the day surgery unit.

Some surgical procedures may also take place in the outpatient department. For example, these may be found in the dental, ophthalmology and dermatology departments. Figure 14.7 shows an example of a letter to patients being admitted for day surgery.

Dear

Your doctor has recommended that you have an ENDOSCOPY. This is an examination of your oesophagus (gullet), stomach and duodenum. The examination is performed as a single procedure using a flexible lighted instrument and is carried out in the Unit by a specially trained doctor. It will help discover the cause of your symptoms or clarify any abnormality seen on X-ray.

*Do not eat or drink anything from midnight before your examination. Medication should also be omitted unless you are a diabetic or on medication for a heart condition. If this is the case please contact the department for instructions.*

Please report to the Day Surgery Unit (sign posted throughout the Hospital). There you will be asked to change into a gown. You may bring your own dressing gown if you wish. Please bring your slippers.

A doctor will take a brief history from you and a small needle will be inserted into your arm or hand. From the DSU you will be transferred to the Endoscopy Unit on a special trolley. Here you will be given something to make you very drowsy. When you are totally relaxed the doctor will pass a tube over the back of your throat and down into your gullet. This will not interfere with your breathing and is not painful. The examination lasts about ten minutes and a nurse will remain with you throughout.

Once the examination is over you will be returned to the DSU to sleep off the effects of the injection. There is a waiting area if your escort wishes to wait for you.

*Please Note: It is essential that you are collected and escorted home by a friend or relative. YOU MUST NOT DRIVE YOURSELF HOME. If there is a problem with a companion taking you home please contact this Department immediately.*

Please note the date and time of your appointment:

DATE: ................................................. TIME: ...............................

Useful information following Endoscopy:

1  Advised not to smoke or take alcohol for 24 hours.
2  You should not drive or operate machinery for 48 hours following Endoscopy.
3  Contact your own doctor two weeks after your Endoscopy for result of examination.
4  Rest for remainder of the day and you should be able to return to work next day.
5  Occasionally some patients experience a slightly sore throat. This will subside without medication.


Yours sincerely,



Day Surgery Unit Manager

**Figure 14.7**  Example of a letter to a patient for day surgery.

DISCHARGE LETTER

| Hospital No.: |
| Surname: |
| First Names: |
| Date of Birth: Sex: |

HOSPITAL: CONTACT TEL No.

Date:

Address:

Dear Dr. .................................................

Your patient, who was admitted on ........................................................................................ to Ward ........................................

was discharged

under the care of ........................................................ was/will be transferred on ................................................ to ................................................

died

DIAGNOSIS (firm (F) or provisional (P)) operations, problems and unexplained abnormal findings

INPATIENT SUMMARY AND RECOMMENDATIONS FOR FURTHER MANAGEMENT

Notifiable diseases only Date notified

ICD coding

HISTOLOGICAL DIAGNOSIS KNOWN/NOT KNOWN. DETAILS

PATIENT WILL/WILL NOT BE SEEN IN OUTPATIENTS. DATE

| Drugs taken home and supply provided | Dose | Frequency | Duration necessary | Supply given wks/days | Drugs taken home and supply provided | Dose | Frequency | Duration necessary | Supply given wks/days |
|---|---|---|---|---|---|---|---|---|---|
| | | | | | | | | | |
| | | | | | | | | | |
| | | | | | | | | | |

DRUGS TO AVOID AND REASONS (including drug sensitivities)

| INFORMATION GIVEN TO PATIENT | Information given to Relative or Friend |
|---|---|
| Diagnosis | |
| Prognosis | |
| Resumption of work | |
| Other | |

SERVICES ARRANGED BY THE HOSPITAL (please tick appropriate box if service has been arranged)

MEALS ON WHEELS ☐ HOME HELP ☐ HOME NURSE ☐

GERIATRIC/HEALTH VISITOR ☐ PART III ACCOMMODATION ☐

OTHER (please state) ☐

Cons.

Yours sincerely,

S. Reg.

A fuller summary will/will not be sent

Copy handed to patient/posted to GP

Please print name Reg.

H.O.

**Figure 14.8** A discharge letter.

| CONSULTANT | | GP: Dr | |
|---|---|---|---|
| ADMISSION DATE: / / | | PATIENT NAME: | |
| DISCHARGE DATE: / / | | HOSPITAL NUMBER: | DOB: |
| WARD: HOSPITAL: | | ADDRESS: | |
| CONTACT TEL NO.: | | POSTCODE: | |

| PRIMARY DIAGNOSIS | MAIN PROCEDURE: | DATE |
|---|---|---|
| 2. | OTHER PROCEDURES: | |
| 3. | | |
| 4. | | |

CLINICAL COMMENTS

A further summary will be sent

| RECOMMENDATIONS FOR FURTHER MANAGEMENT (HOSPITAL, GP) | SERVICES ARRANGED BY HOSPITAL |
|---|---|
| | |
| Date and time of Outpatient Appointment if made:     Transport arranged?: Y/N | |

| DRUGS TO TAKE HOME | ☐ Tick if no drugs required | | ☐ Tick if child resistant closure not required | | Pharmacist Check | |
|---|---|---|---|---|---|---|
| Drugs – Approved Name | Route | Dose | Frequency | Duration necessary | Pharmacy | |
| | | | | | | |
| | | | | | | |
| | | | | | | |
| | | | | | | |
| | | | | | | |
| | | | | | | |
| | | | | | | |
| | | | | | | |
| | | | | | | |
| | | | | | | |
| | | | | | | |
| | | | | | | |

DRUGS TO AVOID AND REASONS (including drug sensitivities):

| Signature: | Grade: |
|---|---|
| Print Name: | Date: |

# INTENSIVE THERAPY UNIT (ITU)/INTENSIVE CARE UNIT

There will be intensive care beds and high dependency care beds for the specialist care and treatment of critically ill patients by a team of staff who generally possess a critical care qualification. All age groups are nursed and ITUs generally provide waiting areas and accommodation for the families. Patients may, for example, have sustained major trauma, require coronary care, burns, sepsis or multi-organ failure.

## Scenario

A patient telephones you and asks you where she is placed on the waiting list and when she can expect to be called for admission. What action should you take and what information can you provide? What variables outside the hospital or your own control may influence the time a patient may spend on the waiting list?

# COMPULSORY ADMISSIONS

It should be noted that whilst the aim is always to advise voluntary admission wherever possible, patients are detained in hospital under the Mental Health Acts in order for a patient's mental state to be assessed and, if necessary, treated. There will be a duty psychiatrist and duty psychiatric social worker available to assist in these cases.

# DISCHARGES

All hospitals will have a discharge policy outlining all matters that *must* be attended to *before* the patient leaves the hospital. This will include, as appropriate:

◆ advice from doctors and nurses on the ward to patients on how best to look after themselves and what to expect
◆ proforma style letter to post or hand to their GP containing information about treatment

and recommendations about future medical care and so forth
◆ any medications the patient may need
◆ medical certificate
◆ arrangements regarding special pension or benefits, with which a hospital social worker may assist
◆ other arrangements, such as social services, meals on wheels, home help, day care, nursing aids, nursing (e.g. Macmillan or others)
◆ date and time of next outpatient clinic appointment, as appropriate
◆ community nursing staff visit date
◆ return of valuables
◆ arrangements for getting home, including transport if necessary (patients may be transferred to another hospital, to a nursing or residential home and arrangements made accordingly)
◆ date of discharge entered on to the PAS
◆ case notes forwarded to the medical secretary
◆ X-rays returned to the X-ray department film stores.

The medical social work department will liaise closely with the ward, primary health care team and the community services regarding the patient's discharge to ensure continuity of care.

To reduce the number of forms in circulation at discharge a self-carbonated form could be used (Fig. 14.8), which can be used in the following way:

◆ the form, completed legibly and clearly by a doctor, can be sent to the pharmacy department in order for drugs on discharge to be prescribed
◆ top copy sent to GP on the day of discharge (or given to patient to deliver)
◆ second copy filed in patient's case notes
◆ third copy sent to the clinical coding department (see below)
◆ fourth copy for pharmacy records.

# PROCEDURES WHEN A PATIENT DIES

When a patient dies in hospital the ward sister usually contacts the nearest relative or personal representative of the deceased. The hospital chaplain will be available and the body will be kept in the hospital mortuary until arrangements are made to have the deceased taken to, for example, a Chapel of Rest.

Deaths are processed by staff in the patient affairs office, generally part of the hospital administration department, together with the doctor concerned with the patient's care. There will usually be a private room available for staff to speak with the relatives of the deceased.

Doctors should inform the patient's GP as soon as possible either by telephone or letter that his/her patient has died.

The doctor responsible for the patient should complete the following paperwork.

**Death certificate.** Unless the case is to be referred to the coroner, this should be issued as soon after the death as possible to prevent further distress to the patients.

The doctor should ensure that all sections of the form are complete and that he/she prints his/her name at the end of the certificate. A register will be kept of all death certificates issued.

The form is sent to the Registrar for Births and Deaths, unless the case is referred to the coroner

The Town Hall Registrar will not accept a certificate if the cause of death is abbreviated or if there is no definite cause of death. Terms such as 'probably' and 'unknown' are not acceptable.

Where there is doubt as to the cause of death, the coroner, who is a doctor or lawyer, will conduct an autopsy. This may be followed by an inquest. Box 14.2 gives examples of circumstances which would necessitate these procedures.

The coroner will send the death certificate to the Registrar of Births and Deaths once a satisfactory conclusion has been reached.

The medical team may also request a post-mortem, with specific consent of the relatives, to:

◆ study the effects of treatment, involving the retention of tissue for laboratory study
◆ remove amounts of tissue for the treatment of other patients and for medical education and research.

**Post-mortem form – to identify the cause of death, if applicable.** If the medical team feel it is

---

**Box 14.2** Circumstances necessitating an autopsy

◆ Patients who have been in hospital for less than 24 hours

◆ Patients whose death may be related to drugs, poison or industrial disease

◆ Accidental death/recent fall/fracture

◆ Suspicious death/circumstances

◆ During a surgical operation/while under anaesthetic

◆ Death is sudden, unexplainable, for example sudden infant death

---

appropriate to request a post-mortem, the patient's relatives must give their permission and a consent form must be completed and a histopathology form submitted by the doctor requesting the post-mortem.

**Medical audit form.**

**Cremation form.** Where appropriate.

**A free from infection certificate for transportation abroad.** If the body is to be transported to another country, this form has to be completed, stating that the body will cause no hazard if transported in a sealed coffin.

Staff in the patient affairs office will also be responsible for ensuring that the correct patient details are forwarded to the patient services department to allow the cancellation of any known appointments, waiting list entries, admissions or transport arrangements and for the case notes to be amended and stored accordingly on their return from the ward. The PAS must be updated as quickly as possible, at least within 48 hours of being notified of a patient's death. Patient affairs staff are also responsible for returning a patient's belongings to the relatives and liaising with the mortuary for the collection of the body.

Failure to provide the correct information may result in the wrong patient appearing on the PAS as deceased, or an ambulance arriving at a deceased patient's home to collect them for an appointment. This action has serious consequences and leads to considerable distress for relatives and friends.

**Reflection point**

When a patient has been discharged the case notes are sent to the medical secretary at the earliest opportunity in order for a fuller discharge summary to be dictated by a nominated member of the medical team and subsequently typed by the secretary for dispatch to the GP. (See Fig. 14.9, Excerpt from an inpatient discharge summary.)

**Reflection point**

Analyse the information which has been recorded in the discharge summary and reflect on the reasons why this information has to be provided before proceeding with the chapter.

# MEDICAL (CLINICAL) CODING

Medical coding involves the abstraction of clinical information from case notes or discharge summaries and the conversion of that information into an alpha-numeric structure so that without additions or personal identifiers, the codes can provide a comprehensive reflection of morbidity and a description of diagnoses and procedures for individual patients. This diagnostic and procedural information can be put into a comparative form which can be analysed for statistical purposes.

There are two coding systems in use.

The International Classification of Diseases and Health Related Problems, currently revision 10 (ICD 10), is published by the World Health Organization. It is a national and international standard through which all clinical activity relating to inpatient diagnoses is measured and is intended to provide a comprehensive list of code numbers to classify all known diseases and injuries. Hospitals produce contract minimum data sets (that is, the demographic, social and clinical information gathered on the PAS) which are coded, and regular central returns made from hospitals to the Department of Health. This information provides users of NHS data with better clinical, social and epidemiological information to improve the planning and running of health services at district, national (e.g. National Audit Office) and international levels (e.g. World Health Organization). Statistics are used to aid decision-making in where to target health promotion in the country, for example where there is a higher than national average for heart disease.

The Office of Population Censuses and Surveys, revision 5 (OPCS 5) provides a further national standard through which all operative procedures are coded in respect of inpatient and day case activity. That is, operations, procedures and their complications will have an identifying code. Revision of the codes is necessary to accommodate changes in medical treatments as they become available.

Each medical firm will have a medical coding officer whose responsibility it is to ensure that coding from each firm is timely, accurate and complete for each inpatient episode. Data is entered onto the PAS and facilitates the production of reports and statistics as well as becoming a vital component for invoice generation and the billing process.

Accurate and timely clinical coding (Box 14.3) is one way of ensuring that medical information is of a high enough quality to reflect accurately the health care practice patterns of doctors and other health care practitioners. As well as ensuring the GP has up-to-date information about the patient's hospital episode, as with patient clinic letters, hospitals can be penalised financially through provider–purchaser contracts when discharge summaries are not sent or delayed. If missing information or disinformation recurs it will have a direct cost implication for the hospital and is therefore closely linked to the other main elements of the delivery of health care, namely contracting, medical and clinical audit and billing.

```
PATIENT'S GP            Dr M. Shah
ADDRESS                 14 Bridge Street, Shackleton, Herts.

HOSPITAL NO             264 299

SPECIALISM              GENERAL SURGERY
CONSULTANT              PETER JONES

SURNAME                 STANLEY
FIRST NAME              QUEENIE
SEX                     F
DOB                     04.06.

PATIENT'S ADDRESS
POSTCODE

ADMITTED       01.05.
DISCHARGED     10.05.
```

**History**
80-year-old lady living in sheltered accommodation. Referred by her General Practitioner.

**Past Medical History**
Congestive cardiac failure and episodic angina. Also suffers from folate deficiency anaemia.

**On Examination**
Referred to us as an emergency with bleeding per rectum. Sigmoidoscopy indicated a malignant tumour of the rectum. Biopsy was reported as rectal carcinoma.

**Diagnosis on Admission**
Admitted for resection of rectal carcinoma.

**Procedure**
Abdominoperineal resection with colostomy.

**Postoperative**
Uneventful postoperative course.

Discharged after 10 days.

**Drug therapy on Discharge**
Nil

<u>**Final Diagnoses**</u>

|  |  | ICD 10 codes |
|---|---|---|
| **Primary** | Cancer of rectum | 000.0 |
| **Secondary** | Folate deficiency anaemia | 000.0 |
|  | Angina | 000.0 |
|  | Adenocarcinoma | M000/0 |

<u>**Procedure**</u>

|  | OPCS 5 Codes |
|---|---|
| Abdominoperineal resection | H00.0 |

**Figure 14.9** Excerpt from an inpatient discharge summary.

◆ Summaries should be legible

◆ Patient identification details should include the following:

registration/hospital number

surname and forename

address and postcode

date of birth, gender and marital status

◆ Consultant and specialty

◆ Date of admission and discharge

◆ Ward

◆ Medical diagnosis should include:

principal diagnosis

subsidiary diagnoses

external cause of condition, if appropriate

histology results

◆ Any operation or procedure undertaken with the dates

◆ Any complications arising

The original function of medical coding was to provide epidemiological data for statistical analysis, by using agreed national and international codes. As contracting develops between purchaser

**Reflection point**

◆ The medical coder relies on the information provided in the discharge summary to code the patient's inpatient episode. A patient with a series of admissions would have several code allocations per admission. With reference to Figure 14.9, the discharge summary, how many of the requirements needed for accurate, timely and complete coding can you identify?

and provider units, Healthcare Resource Groups (HRGs) are used to cost patient care by grouping together comparative costs for treatments.

# DEPARTMENTAL MEDICAL (CLINICAL) AUDIT

In addition to medical coding being entered on to the PAS, computerised departmental audit systems have been introduced to provide medical staff with an opportunity to collect detailed information on every inpatient seen within a firm. Each firm has its own audit aims.

Whilst firms conform to a single standard in the area of diagnostic and procedural coding, they can also access other coding systems, for example Read codes. This is one example of a newly developed comprehensive, hierarchically arranged classification and medical thesaurus of terms used in each medical specialism and structured for use in computers, and cross referenced to ICD 10. Read and other available systems are intended to support the work of doctors with day-to-day patient care and are not designed specifically for wider research purposes or statistical tool outside of the department. The role of departmental audit is viewed as complementary, with Read and the ICD information serving different, if related, purposes. The local audit systems enable doctors to add their own specialist codes to assist them in setting their own standards. They can then measure their local coding practices, in relation to diagnoses, operation and procedure outcomes, for their own patients, against national and international standards.

It should be noted that departmental audit data collected on a local system is of a highly sensitive and confidential nature, as it reflects the performance and activity of individual doctors within a team and is therefore not made more widely available. The success of internal audit to a large extent relies upon the confidence of medical staff that this information will be used positively to assist in improving the departmental standard.

The departmental computerised audit system may also generate GP letters and summaries. Read and other coding systems can be 'mapped up', i.e.

**Box 14.4** How statistics are used

*Local use of statistics*

◆ Number of patients seen by consultant by site and in bed occupancy days

◆ Analysis of referral patterns

◆ Activity for different operations

*National and international use of statistics*

◆ Assessing health needs of the country

◆ Epidemiology

◆ Public health

◆ Population registers

*Successful billing*

*Contracting information*, for example the production of activity reports, are used by providers and purchasers to facilitate planning and to support the contract negotiation process.

converted to, ICD 10 and OPCS 5 computer programs on the PAS, which in turn can be mapped up to other hospital computer systems, including those for finance.

Firms will usually hold regular validation meetings to approve data to be entered on to the departmental database and to ensure the audit data is meaningful. Both you and the coding clerk may participate in these meetings. Figure 14.10 illustrates the coding cycle. Box 14.4 summarises the use of statistics at different levels.

# ACCIDENT AND EMERGENCY DEPARTMENT

The accident and emergency (A&E) department falls outside the usual formality of contract negotiations between purchasers and providers, at least for the first 24 hours of a patient's care. Therefore, treatment must be made available to anyone who presents themselves to the A&E department.

The A&E department provides 24-hour emergency care to a wide cross-section of patients 365 days a year. Its role is to provide clinical assessment and emergency treatment for the full range of specialties and to refer on to their GPs or hospital specialism as appropriate. Designated A&Es will also provide a major incident service for their surrounding area and may keep major incident flying squad stores. There will always be a consultant and/or senior registrar 'on call' in A&E and they must usually be informed in the event of the following:

◆ death in the young (under 40)

◆ deaths where violence may have occurred

◆ seriously ill children/non-accidental injury – known or suspected

◆ significant burns to children and adults

◆ stabbings/shootings/rape/serious assault

◆ episodes with major press or police involvement.

Generally there will be an adjacent fracture clinic consulting area. There may also be clinics held for plastics/minor burns, soft tissue, rheumatology clinic and a weekend dental clinic.

The majority of patients attending A&E are ambulant. There will be a 24-hour reception area where staff take details from patients and register them on the A&E Module on the PAS. Patients are issued with a hospital number and a casualty and incident number. There is also a screen on the computer allowing the hospital staff to request and record a free text summary of the patient's condition. This can be provided by the patient, their relative or the paramedic involved in their case as appropriate.

Patients will then be seen by the 'triage' nurse (triage meaning the order of treatment of the patients being based on clinical urgency). The triage nurse will assess each patient upon their arrival, obtain further history, take baseline observations as required (e.g. blood pressure), carry out first aid and prioritise the more urgent cases.

Patients arriving by ambulance will be taken to treatment, or if seriously ill to the crash room, where the crash team will administer emergency treatment, and the ambulance personnel will pass

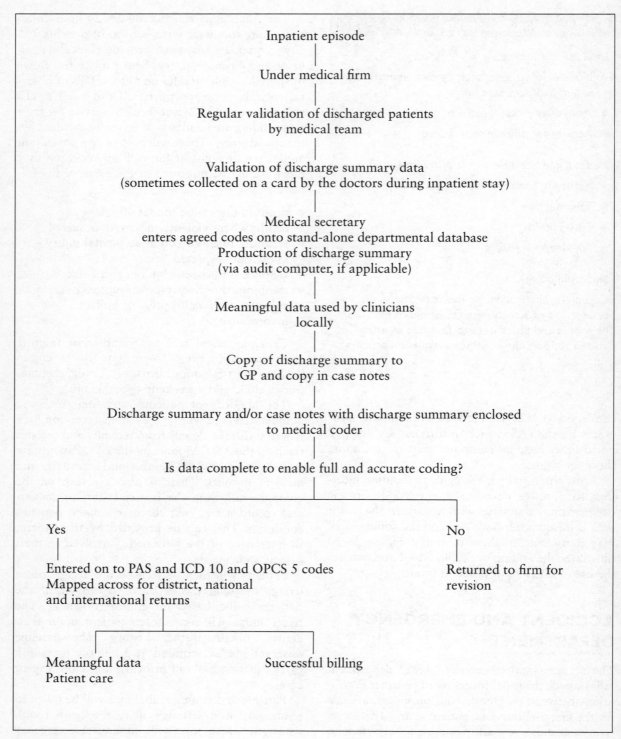

**Figure 14.10** The coding cycle.

on as much information as possible to the A&E reception staff so that the patient can be registered on PAS.

### Reflection point

◆ The Patient's Charter standard for A&E is 90% patients should be seen within 5 minutes of arrival.

All patients who request to see a doctor must see a doctor. The casualty doctor will complete a casualty card, detailing further history, investigations, diagnosis (as far as possible) and will initiate treatment, discharge the patient back to the GP, or refer to a hospital specialist or admit the patient for inpatient care. Patients who are not admitted remain the responsibility of the A&E department, so follow-up arrangements must be made as appropriate. There may also be dedicated A&E beds for stays of 24 hours.

The casualty officer will liaise with the duty registrar of the medical firm 'on take' to find an available bed. Hospital case notes are made up by the admissions department if none already exist and the patient then becomes the responsibility of the consultant's firm who is 'on take'. The consultant's secretary will be responsible for typing the discharge summary to the GP when the patient subsequently leaves the hospital.

The department will include treatment cubicles, X-ray equipment in designated rooms, a fully equipped theatre for urgent surgery and minor procedures, a plaster room, and may have designated paediatric cubicles and paediatric waiting area as well as a relatives' room. There may be doctors' 'on call' rooms nearby, a radiation decontamination unit and isolation suite.

Other staff within the department may include:

◆ porters, with 24-hour cover
◆ liaison sisters, with special responsibilities for the elderly, those with alcohol and drug problems
◆ paediatric liaison nurse

◆ pharmacy, for dispensing small stock of antibiotics and painkillers
◆ duty radiographer for taking X-rays.

As the A&E departmental secretary, you may be required to enter the information from the casualty card onto the PAS and generate the letter to the GP (Fig. 14.11), using free text and a referral letter to the outpatient department for further care as appropriate, or to return to a specialist clinic held in A&E for review or re-dressing.

You may also become involved with the typing of statements for the police, Criminal Injuries Compensation Board reports and solicitors' medical reports and statements. Patient confidentiality is paramount, and permission in writing from the patient should be obtained whenever possible. Requests for patient names and addresses by the police should always be referred to senior casualty staff or the duty administrator.

It should be remembered, however, that the police have a major supporting role in casualty situations, for example in locating next of kin, and they have to supply a report to their superiors when they are first on scene of accident, etc. The doctor may dictate a statement giving information to the police. See Figure 14.12 for an example of a doctor's statement for a police officer.

## CONCLUSION

In this chapter we have looked at the practical administrative issues in running inpatient services including those prior to admission, during an inpatient stay, at discharge and following discharge. By demonstrating the variety of tasks and procedures which must be carried out, the importance of effective communication between all staff groups involved is highlighted. Emphasis should be placed on staff adhering to systems and procedures as this is essential when we consider the number of patients who require inpatient care. It is important for you as a medical secretary to have an overview of the whole system to enable you to resolve queries, or to refer patients to the appropriate department or staff member, as you are often the first point of contact for patients and staff involved in patient care.

---

Dear Dr

Re


The above patient attended the A&E Department of this Hospital on
................................... at ..............

The presenting complaint was LACERATION TO JUST ABOVE WRIST,
LEFT ARM.

Diagnosis:          LACERATION LEFT WRIST.

Treatment:          DRESSING/BANDAGE/SLING.

SUTURING/STERISTRIP.

The patient has been discharged back to your care.


Yours sincerely,



Consultant
Accident and Emergency Department

---

**Figure 14.11**    Example of an A&E attendance letter.

---

'I am a registered medical practitioner currently employed as a senior house
officer in the A&E Department of St Mary's Hospital.

The patient, Joshua Smith, was brought by ambulance to the A&E
Department of this Hospital at 2000 hours on 6th June 19    following an
alleged assault.

I examined him and found him to be suffering from the following injuries: a
2 cm laceration x 1 cm deep on the right cheek of the face and superficial
abrasions to the right hand. The patient's wounds were cleaned and sutured
under local anaesthetic with a total of 5 sutures. The patient was discharged
from the Department at 2200 hours. He was advised to have his sutures
removed in four days....'

---

**Figure 14.12**    Example of a doctor's statement for a police officer.

### Exercises

◆ A patient telephones and says she has been on the waiting list for a long time and wants to know when her operation will be. What information do you require and where and how will you obtain it? What can you tell the patient? How would you go about dealing with this query?

◆ It is a Monday morning. You have just been informed the operating list has to be cancelled for that Thursday morning because the operating theatre your consultant uses has had to be closed for infection control. You have four patients to be admitted on the Wednesday for major or minor surgical procedures. They are to be operated on on the Thursday. You manage the waiting list and sent letters out to the patients some weeks earlier giving them their TCI 'to come in' dates. How will you contact the patients? How do you think this may affect the patients and how may they react to this news? What will you say to them? What administrative procedures and arrangements will need to take place? Are there any other issues this situation may raise?

◆ You are the medical secretary in the accident and emergency department. You receive a telephone call from the police. They say that a man by the name of Paul Johnson, date of birth 10.12.62, has been brought into hospital following a fight. He had allegedly been stabbed. (Paul Johnson is a local celebrity – being a member of a first division football team.) They want to know whether or not they can come in to see him. They would also like a statement from the doctor who is seeing him about his medical condition. How would you deal with this query? What issues does it raise?

BLANK.

# 4

## *Part 4*
## The secretary in general practice

# 15

# General practice and primary care

*Barbara Jones*

## OBJECTIVES

◆ To provide a brief history of general practice

◆ To describe the role of the GP in primary care and involvement in health promotion

◆ To identify the personnel working within primary health care

◆ To give a brief overview of areas used in health centres

◆ To stress the importance of standards within premises, maintenance and security.

## INTRODUCTION

This section deals with general practice within the National Health Service and the wide-ranging areas of primary care. The present direction of health care focuses on general practice, allowing and encouraging GPs to take a major part in the standard of primary health care of their practice population and to take an active part in the motivation of the primary health care team.

Before you begin to study this chapter, you may find it useful to obtain a copy of a practice leaflet.

## BRIEF HISTORY

The National Health Service (NHS) as we know it today came into being with the introduction of the NHS Act in 1946. Prior to that, the National Health Insurance Scheme had been instituted in 1911 and all employed and self-employed people were obliged to pay contributions that entitled them to receive free medical care from a general practitioner. The introduction of the NHS Act extended this obligation to the whole population – 'A free Health Service for all'. There have been several changes made over the years and Acts of Parliament have been issued in order to carry out these changes. The NHS Act of 1977 requires that the Secretary of State continues to monitor and promote improvements in the health of the nation, not only in the diagnosis and treatment of illness but also through prevention measures. The NHS (General Medical Services) Regulations 1992 set out the terms and services which give a framework within which all general practitioners must work and list specific duties to be carried out. Payments made to general practitioners for this work are paid in accordance with the 'Statement of Fees and Allowances' most often referred to as the 'Red Book'. All doctors who wish to practise in the UK must, by law, be registered with the General Medical Council.

The introduction of fundholding in 1991 allowed some practices to purchase directly from hospitals the health care needed for their patients. They hold their own budgets for various areas of health and are free to purchase from whichever 'provider' (hospital or Trust) they feel will supply the best service and value for money, for their patients. Practice budgets are initially based on the total capitation size of the practice, and the activity data collected during the 'preparatory year' of fundholding, before the practice actually goes 'live' and begins managing the allocated budget. The data will include the number of patients referred to hospitals for treatment, every initial and review consultation that takes place, all laboratory tests and X-rays and all community services.

The present government is implementing changes to abolish the 'internal market' within the NHS and base patient care on need and not on the practice's fund availability. Commissioning care groups are to be set up in 1999 to replace fundholding and manage patient care. This may entail groups of practices totalling approximately 100 000 patients developing and managing the needs of patient care within that area and so delivering a service which is relevant and effective.

It is intended that this new system will abolish the implication of a two-tier system of health care, whereby the best service was apparently available only to those who have budgets and money available within those budgets to pay for treatment.

## THE ROLE OF THE GP IN PRIMARY CARE AND HEALTH PROMOTION

Most GPs practise within the National Health Service. They are not employed by the NHS but work under contract as *independent contractors* for the health authorities in their area. Details of their

---

> **Box 15.1**  Terms of Service for Doctors in General Practice (DoH)
>
> ◆ *Provision of services to patients* – covering health checks and advice, diagnosis and treatment of the patient.
>
> ◆ *Obligations to the Health Authority Committee* – to inform them of their hours of availability, regulations governing the employment of deputies and their ability to practise.
>
> ◆ *Acceptance of fees* – rules and regulations governing the NHS fees payable for *General Medical Services (GMS)*.
>
> ◆ *Practice leaflet* – information about the personnel and services available and keeping this up to date.
>
> ◆ *Prescriptions and referrals* – obligations to prescribe and refer patients for treatment.
>
> ◆ *Annual Reports* – to provide Annual Reports for the Health Authority on the activity and progress of the practice workload and employees.

---

obligations as a GP working as part of the health service are laid out in the Department of Health 'Terms of Service for Doctors in General Practice' (Box 15.1).

Registered GPs have a list of patients who have chosen to be treated by them and for whom they are responsible. Should a GP accept a new patient or remove a patient from his or her list, the relevant Health Authority must be informed immediately so that accurate details of the list size and the patients the doctor is responsible for are maintained.

The Terms of Service for Doctors in General Practice cover the wide-ranging areas of health care a doctor needs to provide and specific duties doctors must carry out. Besides treating patients who attend surgery, prescribing medication and making necessary home visits, they also have to carry out an active health promotion role within their practices. They are obliged to give advice on the patient's health status in the following areas.

◆ *Obesity/exercise/smoking/alcohol and drugs* – offering appropriate services to identify, control or reduce the risk of disease by giving advice on suitable lifestyle changes.

◆ *Over 75-year-old health checks* – offering and providing health checks for elderly patients.

◆ *New patient health checks* – providing health checks for new patients in order to give a basic insight into their health status.

◆ *Vaccination and immunisation* – offering and providing the necessary vaccinations against measles, rubella, pertussis, Hib, polio, diphtheria and tetanus.

◆ *National screening* – taking part in the national cervical cytology screening, diabetes, asthma and chronic/ischaemic heart disease as required by the government.

These priorities may change as information is collected and analysed highlighting other areas that need to be targeted. The government is constantly reviewing health promotion targets in order to address the wider influences on health such as the environment and poverty. Cytology and immunisation and health promotion targets are linked to income for the practice and the medical secretary's role in collecting accurate information and managing clinics is very important (see Chapter 16).

**Reflection point**

◆ How do practices encourage patients to participate in health screening?

# PERSONNEL WORKING WITHIN PRIMARY HEALTH CARE

The personnel you will find working in primary care may vary depending on the size and type of surgery you work in. In a small non-fundholding *single-handed* practice, although having the district nurse, health visitor and midwife working with them, any additional services may have to be referred to the local hospitals. A larger, *group*

*practice*, of two or more doctors working together to look after patients registered with them, would have bigger premises and the resources to hold several in-house services for patients, including chiropody and physiotherapy facilities.

This section provides a brief description of the people you may work with in general practice.

## Medical staff

Obviously these are the main core of general practice and patients will consult with them for medical advice and diagnosis of their symptoms. From this consultation they may be referred for specialist treatment at hospital or to one of the in-house services available to the patients, should the doctor feel this necessary.

Working arrangements will vary from practice to practice but depending on whether the doctor is employed on a full-time or part-time basis the number of hours he or she is available for surgeries and patient care will be set in a regular pattern. Rotas will be in place to cover weekend on call work, out of hours call out and holiday cover. Often in a group practice when a doctor is off for holiday, sickness or study leave there is flexibility in the surgery rota to allow the other doctors in the practice to cover the surgeries or a *locum doctor* is employed.

### The locum doctor

Locums are fully qualified doctors who have also completed 12 months in general practice as 'trainees', which gives them the qualification to work in general practice.

Often they are looking for permanent work as full partners within a partnership of doctors but carry out temporary work until they find a suitable position. *Partnerships* are groups of doctors who work together from one main surgery (plus small branch surgeries in some rural or large practices) to care for patients. As they are working as a small business and have overheads and responsibilities relating to this, *partnership agreements* which bind them legally to fulfil their part of the commitments of the practice are necessary. Carrying out locum work provides a valuable insight into the surgeries in the area and how they are run.

Locums can provide their services for one session only or longer periods if required and are paid by the hour or session at BMA rates. The GP remains contractually responsible for the services given by a locum to their patients, unless the locum is on the Local Health Authority's medical list.

### General practice registrars

These are fully qualified doctors who are carrying out training to become general practitioners. They have to complete 12 months' training under the guidance of an approved GP trainer before they can apply to be general practitioners in their own right. Very often they have considerable hospital experience in medical fields other than general practice.

### Retainer doctors

These are doctors, generally female, who work a reduced commitment of up to two sessions per week on the government-sponsored retainer scheme. This scheme allows women with family responsibilities to keep up to date and use their medical skills until they are able to increase their commitments to general practice.

### Assistants

These are qualified doctors, the same as GPs, but they are employed directly by the GPs on a salaried basis. They often work part-time for just two or three sessions per week. They have the final clinical responsibility for the patients they treat but do not have a say in the running of the practice as they are not full partners.

### On call agency doctors

There are agencies that work locally and nationally to provide on call cover services. Surgeries are able to book doctors from the agency for short notice emergency rota cover.

Out of hours cover for night visits for patients is often covered by a cooperative of doctors in an area. A rota sharing the 'on call' nights is distributed and each surgery carries out its part in the rota. Whoever is on duty will see or speak to all the patients who request night visits irrespective of which surgery they are registered with.

## The practice nurse

The practice nurse assists the doctor in delivering medical care to the patients. They hold health promotion clinics including asthma, diabetes, family planning, holiday vaccine, heart disease and stroke clinics, besides carrying out basic nursing procedures such as dressing wounds, taking blood pressure, cholesterol and blood tests, giving injections and carrying out registration health checks. The practice nurse also has to keep up to date with training and additional courses. The intention is that the practice nurse can take all routine medical work from the doctor, freeing him or her to concentrate on more complex work and diagnosis. The practice nurse's training enables her or him to inform the doctor and highlight any concerns regarding patients. The role is gradually changing and expanding. The government is promoting the development of nurse practitioners who may become even more important in general practice as they will be allowed to diagnose and prescribe certain groups of medicines. Practice nurses will also work on applying and structuring health promotion protocols and guidelines.

## Ancillary staff

### Practice manager

Most practices today employ a practice manager to supervise and implement the smooth running of the practice. They take the workload from the senior partners and allow them to concentrate on patient care. The practice manager will be responsible for all staff personnel matters and the selection and training of administration staff.

They will meet with the partners and discuss practice policies and systems, manage the practice accounts and staff payroll, liaise with the Health Authority on behalf of the practice and organise primary health care team meetings. They will also ensure that procedures are in place to maximise the practice income from item of service claims and check all quarterly payments from the Health Authority for accuracy. They will be responsible for the execution of health and safety procedures within the practice and the implementation of the practice complaints procedure.

### Office manager/administrator

Sometimes the practice manager has the help of an office manager or administrator who will monitor and control the work carried out with item of service claims and the basic smooth running of the administration side of general practice. This is often a role taken over by the senior receptionist or medical secretary. Depending on the type of practice you work in, if you are able to develop your skills and knowledge to cover all aspects of general practice work, then a career progression towards management is appropriate.

### Budget or fund manager

The fund manager will manage the fund budgets in a fundholding practice. They will negotiate contracts on behalf of the practice, or in conjunction with the lead-partner for fundholding, with the various hospitals and Trusts who are able to supply services to the practice and manage the fund budget. They will prepare statements and reports for the practice and Health Authority and prepare accounts for the internal and external auditors of the fund. In some practices the fund manager and practice manager are the same person and carry out both duties. As fundholding is being phased out under changes in the NHS, this role will change, although budgetary control will remain an important function within general practice.

### Computer staff

Some surgeries employ data input clerks to ensure all health promotion details are entered on the computer. They may carry out only these duties or also be involved in medical audits and development of the full use of the computer system, setting up templates for the accurate and appropriate

capture of information for inclusion in the health promotion targets and Item of Service fee claims. Efficient collection at this time of data adds to the income of the practice. See also Chapter 16 for more information.

### Receptionists

Most receptionists are employed on a part-time basis. Their duties cover not only basic reception desk duties and first line patient contact but also filing, processing repeat prescriptions, giving out test results to patients once they have been checked by the doctor (the doctor usually contacts the patient where results are abnormal or indicate that an appointment should be made for the patient to discuss the result), booking ambulance transport, X-rays, appointments, home visits, pulling records for surgeries and countless other tasks which are essential parts of the job. Often there is a full-time senior receptionist who has a supervisory role in addition to reception duties and ensures the smooth running of reception and efficient processing of item of service claims.

### Medical secretary

Depending on the type of surgery you are working in, your duties may vary from basic audio typing of referral letters and booking hospital appointments to working with the doctors and nursing staff to implement the surgery cervical recall system, medical audits, taking minutes of primary health care meetings, developing the practice computer system to maximise its use.

In a single-handed doctor practice you would most probably be carrying out reception, secretarial and, if the practice is a dispensing one, dispensing duties which would give you an excellent foundation of experience to develop your career.

In a larger practice there would be more staff available to specialise in different areas of administration. As a medical secretary you could be working with the practice manager on improving inefficient work processes, improving working conditions and ensuring the smooth running of the practice. Box 15.2 provides a sample job description.

**Box 15.2** Job description for a medical secretary

JOB TITLE:                          *SECRETARY*

MAIN PURPOSE OF THE POST:           *To provide a wide range of duties including secretarial, clerical and computer input to facilitate the administration work required to provide an efficient medical service to the patients.*

RESPONSIBLE TO:                     *Practice manager.*

### MAJOR DUTIES AND RESPONSIBILITIES

1. Secretarial duties.
2. Clerical duties.
3. Computer duties.
4. Monitor of stationery stock levels.
5. Any other delegated duties considered appropriate to the post.

### SPECIFIC TASKS

1. Secretarial duties
   — All hospital referrals (5 partners, retainer doctor, locum doctors).
   — Typing miscellaneous letters.
   — Hospital enquiries – results, appointments, etc.
   — Deal with enquiries/requests from solicitors, consultants and hospitals relating to patients.

2. Clerical duties
   — Sorting insurance reports, DSS forms, filling in tracer card to obtain records ready for the doctor.
   — Monitoring all inadequate/abnormal smears and sending appropriate letters to patients.
   — Sorting the morning post and allocate to the correct partner.
   — Selecting appropriate mail for the computer operator.

3. Computer duties
   — Entering date of receipt of insurance reports, etc.
   — Using the Medical System word processor to record referral letters.
   — Using the Medical System word processor to produce smear repeat letters.

4. Monitor of stationery stock levels
   — On a regular basis monitor general usage and request requirements for stationery orders.
   — Liaise with the practice manager for order/purchase of requirements.

## Other primary health care team members

The primary health care team consists not just of the general practice staff but of all the additional medical disciplines that work together to provide a complete and caring service to the patient. They are all qualified in their own fields of work and are attached to the practice. They are not employed directly by the practice but through the Health Authority or through the contract set up with the Trust who employs them.

*District nurses* carry out their work with house-bound patients who need clinical assistance to cope with their illness. Their work may also cover running clinics, for example a diabetic clinic, which monitor the disease and give lifestyle advice to patients.

*Health visitors* are well known for involvement with child care development but this is only one area of their work. They can be involved with health clinics, parenthood classes, 'Look After Yourself' lifestyle clinics and links with the elderly – not just the baby clinic and childhood immunisation programme. Patients do not have to be referred to the health visitor by the doctor, they can refer themselves.

*Midwives* carry out visits to patients before and after the birth of their babies, hold antenatal clinics including relaxation and child care instruction within the surgery to monitor the pregnancies and, as part of the 'named-nurse' continuing care policy, are present for the birth of the baby whether the delivery is at home or in the hospital. They visit the mother for a specified length of time after the birth to ensure that mother and baby are well and there are no problems.

*Physiotherapists* work in-house supplying a rapid-access physiotherapy service for patients and can also continue the treatment at the hospital should more complex equipment be required to treat the patient.

*Chiropodists* work in-house or at health centres or hospitals usually looking after the foot care of diabetic patients or the elderly, children with foot problems, pregnant women and disabled patients.

*Counsellors* work for the practice on a sessional basis counselling patients referred to them by the doctor. By employing a counsellor the practice can benefit in many ways. Practices have counsellors to help people deal with their personal problems and counselling of this nature cannot be carried out in a normal surgery appointment time. The counsellor is trained to listen to patients and help them come to terms with personal problems in a positive way. The prescribing of antidepressants and tranquillisers can be greatly reduced when patients are able to cope with their problems. Patients have to be referred by the GP to the surgery counsellor. Patients can self-refer to a private counsellor and would pay any fees for this service.

*Community psychiatric nurses* are named nurses attached to the surgery and they use their

---

**Box 15.3**  Reasons for contacting the social services department

1. *Fostering and adoption of children* – the GP will be involved in giving medical opinions about the adopters, fosterers and the children if they are registered with the practice.

2. *Accommodation for the elderly* – Should it become increasingly difficult for an elderly patient to look after themselves, or close relatives of the elderly patient are unable to cope with looking after them, the doctor may contact the social services for their help in arranging full-time care for the patient, or various in-house help or aids such as additional stair rails, equipment to help the patient bathe easily, cooker adaptations, meals on wheels and home helps.

3. *Respite care* – Some relatives who care for elderly patients in their own homes can have short periods when the patient can go into nursing home care for respite care. This gives the carer a few weeks 'holiday' and eases the strain of caring for an invalid or sick relative.

4. *Accommodation for patients* – Poor housing conditions often aggravate some health problems and the GP may recommend better housing as a clinical priority for these patients.

skills and training to treat more complex mental problems than the counsellor. Often they carry out rehabilitation work with patients discharged from psychiatric units to live in the community and with drug addicts, working closely with the GP.

*Social workers* are attached to the practice and they are the link doctor's contact when patients need additional care or services beyond medical assistance.

You may have to contact the social services department for a variety of reasons (Box 15.3).

*Macmillan nurses* are nurses especially concerned with the care of cancer patients and are often linked with hospices in the locality.

*Alternative medicine practitioners* may include aromatherapist, acupuncture, homeopathy, reflexology. These services are not commonplace and you will find that most practices do not hold them in-house and in these cases patients would have to pay privately for consultations.

It is important that you get to know the members of the primary health care team and all the practice staff as you will be working with them as part of the team. Knowledge of each role and the part they play within the organisation helps strengthen your ability to work as an efficient and valued team member.

**Reflection point**

◆ Make a note of all the professionals you come into contact with at work or on your GP placement. How does the practice encourage a feeling of team participation?

**Our responsibilities**
1. You will be treated sympathetically and politely by Practice Staff.
2. Your privacy and confidentiality will be respected at all times.
3. We will do everything possible to ensure that our systems for providing a health care service to you are reliable and effective.
4. Patients are at liberty to see any of the partners irrespective of the doctor they are registered with.
5. You will have a right to information about your own health, treatment and its likely outcome.
6. You will be offered a Health Check on joining the Practice and given information and advice on maintaining good health and avoiding illness.
7. All patients of 75 years and over will be offered an annual health check.
8. Urgent emergency cases will be seen the same day in the surgery.
9. You will be seen within 30 minutes of your appointment time unless some unforeseen emergency delays the doctor. In such a case the receptionist will keep you informed.

**Your responsibilities**
1. To be polite to doctors and staff.
2. To give the practice adequate notice if you wish to cancel an appointment.
3. To request home visits before 11.00 a.m. and only if they are medically necessary and you are too ill to attend the surgery.
4. To give at least 24 hours' notice for a request for a repeat prescription. These should be collected within one month.
5. When you are notified that a repeat prescription is due for a review you should make an appointment to see the doctor before your next request.
6. If you need to speak to a preferred named doctor you must wait until after booked surgery appointments.
7. No smoking on the premises.
8. To inform the surgery straight away if you change your address.

**Figure 15.1**  A practice charter. (Reproduced by permission of Elms Medical Centre, Chester.)

## ENSURING GOOD SERVICE

All general practices today have to have a *practice charter* listing items and standards the practice provides to its patients and also what is expected from the patients (Fig. 15.1).

A *complaints procedure* is another requirement and Health Authorities have standard information packs with guidelines to help practices put together their own procedures. Samples of these are given Figs 15.2–15.6. The Community Health Council also contacts and visits surgeries to discuss services and complaints procedures.

**Reflection point**

◆ Are these notices available in languages other than English? Consider the local population using the practice. Is this and other sources of information clear and accessible to everyone?

## OVERVIEW OF AREAS IN HEALTH CENTRES

The basic layout required in health centres includes a reception desk, patients' waiting area and a consultation room for the doctor. Not many years ago this was the norm. Today, with all the additional services doctors are obliged to provide and the services they want to provide for their patients 'in-house', much larger accommodation is required. Not only does the waiting room provide a seating area with magazines for patients and various health leaflets, you may also find areas set aside specifically with children in mind with several choices of toys and games. The in-house services supplied speed up the delivery of treatment and you will find rooms for practice nurses, counsellors, physiotherapists, chiropodists, midwives, alternative medicine practitioners and some surgeries supply an area office for district nurses and health visitors to use as a base. These additional in-house clinics allow the patient to be treated quickly, close to home, so providing better health care. There are usually additional offices for the practice manager and secretarial and computer support staff, and a library or common room where team meetings, training sessions and study can take place.

## THE IMPORTANCE OF PREMISES PRESENTATION

As previously mentioned, the premises of today's surgeries are much larger and kept to a higher standard. From the patient's point of view it is important that the waiting room is pleasant in appearance, clean and well organised with useful, informative leaflets and information to hand – and of course a good supply of recent magazines. Any notice boards should be well maintained with posters neatly and clearly laid out – not pinned up in a cluttered and disorganised manner so that patients cannot read them clearly. A badly laid out information notice board is worse than useless to patients or the surgery attempting to inform them.

Some surgeries may have piped music in the waiting room, which is pleasant to listen to and relaxing for the patient, or perhaps a television screen with video presentations of health information.

A play area or corner for young children with simple toys and children's books is usually available, but again this should be kept tidy and all toys should be in a clean condition and washed regularly. Care needs to be taken in this area with regard to age suitability, hygiene and space required.

**Reflection point**

◆ List the toys you think are suitable and unsuitable.

Seating should be in good condition and not torn and dirty. First impressions are very important and simple measures of regular maintenance

# THE ELMS MEDICAL CENTRE

## Complaints Protocol

1. All complaints concerning the practice should be referred immediately to the Practice Manager.

2. The Practice Manager will reply to/contact the complainant within two working days and investigate the complaint.

3. All details of the investigation will be recorded.

4. Once the investigation is complete the Practice Manager will report back to the Practice.

5. The Practice Manager together with the partnership will decide how best to report back to the complainant.

6. An explanation will be sent to the complainant within ten working days. *(If this is not possible, the Practice Manager will contact the complainant to explain the delay and set a revised time scale for the conclusion of the procedure.)*

7. If, following the practice's explanation, the complainant remains dissatisfied, they will be informed of their rights to pursue the complaint via the Health Authority.

   The Health Authority number is 01244 650300

   (Freephone Number 0800 132996)

**Figure 15.2** A complaints protocol. (Figs 15.2–15.6 reproduced by permission of Elms Medical Centre, Chester.)

---

## THE ELMS MEDICAL CENTRE

### <u>Notice to Patients</u>

*In this Practice we operate a
Practice Complaints Procedure as
part of the N.H.S. system for dealing
with complaints.*

*Our aim is to provide you
with a high standard of care and we
will try to deal swiftly
with any problems that may occur.*

*Our Practice Manager or Senior
Receptionist can give you further
information.*

---

**Figure 15.3**  A notice to patients about the practice complaints procedure.

in these areas will keep your surgery welcoming and efficient.

### Reflection point

◆ If you were planning to redecorate and replace items in your surgery, what would be the most important points to take into consideration?

Cleanliness in the surgery is obviously very important. Surgery cleaners or contract cleaners should ensure that treatment rooms are thoroughly cleaned to avoid any possibility of infection being spread from unhygienic standards. The waiting room areas, reception and toilets should be cleaned daily and all rubbish placed outside in appropriate containers ready for collection. All treatment room and consultation room clinical waste is classed as *hazardous waste* and should be placed in yellow waste collection bags ready for collection with the yellow sharps polythene

*This leaflet explains how you can share your views or concerns about any aspect of the service you receive from us.*

If you would like more information about this you can telephone
The Complaints Manager on
FREEPHONE 0800 132996

If you prefer you can write to

The Chief Executive
South Cheshire Health
Authority
FREEPOST (no stamp required)
1829 Building
Countess of Chester Health Park
Liverpool Road
Chester CH2 1YZ

You can also obtain independent advice from the Local Community Health Council at Chester
Tel: 01244 318123

# The Elms Medical Centre

*Your views – good or bad – are always welcome.*

Our simple procedure can resolve concerns quickly and confidentially by giving you an opportunity to express your views – *good or bad*.

The person responsible for dealing with your comments and complaints is the Practice Manager.

If you have discussed an issue with her and are still unhappy we respect your right to make a complaint.

We have forms available for you to fill in with details of your complaint.

Your complaint should be made as soon as possible, ideally within a matter of days, so that we can investigate accurately while things are still fresh in everyone's mind.

If, for some reason this is not possible you should let us have details of your complaint:

– within 6 months of the incident

## OR

– within 6 months of discovering that you have a problem, provided this is within 12 months of the incident.

We will send you a written acknowledgement within two working days of receiving your complaint and will do all we can to complete our investigation within ten working days.

We will then write to you again with an explanation or suggest a meeting with those involved.

If you are still dissatisfied or perhaps you don't want to raise the problem directly with us, you have the right to raise the matter with South Cheshire Health Authority.

**Figure 15.4** Excerpt from a leaflet explaining the complaints procedure.

# COMPLAINTS FORM

## Complainant Details

Surname _____     Forenames _____

Address _____

_____

_____

Telephone _____     Date of Birth _____

### Patient's Details (where different from above):

Surname _____     Forenames _____

Address _____

_____

_____

### Details of Complaint

*(including date(s) of events and persons involved)*

_____

_____

_____

_____

_____

*(Continued on next page)*

Date: _____     Complainant's Signature: _____

### Where the complainant is not the patient:

I authorise the complaint set out above to be made on my behalf (name) _____
and I agree that the practice may disclose to (name) _____ (only
in so far as is necessary to answer the complaint) any confidential information about me which I
provided to them.

Patient's Signature: _____     Date: _____

**Figure 15.5** A complaints form.

# COMPLAINT ACTION SHEET

**Complainant Details**

Surname _____ Forenames _____

Name of Patient (if different)_____

Consent required:    YES/NO                    Date of Birth: _____

Contact Telephone Number: _____

First Contact made by:   Telephone _____    Letter _____ Personal Contact_____

Date of Incident: _____    Complaint Received: _____

Received by: _____

---

**Summary of Complaint:**

_____
_____
_____
_____
_____
_____

Action Taken: _____
_____

---

**DETAILS OF RESPONSE**

By (name): _____

First Contact made by:   Telephone _____    Letter _____ Personal Contact _____

Date:
_____
_____

Outcome:     SATISFIED/DISSATISFIED

If dissatisfied has the complainant been informed of Health Authority contacts    YES ☐    NO ☐

**Figure 15.6**  A complaint action sheet.

box containers that hold used syringes. These are collected separately by a Health Authority authorised contractor and are incinerated, for they are governed by the Control of Substances Hazardous to Health Regulations 1989. (See Chapter 17.)

## Stationery stock items

The doctors' surgeries should be well stocked with relevant forms and information that are used regularly and the medical secretary should check these stocks weekly and ensure they are restocked and arranged tidily. The doctor does not want to have to search for regularly used forms in the middle of a consultation.

General stationery stocks should be monitored and a list of stock requirements given to the practice manager for reordering; often this is the responsibility of the secretary. Postage costs and postage stamps will be recorded and a record kept.

**Reflection point**

◆ What other stocks should be checked?

## SECURITY

A great deal of equipment and confidential information is held in surgeries so security is of prime importance. Not only the commitment every employee makes to confidentiality of patient details and information but the need to safeguard the building that houses this information is of prime importance. You may be asked to sign a notice of confidentiality, as shown in Figure 15.7. Burglar alarms and security lighting are additions to robust locks and sometimes, depending on the area the premises are in, and insurance requirements, metal shutters are installed.

Personal safety is obviously important. Although very few patients are aggressive or

---

### CONFIDENTIALITY

In the course of your duties you may have access to confidential material about patients or other health service business. On no account must information relating to identifiable patients be divulged to anyone other than authorised persons.

Failure to observe these rules will be regarded by your employers as serious misconduct which could result in serious disciplinary action being taken against you, including dismissal.

Signed _____

Date _____

**Figure 15.7**   A notice of confidentiality.

disruptive to the general running of the surgery, there are a small number that have to be carefully managed. The experienced receptionist will cope relatively easily with these patients and it would be an advantage to spend part of your induction period to the practice in reception observing these skills. Keeping calm, not taking any verbal abuse personally, quietly but positively dealing with the situation will often keep the agitated and abusive patient under control – at least until the practice manager or a doctor is available. (See also Chapter 5.)

Violent patients are a similar concern and obviously your safety and the safety of other patients in the waiting room are of paramount importance. Some surgeries have alarm buttons to press when staff are in threatening situations. For uncontrollable patients calls should be made directly to the police station to have them removed from the premises. Very often doctors will refuse to treat patients who are violent or abusive to staff and have them removed from the list if incidents occur repeatedly. The Health Authority or various private training companies hold courses in dealing with this type of patient.

**Reflection point**

◆ Find out if there is any training available in your surgery.

## Computers

Computers and medical equipment need to be security code marked and computer file servers should be enclosed in security casing and secured to the floor.

## Building maintenance

GPs by law have a duty to ensure the safety of anyone who enters the surgery and may be liable if there is an accident. Therefore it is extremely important to keep the building and all equipment in good repair. All maintenance to the fabric of the

building, equipment and security systems is organised by the practice manager. Yearly maintenance checks are made on equipment and the building security system and any repairs are carried out immediately.

## CONCLUSION

This chapter has provided you with an overview of general practice and the people who work there, and the roles and functions they fulfil. It has also provided you with an introduction to your role as a medical secretary within general practice. The most important thing to remember is that in general practice you are part of a team that ensures the effective running of the practice. Do take the opportunity to find out as much as possible about the practices you have been involved with either as a medical secretary or as a patient.

**Exercises**

◆ Compare different practice leaflets if available. Try to think of them from the perspective of the patient. Are they helpful? Could they be improved?

◆ Find out more about other personnel involved. Talk to them about what they do.

◆ All practices are different. While on work placements compare notes on the variety of provision and collect material to help you build a full picture of your surgery's methods of ensuring good service.

## FURTHER READING

National Health Service. General Medical Services. Statement of Fees and Allowances (The 'Red Book') NHS Executive

National Health Service 1996 Practice-based complaints procedures. HMSO, London

Quinn NE, Simon P 1996 The GP Receptionists Handbook. Baillière Tindall, London

# 16

# The working practice

*Barbara Jones*

## OBJECTIVES

◆ To provide a broad outline of the numerous tasks carried out daily in general practice

◆ To explain the uses of computer systems in general practice

◆ To give an overview of procedures carried out in general practice and associated claims

◆ To emphasise the importance of accurate storing and retrieval of information

◆ To give a brief description of the various rotas and protocols used to ensure good practice.

## INTRODUCTION

This chapter explains how general practice works and the medical secretary's role in assuring the smooth running of the practice. There are a vast range of tasks performed in general practice and teamwork and accuracy when carrying out your part are essential.

## GENERAL PRACTICE TODAY

High standards are needed in today's general practice. Not only are there high levels of skills and services available for patients, patients themselves have high expectations of health care professionals and are far more demanding of the services they receive.

### Practice charter

Guidelines for your surgery will be contained in the practice charter and it will state the maximum length of time patients are expected to wait until they are seen. They should be informed if the doctor is delayed and offered another appointment on another day if they cannot wait. Patients need to know what basic standards they can expect from their surgery and the practice charter provides this. In order for the standards to be met there should also be some commitment from the patient and many surgeries have patient's charters to give guidance on the basic expectations the surgery has of its patients. When patients and doctors work together in this way standards and services can be delivered in a positive and effective manner. (See Figure 15.1 in the previous chapter for an example of a practice charter.)

# COMPUTERS IN GENERAL PRACTICE

In order to keep pace with the many changes and provide a caring yet efficient service in general practice use of modern technology is essential (see also Chapter 8). There are several computer medical systems developed especially for use in the doctor's surgery such as Vamp, EMIS, Meditel and Genisyst. These systems provide quick and efficient retrieval of information. Whichever system you are working with, it will be networked throughout the surgery. This allows doctors, reception and the medical secretary access to enter their specific work onto the patients' files at the same time. The computer stores all this information and it can be searched, audited or retrieved at any time within minutes. All the clinical systems have a basic word-processing program which enables the medical secretary to type referral letters and process bulk recall letters to groups of patients by mail merging quickly and efficiently.

Most practices will also have various software on additional computers which enable them to carry out word processing with advanced capabilities for producing professional posters, newsletters and leaflets. Spreadsheet software is also invaluable for producing activity statistics, rotas, financial forecasts, etc. The practice accounts system and payroll, whether they are specific software packages purchased for the task or in-house spreadsheets, are also quick, easy and accurate in producing the financial records of the practice.

Medical systems in general practice are fast becoming indispensable. All the information required on all aspects of the work carried out in the practice once entered on the computer can be easily retrieved in a variety of ways and statistics can be produced to give a simple picture of the facts you are looking at. Entering patients on the medical database dispenses with the necessity to compile an age/sex register.

The manual age/sex register consisted of writing out two identical index cards containing basic details of patients when they registered. They were then filed into two sections of male and female and one set filed alphabetically and the other in date of birth order.

Once entered on the computer details from the database can be searched rapidly on many areas, not just name and date of birth. Addresses, families, streets or roads or even postcodes depending on the information you need to match can be obtained with just a few key strokes, not an afternoon or days checking through thousands of cards.

As long as you have adequate back-ups for the daily input of data you need never worry too much should the computer go down or 'crash'.

Details entered on the practice computer can be accessed from any computer in the building as long as it is networked to the main file server. Claims, medical histories, health promotion details and also referral letters can be viewed quickly and easily from anywhere in the building without having to check files, folder or log books in reception, the practice manager's room, or treatment room.

**Reflection point**

◆ What are the security and confidentiality issues concerning the increased use of computers in general practice?

## Fundholding software

With the introduction of fundholding in 1991 medical software companies had to develop accounting systems that could link with the medical systems and store information to cost the services requested by the practice for their patients. Referral letters processed on the medical system would be automatically linked to the fundholding. The systems had to produce accountancy reports and balances for large budgets allocated to practices to pay for the hospital services and specialties needed for their patients. All hospital services including laboratory tests, X-rays, physiotherapy (in-house and at the hospital), operations and initial and follow-up consultations with hospital clinicians were chargeable to the practice budget. It would be the practice's responsibility to get the best service and value for money and keep within their allotted budgets. Reports and statements had to be sent to the Health Authority each month and accounts would be audited at the end of the financial year. Some fundholding practices purchased a separate fundholding system and entered all fundholding data onto that computer separately from the main medical system.

With the changes in the pipeline for the internal market of health care the use of commissioning groups appears to be the preferred route for general practice. This allows the continuing development of primary health care and also area needs or localities are taken into consideration when deciding on the services required from hospitals. The need for computerised systems to provide quality information will remain.

### Pathology tests – laboratory links to practice

Another development that is gaining momentum in general practice is the linking up of hospital computers with the general practice computer to provide fast and efficient service in supplying the results of patients' laboratory tests. Tests are carried out at the pathology laboratory and the results entered on the hospital computer. These are sent down the modem line to the practice 'mail box' at a certain time during the night and the practice computer 'picks up' information placed in its mail box at a set time during the night or early morning. When the computers are switched on in the morning the patient's results are already on computer for the doctor to view and assess.

Health Authorities are in the process of developing these links even further, so that hospitals and surgeries can send referral letters via links and actually book appointments for patients at the hospital on the same day they visit surgery. Information links with Health Authorities would certainly cut down on the amount of paper that is passed via surgery delivery services informing practices of courses, item of service updates, and the mass of information that is churned out weekly in order to keep communications between

Health Authority and surgery up to date. Once these advances have been perfected the benefits of computer networks can be fully appreciated.

## REGISTERING NEW PATIENTS

The use of the computer with GP/HA Links in processing registrations and claims forms is another area where time and efficiency has been applied. Managed well, this system has been a great success for improved accuracy of claims and prompt payment.

The medical computer system is used in all aspects of general practice. If we begin at the beginning, the first contact a patient makes at a surgery to register is logged on the computer. The details from this medical card, form FP4 or a purple registration form FP1, are checked through with the patient to ensure all entries are completed. There is a section on the back of the FP1 form which allows patients to give consent for their inclusion on the Organ Donor Register. The details are then entered on the computer system and sent through a modem line via GP Links to the Health Authority and are acknowledged within 48 hours. Once acknowledged, the patient is included on the list of the practice and the doctor begins receiving a payment each quarter for supplying medical services.

Once the patient is accepted onto the list, the Health Authority requests the medical records from the patient's previous doctor and usually within 4 to 6 weeks the full medical notes are with the practice. If the doctor requires the records immediately the Health Authority will request them from the previous doctor or if they are moving into the area from another Health Authority they will contact them to obtain the records urgently.

Patients registering with the practice must be living within the practice boundary. The doctors define their practice area in the practice leaflet and patients living outside this should not be registered. When patients register with the doctor they are usually asked to make an appointment with the practice nurse for a registration health check. This allows the practice to obtain information from patients on their medical history and details of any medicines they are presently taking. Details from the health check are valuable ways of obtaining the health promotion data which is requested each year.

Basic instructions on how to register patients and when to fill in the various claims forms are usually available in all practices (Figs 16.1–16.3). These help staff learn new procedures and are invaluable when new staff or college students begin work in the practice. Although the forms and regulations governing them are the same you will find that each practice has its own way of implementing them.

## PATIENTS LEAVING THE PRACTICE

When patients leave the practice the Health Authority requests the patient's records and it is the practice's duty to return these records immediately. The patient's new doctor may require urgent access to the medical history; therefore it is a responsibility that must be fulfilled. Medical records are the property of the National Health Service and therefore belong to the government. The doctors are responsible for them during the time the patient is registered with the practice and strict confidentiality rules must be adhered to by practice staff.

## CHANGING DOCTORS

Patients have a right to change doctor without giving a reason and therefore they can move from practice to practice if they are not satisfied with the service they are receiving. In cases like this their medical records will be requested via GP Links if you are computerised or from a computer printout sheet from the Health Authority called the FP22.

## DECEASED PATIENTS

If a patient dies the Registrar of Births and Deaths notifies the Health Authority and they will then remove the patient from your list and request the return of the medical records. More internal work within the practice has to be carried out when a patient dies as they may be on a consultant's list at the hospital or on a practice recall list (Fig. 16.4). If this is the case the hospital has to be contacted so that no future appointments will be sent to the patient's home. It can be very distressing for relatives if this happens. It is usually the medical secretary's job to contact the hospital and inform the necessary department of the death.

## FORM FP69

This is a green card which is issued to the surgery when an item of mail has been sent from the Health Authority to the patient and been returned by the Post Office as not living at that address anymore. The Health Authority then put a tag on the patient's computer details, produce and send the green card to the practice. If it is not returned with the patient's new or confirmation of the address within six months the patient is taken off the list. The records are returned and stored at the Health Authority until the patient registers elsewhere in the same area or the United Kingdom and then the notes are passed on to the new doctor.

## REMOVAL OF A PATIENT FROM THE PRACTICE LIST

A doctor can remove a patient from his or her list without giving a reason. This may be because the patient has moved outside the practice boundary or because there has been an irretrievable breakdown in the relationship between the doctor and patient. Patients who behave badly at the surgery by being violent or abusive to staff, or make inappropriate demands upon the practice by making frequent request for home visits for minor issues, can be removed from the list at the doctor's request.

**Reflection point**

◆ Patients don't have to give a reason when they change doctors. Should doctors have to give a reason when they remove patients from their practice list?

# APPLICATION TO GO ON A DOCTOR'S LIST
## (Form FP1)

### General Information

Applications to go on a doctor's list are filled in and used when the patient wishes to register with the practice but does not have his NHS medical card available.

### FILLING IN THE FORM

1.  Ensure the form is filled in completely with:

    a)  The **patient's Surname, Forename, any previous Surname.**
    b)  **Date of birth** and **whether male or female** (this is particularly useful when accepting foreign patients with unusual names).
    c)  Their **full permanent address with Postcode.**
    d)  Enter **the NHS number**, if known.
    e)  Their **previous doctor** and his **address.**
    f)  The **patient's previous address, town or country of birth.**

2.  *If the patient has been abroad* and is returning to reside in this country *or moved from abroad to live here*, ensure that:

    a)  The **date of arrival** is filled in and the **date when the patient left this country.**

3.  **Ensure the patient signs the form and dates it.**

4.  On the reverse of the form **the parent** of a child applying to go on the doctor's list should **tick the box for child health surveillance.**

    The patient can also indicate whether or not they would like to be an organ donor.

5.  On the reverse of the form you should also **ensure the doctor's name, code number and signature with date are entered.**

    *It is essential that all new patients over 5 years old MUST BE OFFERED AN APPOINTMENT TO SEE THE PRACTICE NURSE FOR A HEALTH CHECK.*

**Figure 16.1**    Instructions for filling out Form FP1 (application to go on a doctor's list).

# BASIC REGISTRATION PROCEDURES

When a patient comes to the Reception Desk to register with the Practice they should be asked to fill in an FP1 (purple form) if they do not have their Medical Card.

Ask them to go to the side of the Reception Desk if reception is busy to fill in the form.

When they have completed the form the receptionist should check that all the details have been filled in correctly.

An appointment can then be made for the patient with the nurse for a registration health check *(or an appointment with the doctor if the patient needs to be seen)*.

The FP1 or Medical Card should then be placed in a doctor's tray ready for the doctor's signature. (Applications should be signed daily.)

The Senior Receptionist will make out the Provisional Record folders with the necessary basic continuation sheets for each new application and the folder will be filed with the Provisional Records awaiting full records from the Health Authority.

Once the applications have been signed by the doctor they should be forwarded in the bag to Pen y Bont Surgery to be processed on the GP Link computer.

When the full notes arrive at Pen y Bont surgery from the Health Authority they will be summarised and sent out to the branches.

The provisional notes at the branch will be matched and added to the full notes and the complete file will then be stored in the main records filing system.

The empty Provisional Folder can then be re-used for another patient.

Keeping provisional files separately not only prevents duplication of files and applications but it is a good check on any outstanding medical records.

The Senior Receptionist should check each week if any Provisional Files are over six weeks old. If there are any, a list should be drawn up with the patient's name, date of birth, address and date of registration and forwarded to the Practice Manager who will arrange contact with the Health Authority requesting the notes.

**Figure 16.2** Instructions relating to basic registration procedures.

## Procedure for Completing a Temporary Resident/ Immediately Necessary/Emergency Treatment Form

1. Obtain relevant details to complete the form (over the telephone or at the desk).

3. Make the appointment entering TR by the name of the patient in the Appointment Book.

4. **Write the date and time of the appointment at the top of the form.**

5. **Place the form at the front desk** – to await the appointment.
   *(This will prevent any TR forms being lost/duplicated or incomplete forms being sent to the doctor for signing and notes can be kept on those who did not attend.)*

6. When the patient arrives for the appointment carry out the following:

   a) Quickly **check the form** *to ensure we have all the necessary information filled in.*

   b) **Give the form to the patient** *to confirm that all the details entered are correct.*

   c) *When satisfied the form has been completed correctly give the patient the form and* **ask them to take a seat and hand it to the doctor/nurse when they are called in.**

7. Once the patient has been seen the doctor/nurse will then fill in the consultation details. The doctor will sign and date the form and it should be placed with the records and returned to reception at the end of surgery. **N.B.** *(Practice Nurse appointments will only have consultation details and should be placed in a doctor's tray for the doctor to sign once they have been seen and have been returned to reception with the other surgery records.)*

8. Staff filing records should remove any TR forms and place them in the TR box, and file them alphabetically.

9. The Senior Receptionist will check them weekly and return all TRs that have expired to Pen y Bont. There they will be checked and forwarded to the Health Authority.

**Figure 16.3** Instructions for completing a temporary resident form.

---

## Deceased Patient Protocol

When the surgery is informed that a patient has died at home:

1. **Pass the message on to the Doctor** together with the patient's Medical Record.

2. **Write** the **name of** the **patient** on the **Notice Board** in reception.

3. **Doctor** will **inform the District Nurse** if it was a terminally ill patient.

4. **Secretary** will **inform** the **hospital** by telephoning.

5. Ensure the **cause of death** is **entered** in the **Medical Record** and on the **computer**.

---

**Figure 16.4** A deceased patient protocol.

## APPOINTMENT SYSTEMS

Each doctor, nurse or in-house specialty will have their own schedule of surgeries. Doctors will normally have two surgeries per day – morning and afternoon/evening. Consultation times may vary from doctor to doctor, with one allowing 10 minutes per consultation and another 7 minutes, another only 5 minutes, another less but with a block every few patients to allow for 'catch up' time. Check the appointment system where you are and analyse how it is worked out and what types of things have been taken into consideration when setting it up.

### Reflection point

◆ A patient is demanding an immediate appointment – consider ways of coping with this demand and a full appointments schedule.

Consultation statistics can be compiled easily from computerised appointment systems but practices usually have an adequate manual system in place to monitor the workload and home visits made by the doctors (Fig. 16.5).

The various clinics held in the practice, e.g. diabetic, asthma, antenatal, child health, minor surgery, will all be set in a regular pattern and the correct length of time allowed for each type of consultation.

The community midwife will hold her clinics to monitor the progress of the mother and developing baby and gradually build a relationship with the mother-to-be to give her confidence to discuss any problems or worries. Should the mother wish to have a home delivery then this relationship is paramount. The shared-care system of midwife, doctor, health visitor and members of the primary health care team all working together for the benefit of the patient is highlighted in the antenatal and child health clinics, where several disciplines of medical care are pulled together.

| APRIL '98 | Doctor | Branch A | Branch B | Branch C | Home Visits | Total Consultations |
|---|---|---|---|---|---|---|
| | DR A | 62 | 280 | 91 | 49 | 482 |
| | DR B | 194 | 259 | 183 | 65 | 701 |
| | DR C | 122 | 219 | 129 | 46 | 516 |
| | DR D | 112 | 72 | 165 | 47 | 396 |
| | DR E | 97 | 192 | 65 | 21 | 375 |
| | DR F | 193 | 212 | 102 | 49 | 556 |
| | | 780 | 1234 | 735 | 277 | 3026 |

| MAY '98 | Doctor | Branch A | Branch B | Branch C | Home Visits | Total Consultations |
|---|---|---|---|---|---|---|
| | DR A | 194 | 188 | 189 | 40 | 611 |
| | DR B | 191 | 217 | 81 | 55 | 544 |
| | DR C | 150 | 303 | 99 | 60 | 612 |
| | DR D | 151 | 140 | 175 | 54 | 520 |
| | DR E | 107 | 180 | 42 | 45 | 374 |
| | DR F | 163 | 91 | 89 | 21 | 364 |
| | | 956 | 1119 | 675 | 275 | 3025 |

| JUN '98 | Doctor | Branch A | Branch B | Branch C | Home Visits | Total Consultations |
|---|---|---|---|---|---|---|
| | DR A | 310 | 176 | 97 | 47 | 630 |
| | DR B | 179 | 179 | 123 | 56 | 537 |
| | DR C | 217 | 201 | 104 | 45 | 567 |
| | DR D | 108 | 131 | 175 | 41 | 455 |
| | DR E | 258 | 261 | 136 | 53 | 708 |
| | DR F | 150 | 149 | 42 | 38 | 379 |
| | | 1222 | 1097 | 677 | 280 | 3276 |

| JUL '98 | Doctor | Branch A | Branch B | Branch C | Home Visits | Total Consultations |
|---|---|---|---|---|---|---|
| | DR A | 214 | 174 | 99 | 44 | 531 |
| | DR B | 180 | 189 | 191 | 67 | 627 |
| | DR C | 110 | 334 | 121 | 46 | 611 |
| | DR D | 96 | 55 | 37 | 27 | 215 |
| | DR E | 191 | 209 | 175 | 52 | 627 |
| | DR F | 220 | 251 | 91 | 55 | 617 |
| | | 1011 | 1212 | 714 | 291 | 3228 |

| AUG '98 | Doctor | Branch A | Branch B | Branch C | Home Visits | Total Consultations |
|---|---|---|---|---|---|---|
| | DR A | 175 | 197 | 79 | 50 | 501 |
| | DR B | 159 | 168 | 106 | 42 | 475 |
| | DR C | 122 | 261 | 72 | 55 | 510 |
| | DR D | 147 | 95 | 97 | 47 | 386 |
| | DR E | 91 | 140 | 137 | 45 | 413 |
| | DR F | 166 | 120 | 75 | 37 | 398 |
| | | 860 | 981 | 566 | 276 | 2683 |

| SEPT '98 | Doctor | Branch A | Branch B | Branch C | Home Visits | Total Consultations |
|---|---|---|---|---|---|---|
| | DR A | 189 | 265 | 53 | 47 | 554 |
| | DR B | 181 | 196 | 185 | 53 | 615 |
| | DR C | 123 | 152 | 126 | 42 | 443 |
| | DR D | 103 | 249 | 117 | 32 | 501 |
| | DR E | 157 | 114 | 149 | 39 | 459 |
| | DR F | 152 | 177 | 46 | 34 | 409 |
| | | 905 | 1153 | 676 | 247 | 2981 |

**Figure 16.5**  Consultation statistics.

## Home Visit Totals 1998–99

| Doctor | Apr-98 | May-98 | Jun-98 | Jul-98 | Aug-98 | Sep-98 | Oct-98 | Nov-98 | Dec-98 | Jan-99 | Feb-99 | Mar-99 | Year Total |
|--------|--------|--------|--------|--------|--------|--------|--------|--------|--------|--------|--------|--------|------------|
| DR A | 49 | 40 | 47 | 44 | 50 | 47 | 43 | 0 | 0 | 0 | 0 | 0 | 320 |
| DR B | 65 | 55 | 56 | 67 | 42 | 53 | 56 | 0 | 0 | 0 | 0 | 0 | 394 |
| DR C | 46 | 60 | 45 | 46 | 55 | 42 | 61 | 0 | 0 | 0 | 0 | 0 | 355 |
| DR D | 47 | 54 | 41 | 27 | 47 | 32 | 53 | 0 | 0 | 0 | 0 | 0 | 301 |
| DR E | 21 | 45 | 53 | 52 | 45 | 39 | 39 | 0 | 0 | 0 | 0 | 0 | 294 |
| DR F | 49 | 21 | 38 | 55 | 37 | 34 | 67 | 0 | 0 | 0 | 0 | 0 | 301 |
| Total | 277 | 275 | 280 | 291 | 276 | 247 | 319 | 0 | 0 | 0 | 0 | 0 | 1965 |

## Doctor Consultation Totals

| | Apr | May | Jun | Jul | Aug | Sept | Oct | Nov | Dec | Jan | Feb | Mar | Total |
|------|------|------|------|------|------|------|------|------|------|------|------|------|-------|
| Dr A | 482 | 611 | 630 | 531 | 501 | 554 | 0 | 0 | 0 | 0 | 0 | 0 | 3309 |
| Dr B | 701 | 544 | 537 | 627 | 475 | 615 | 0 | 0 | 0 | 0 | 0 | 0 | 3499 |
| Dr C | 516 | 612 | 567 | 611 | 510 | 443 | 0 | 0 | 0 | 0 | 0 | 0 | 3259 |
| Dr D | 396 | 520 | 455 | 215 | 386 | 501 | 0 | 0 | 0 | 0 | 0 | 0 | 2473 |
| Dr E | 375 | 374 | 708 | 627 | 413 | 459 | 0 | 0 | 0 | 0 | 0 | 0 | 2956 |
| Dr F | 556 | 364 | 379 | 617 | 398 | 409 | 0 | 0 | 0 | 0 | 0 | 0 | 2723 |
| TOTAL | 3026 | 3025 | 3276 | 3228 | 2683 | 2981 | 0 | 0 | 0 | 0 | 0 | 0 | 18219 |

## Branch Totals

| | X | Y | Z | TOTAL |
|---------|------|------|------|-------|
| APRIL | 780 | 1234 | 735 | 2749 |
| MAY | 956 | 1119 | 675 | 2750 |
| JUNE | 1222 | 1097 | 677 | 2996 |
| JULY | 1011 | 1212 | 714 | 2937 |
| AUG | 860 | 981 | 566 | 2407 |
| SEPT | 905 | 1153 | 676 | 2734 |
| OCT | 917 | 1037 | 720 | 2674 |
| NOV | 0 | 0 | 0 | 0 |
| DEC | 0 | 0 | 0 | 0 |
| JAN | 0 | 0 | 0 | 0 |
| FEB | 0 | 0 | 0 | 0 |
| MARCH | 0 | 0 | 0 | 0 |
| TOTAL | 6651 | 7833 | 4763 | 19247 |

**Figure 16.5**   (continued)

Child health clinics run by the health visitor in conjunction with a doctor from the surgery monitor child development and immunisation status. These clinics are usually noisy, relaxed and welcoming. Mothers with babies and toddlers attend to have the baby weighed and discuss with the health visitor any queries they may have about feeding or concerns about their child. As their baby grows regular development checks on height/length, weight, hearing and eyesight, movements, etc., are carried out by the doctor at various ages, usually 6 weeks, 4 months and 3 years. Some Health Authorities have additional checks. If the child does not seem to be developing to the standard levels required, the doctor can refer the child to a relevant hospital consultant for appropriate treatment or diagnosis at an early stage.

The practice nurse will be responsible for holding clinics in the surgery with direct access to the doctor if any urgent treatment is required. The nurse's rotas may be set for different types of clinics, e.g. asthma, well woman, or a general clinic is held which covers all areas and opportunistic screening or monitoring is carried out. As various checks and procedures take different lengths of time, basic timetables have to be made available for the receptionist when booking appointments and written instructions should also be in place (Figs 16.6 and 16.7). This avoids overbooking appointments and allows a greater understanding of the procedures being carried out.

You should speak to the practice nurse in your surgery and find out how tests and checks are carried out and how the way you carry out your job could help improve the system or communications.

---

## PRACTICE NURSE APPOINTMENTS

1. **09.00 a.m. Appointments**

   (i)  These are for **3 blood tests only.**

   (ii) Patients for blood tests after fasting may have **water only** from **9.00 p.m.** the previous evening.

   *N.B. Non-fasting blood tests may be done at any time **before 3.00 p.m.** in ordinary sessions.*

2. **Telephone Calls**

   Only urgent calls are to be put through during clinic sessions.
   Non-urgent calls, e.g. Reps or patients requesting advice will be taken between
   12.30 p.m.–1.00 p.m. and 5.30 p.m.–6.00 p.m.

   *N.B. Some calls are not appropriate for the Practice Nurse to deal with, e.g. questions about contraception, medication and illness.*

3. **Drug Company Representatives**

   From September **Reps** will be seen by appointment only at **12.30 p.m. on Tuesdays.**

4. **Reasons for Patient Appointments**

   When making appointments please state reason.

**Figure 16.6** Instructions for practice nurse appointments.

## PRACTICE NURSE CLINICS

| CLINIC | TIME | URINE SAMPLE | DOCTOR ON PREMISES | NOTES |
|---|---|---|---|---|
| **ASTHMA** | Monday 3.00–5.30 p.m. | 1st Appointment | YES | NEW PATIENTS – 30 minute appointments (i.e. 1st Appointment) Patients may be seen at other times by Jenny. Patient must bring inhalers, etc., with them. |
| **BABY IMMUNISATIONS** | Tuesday 2.00–3.30 p.m. | NO | YES | *NB. Not carried out if baby unwell.* Appointments may be made during ordinary sessions if unable to attend clinic. |
| **BLOOD TESTS** Fasting Blood Tests | 9.00 a.m. | NO | NO | **3 only at 9.00 a.m. (none Wednesday)** For Fasting Blood Tests – Patients are allowed only water for 12 hours before the test is taken. |
| Non-fasting | Before 3.00 p.m. | NO | NO | For Non-fasting Blood Tests appointments can be made anytime before 3.00 p.m. |
| **CORONARY HEART DISEASE SCREENING** | Wednesday 3.00–5.15 p.m. | YES | NO | 30 minute appointments. ECG appointments can be made during CHD Clinics (30 minute appointments). |
| **DRESSINGS** | Anytime | NO | YES | |
| **EAR SYRINGING** | Anytime | NO | YES | ONLY patients who have been referred by the doctor or have had their ears syringed before can make an appointment. Drops (e.g. Olive Oil or Sodium Bicarbonate) to be used in ear twice a day for four days before appointment. |
| **ECG** | CHD Clinic or 11.45 a.m. | NO | NO | 30 minute appointment. |
| **HOLIDAY IMMUNISATIONS** | Anytime | NO | YES | APPOINTMENT to be made to discuss requirements and start immunisation programme. |
| **INJECTIONS** | Anytime | NO | YES | ZOLADEX, MYOCRISIN, B12, SUSTANON given by nurse. *NB. NOT the contraceptive injection.* |
| **NEW PATIENT HEALTH SCREEN** | Anytime | YES | NO | 15 minute appointment. |
| **OVER 75 YEAR CHECK** | Anytime | YES | NO | 30 minute appointment. |
| **REMOVAL OF SUTURES** | Anytime | NO | YES | |
| **SMEAR ONLY** | Anytime | | | Repeat smears – 15 minute appointments. |
| *DIABETIC CLINIC* | *Tuesday 9.30–10.30 a.m.* | YES | YES | *Carried out by District Nurse* |

**NB.** The Well Woman Clinic has now been cancelled. Patients requiring smears can make appointments at any time with the nurse using a 15 minute appointment.

**Figure 16.7** A timetable for practice nurse clinics.

## Advance booking of appointments

Surgeries will all have their own set ruling on advance bookings. Some have no limit, others only allow booking one month ahead, some only next day appointments. Often there is a high percentage of non-attenders in the surgeries which book ahead. Perhaps this is a reason for next day only appointments. Doctor time wasted when patients do not turn up is very annoying, especially when receptionists are having to tell other patients there are no appointments available. The education of patients in this area would be a great advantage for the busy practice.

Advance appointments are usually made for courses of immunisations, recalls for cytology screening, blood pressure monitoring, specific review requests by the doctor. Minor surgery clinics usually have a waiting list and advance bookings are needed here. When a person is to have a minor operation in the surgery, no matter how small, he or she should sign a basic consent form agreeing to the procedure to be carried out. In some cases, for example elderly patients, it is wise to inform patients that they may like to have someone with them or arrange transport home after the surgery.

There is also the 'Open Surgery' where no appointments are made and patients turn up and sit and wait and take it in turn to see the doctor. In this case, systems have to be in place to provide a smooth and orderly running of the session to avoid patients jumping the queue and causing disruption. Medical records have to be retrieved quickly as patients arrive in order that the doctor will have all the necessary information or recent laboratory tests to hand when seeing the patient.

Receptionists normally book all appointments but the medical secretary may be asked by the doctor to contact the patient and book a suitable appointment with the nurse, a doctor, counsellor, physiotherapist, etc. Ensure you know how to use the system whether it is computerised or manual.

## HOME VISITS

Home visits are intended for the elderly, housebound or very sick patients too ill to come down to surgery. Some people abuse this service and request home visits for trivial reasons – sometimes simply because there have been no free appointments available for that morning. Requests for home visits usually have to be made before 11.00 a.m. Staff taking requests for home visits have to be accurate in obtaining and passing on information. The patient's name, address and telephone number if they have one and, should someone else be phoning in for them, that person's details would also be useful in case the doctor wishes to contact them for further details of the sick patient. A brief description of the reason for the call will give the doctor insight into the urgency of the visit and also alert the receptionist. Obviously a patient with a pain in the chest or left side, difficulty breathing, having a fit, collapsing, etc., would ring alarm bells for the receptionist to pass the message immediately to the duty doctor. It is not the receptionist's job to diagnose the severity of the illness – this is solely the doctor's responsibility. Should you take a call of this nature do not hesitate to pass it on to a doctor or in his absence the nurse for further medical advice. The receptionist should get the patient's medical records out ready for the doctor and ensure the correct address is on the record. Sometimes patients could be staying with friends or relatives while they are ill or perhaps could have moved and not informed the practice. Always check these details as delays in finding the patient's home in urgent requests could be fatal.

Patients should always be asked if they can get down to surgery, as doctors can see more patients in the surgery in the time that it takes travelling out and visiting just one patient. Sometimes requests are made for home visits for very minor symptoms and each surgery will have its own standard procedure of accepting and filtering these calls.

**Reflection point**

◆ Discuss the most professional and tactful ways of finding out the details needed for a home visit.

## REPEAT PRESCRIBING

The use of the computer with repeat prescribing is again invaluable. Computers record all processed requests for medication and can be set to limit the number of prescriptions issued in order that the doctor can monitor the progress of the drug. If this has been done or the practice has a protocol then most patients on repeat medication will have to see their doctor within a set time for review. Good practice dictates that regular monitoring of repeat prescribing is a necessity. Most practices will have a protocol to cover this which will include setting limits on the computer to indicate when a patient needs to see the doctor before another repeat can be issued (Fig. 16.8).

Computerised scripts also give a quick method of checking if a patient is over-using a certain drug and it can be brought to the attention of the doctor immediately. Often there is a simple reason for it but if a patient is over-using a prescribed drug it could be doing more harm than good and the doctor needs to assess the situation.

**Reflection point**

◆ What guidelines do you have in place for monitoring repeat prescribing? What advantages do prescribing protocols give the practice?

When repeat prescriptions have been run off they also produce an attached side slip of paper listing all the medications the patient has on repeat. The patient then selects the items he or she requires and returns the slip to the practice a few days before the medication runs out. The receptionist then processes the request and the doctor signs it. The script is then placed ready for collection at the surgery or, as is increasingly popular, a named chemist of the patient's choice can collect it. Often these chemists provide a delivery service, which is ideal for housebound or elderly patients.

## Controlled drugs

These are drugs which cannot be included in a repeat prescribing list but have to be handwritten by the doctor. They include drugs used by addicts and they have to be issued on a special prescription which gives the chemist authority to dispense the drug on a daily basis.

## Drug audits

Information from the repeat prescribing can give insight into the prescribing patterns of doctors and highlight areas where expensive drugs are being used inappropriately. A practice formulary will help standardise this but very often the formulary is an ongoing process. Regular searches on the computer for specific drug usage and meetings to discuss the drug budget can help control the amount of spending in this area.

## PROCESSING ITEM OF SERVICE CLAIMS

The use of the computer system for other transmitted paperwork such as claim forms for contraceptive care, minor surgery, vaccination and immunisation, temporary residents, registration health check, night visits, maternity services can all be claimed quickly and efficiently via GP Links. If the surgery is not linked via a modem to the Health Authority then claims forms for each item of service have to be completed and sent each week via the internal delivery/collection service. The manual paper system is far more time consuming for staff and payments for the claims are delayed while the Health Authority enter them on their computer and return any incomplete forms before processing of the payments.

As a medical secretary you may be responsible for some of the item of service claims, for example maternity claims or for the cytology or vaccination and immunisation targets. This involves accurate record-keeping of women eligible for cervical cytology screening, informing the Health Authority of all women who have had hysterectomies, who are pregnant and are unable to attend for

# Repeat Prescribing Protocol

This protocol sets out the procedures used for dealing with requests for repeat prescriptions at the main surgery and branch surgeries in order to provide a rapid, accurate and safely monitored service to the patient.

### Authorisation

Repeat prescriptions are computer-generated. The items are put on the computer only with doctor authorisation and the following standards apply.

No controlled drugs are included.

Drugs with an abuse potential are only included at the doctor's discretion.

The number of prescriptions to be issued is authorised by the doctor, entered on the computer and the computer will then indicate 'expired' once this number is reached. Any additional requests made after this can only be processed after obtaining authorisation from the doctor to update the computer to allow further issues of repeat prescriptions.

This information will also show up on computer generated surgery lists which are used for all surgeries. Drugs can be added or omitted by the doctor writing the drug dose and quantity on the surgery list.

There is a liaison slip which is attached to the manual record when hospital requests for drugs are made via discharge letters or clinic letters. The doctor fills in the information he requires on the computer prescription. This is on approved FP10 computer forms and comes complete with counterfoil which lists numerically the drugs which can be repeated.

### Requesting a Repeat Prescription

Ideally, the patient will present the counterfoil from his previous prescription to the reception staff with the requested items endorsed. They will accept it and inform the patient that the repeat prescription will be available in 24 hours.

In the case of postal requests a stamped self-addressed envelope is required in order to return the prescription by post.

The patient may request prescriptions to be collected from the branch surgeries. A daily processing of prescriptions at the branch surgery ensures they are available for collection.

### Telephone Requests

We encourage the patient not to telephone for repeat prescriptions yet sometimes this is unavoidable. Telephone requests are accepted between 11.00 a.m. and 12.00 noon in the morning and from 2.00 p.m. to 3.00 p.m. in the afternoon. These should be emergency calls only and patients are told the prescription will be ready after 2.00 p.m. the following day.

**Figure 16.8**   A repeat prescribing protocol.

### Generating a Prescription

The repeat prescription requests are entered into the computer and one member of staff and one terminal are dedicated to this task in the mornings. (Urgent requests during the afternoon are processed by the receptionist on duty.)

All patients who are on repeat medication have a repeat prescription request limit on their computer file. Each request is entered on the computer and attention is drawn to the number of repeats that have been issued.

Once the number allowed has been reached the computer indicates that authorisation has 'expired'. This alerts the receptionist to gain further authorisation from the doctor before further repeats are issued.

The receptionist enters all the requests for prescriptions received that morning into the computer and once completed the computer will print out a batch of all of the morning's requests. This is usually completed by 12.00 noon.

The prescriptions are then separated for the individual doctors and are presented for signing.

By 1.00 p.m. each day the process is completed by the reception staff. The prescriptions are sorted for posting to the patient or collection.

### Generic Prescriptions

When the doctor changes a patient's prescription from a brand named drug to the generic equivalent a short letter is attached to the prescription explaining the change to the patient.

This avoids causing the patient concern when they collect the prescription from the chemist.

### Exclusions

The computer will not print out a prescription if it has expired and will only prescribe the amount of drug authorised.

Any amendment has to be made by the doctor of the patient and the patient may be required to make an appointment for a review of his medication.

### Non-Computer Generated Repeat Prescriptions

Under certain circumstances patients request repeat prescriptions which they have had previously but they are used infrequently or for other reasons are not on the computer repeat prescribing system, e.g.

> Hayfever tablets
> Paracetamol for infants
> Preparations for head lice.

Under these circumstances the staff will accept the request but inform the patient that it cannot be issued until after surgery when the doctor will authorise the prescription whilst he is signing the computer printed repeats.

**Figure 16.8** (continued)

their screening until after the birth, or who are having some type of treatment which prevents them having their smear test at that time. The Health Authority, once notified, will then take them off the target list until the agreed time. A search on the computer of all those females who have not had their smear test and a mail merge of their addresses with a standard letter should be a job suited to the medical secretary. Keeping details of the immunisation status of children under 5 years and sending out appointment letters for them to attend the baby clinics for their immunisations when they are due may be a combined task for reception and secretary. However it is processed in your practice, inaccurate records of the cytology and immunisation registers can lose the practice a great deal of money. Computerisation of these details gives quick and accurate information, helping you to keep ahead of the necessary target levels.

# FEES PAID DIRECTLY TO DOCTORS

## Insurance medical reports

These are requests by insurance companies for medical reports on the patients. A full medical is not usually required but a standard form is supplied to obtain the necessary information for the report on the patient's health status. A patient's consent sheet or section will always be included with these requests as a report should not be processed without it. If the patient signature on a consent form is not included with the paperwork you should contact the company requesting the patient's consent and hold the application on file until it is received. Copies of these reports should be kept on file for 6 months. A patient has the right to see the report before it is sent off to the company. A place on the application form indicates this by selecting the option to see the report. If this is the case you must hold back the report for 28 days to allow the patient to contact the surgery to make an appointment with the secretary or practice manager to see the report. Once the report has been seen it can be sent off. If the

patient has not contacted the surgery within 28 days the report can be sent off. The income to the practice varies depending on the amount of information required. If a full medical is needed then the fee payable is greater. The BMA provides guidelines on appropriate and acceptable levels of charges for the doctor's work.

Sometimes a company will request a full medical and report on a person who is not registered with the practice. This is usual as some companies prefer to have an independent doctor's opinion and it may be part of your duties to contact the person and arrange a suitable time when the doctor can carry out the examination.

## Private sick notes

Sometimes patients require a private sick note for their employer or for a sickness insurance policy. A fee is charged for this and is payable by the patient.

## Travel insurance forms

Patients travelling abroad for their holidays often take out travel insurance. If they should have to claim on these policies for medical reasons they require medical evidence to support their claim. A fee is claimable from the patient or the insurance company, whoever is requesting the details.

## Death certificates

After a patient has died the doctor attending the patient issues a death certificate and seals it in the envelope provided ready for collection at the reception desk by a member of the deceased's family. A fee is charged for this.

## Cremation fees

If the deceased is to be cremated the undertaker will ask the doctor to complete Form B of the cremation forms. The doctor completing Form B asks a second doctor to complete Form C. These doctors must not be in partnership or related and they will receive the appropriate fee from the undertaker.

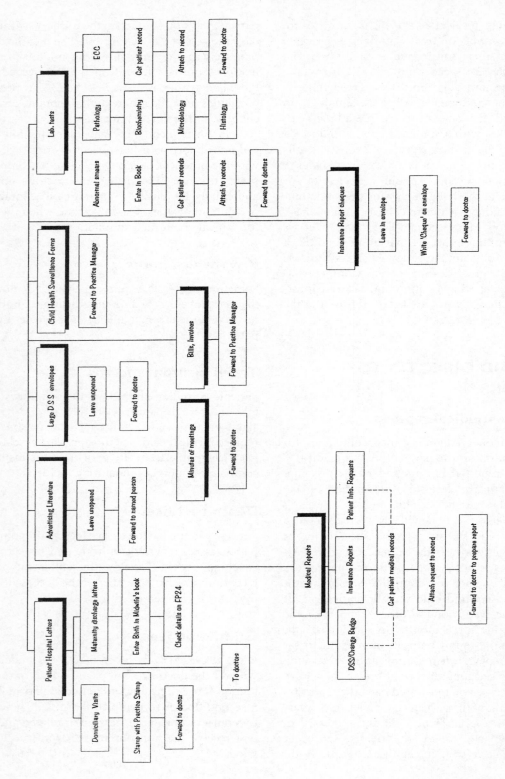

**Figure 16.9** Types of mail.

## CORRESPONDENCE AND PAPERWORK IN GENERAL PRACTICE

Letters, advertising circulars, forms, laboratory tests are part of the incoming mail that has to be dealt with in the practice and it is important that the mail is forwarded to the correct person or section to process it. Practices will all have their own system of processing the mail in the most efficient way and you should familiarise yourself with the responsibilities of the members of the practice team so that you can play your part in directing the mail to the correct person. Figure 16.9 gives an example of the types of incoming mail and how it is processed in one surgery.

## FILING

One job in general practice that is vast and never ending is the filing. Each day more hospital letters and laboratory tests come into the practice and once seen by the doctor need to be filed quickly in the patient's medical record. It is a never ending task but a most important one that should never be carried out casually or in a haphazard manner.

If clinical correspondence is filed in the wrong patient's record time will be wasted searching for it, and there will be annoying embarrassing delays for the doctor and patient while staff search for the missing item. Should a copy be requested from the hospital or laboratory it could take days to find and it does not give a very good impression of the professionalism and efficiency of the staff. A filing system that is not accurate and up to date is worse than useless.

In general practice the patients' notes will be filed in small 'Lloyd George' folders. These were produced when the NHS was first implemented and at that time there was less access to all the consultants' and laboratory tests and X-rays that can be carried out today. Over the years they have served the system well but increasingly some practices are changing over to the larger A4 size folders. They do require more space for storage but give a far easier access for doctors to see at a glance the latest test or letter. In the Lloyd George

| | | | | | |
|---|---|---|---|---|---|
| May | 3rd | Dr A | September | 6th | Dr D |
| | 10th | Dr B | | 13th | Dr E |
| | 17th | Dr C | | 20th | Dr A |
| | 24th | Dr D | | 27th | Dr B |
| | 31st | Dr E | October | 4th | Dr C |
| June | 7th | Dr A | | 11th | Dr D |
| | 14th | Dr B | | 18th | Dr E |
| | 21st | Dr C | | 25th | Dr A |
| | 28th | Dr D | November | 1st | Dr B |
| July | 5th | Dr E | | 8th | Dr C |
| | 12th | Dr A | | 15th | Dr D |
| | 19th | Dr B | | 22nd | Dr E |
| | 26th | Dr C | | 29th | Dr A |
| August | 2nd | Dr D | December | 6th | Dr B |
| | 9th | Dr E | | 13th | Dr C |
| | 16th | Dr A | | 20th | Dr D |
| | 23rd | Dr B | | 27th | Dr E |
| | 30th | Dr C | | | |

**Figure 16.10**  A doctor Saturday morning rota.

| | May 1997 | | | | | | | | | | | | | | | | | | | | | | | | | | | June |
|---|---|---|---|---|---|---|---|---|---|---|---|---|---|---|---|---|---|---|---|---|---|---|---|---|---|---|---|---|
| | 5 | 6 | 7 | 8 | 9 | 10 | 11 | 12 | 13 | 14 | 15 | 16 | 17 | 18 | 19 | 20 | 21 | 22 | 23 | 24 | 25 | 26 | 27 | 28 | 29 | 30 | 31 | 1 |
| | M | T | W | T | F | S | S | M | T | W | T | F | S | S | M | T | W | T | F | S | S | M | T | W | T | F | S | S |
| Dr A | | | | | | | | | | | | | | | | | | | | | | | | | | | | |
| Dr B | | | | | | | | | | | | | | | | | | | | | | | | | | | | |
| Dr C | | | | | | | | | | | | | | | | | | | | | | | | | | | | |
| Dr D | | | | | | | | | | | | | | | | | | | | | | | | | | | | |
| Dr E | | | | | | | | | | | | | | | | | | | | | | | | | | | | |

| | June | | | | | | | | | | | | | | | | | | | | | | | | | | | |
|---|---|---|---|---|---|---|---|---|---|---|---|---|---|---|---|---|---|---|---|---|---|---|---|---|---|---|---|---|
| | 2 | 3 | 4 | 5 | 6 | 7 | 8 | 9 | 10 | 11 | 12 | 13 | 14 | 15 | 16 | 17 | 18 | 19 | 20 | 21 | 22 | 23 | 24 | 25 | 26 | 27 | 28 | 29 |
| | M | T | W | T | F | S | S | M | T | W | T | F | S | S | M | T | W | T | F | S | S | M | T | W | T | F | S | S |
| Dr A | | | | | | | | | | | | | | | | | | | | | | | | | | | | |
| Dr B | | | | | | | | | | | | | | | | | | | | | | | | | | | | |
| Dr C | | | | | | | | | | | | | | | | | | | | | | | | | | | | |
| Dr D | | | | | | | | | | | | | | | | | | | | | | | | | | | | |
| Dr E | | | | | | | | | | | | | | | | | | | | | | | | | | | | |

| | | July | | | | | | | | | | | | | | | | | | | | | | | | | | |
|---|---|---|---|---|---|---|---|---|---|---|---|---|---|---|---|---|---|---|---|---|---|---|---|---|---|---|---|---|
| | 30 | 1 | 2 | 3 | 4 | 5 | 6 | 7 | 8 | 9 | 10 | 11 | 12 | 13 | 14 | 15 | 16 | 17 | 18 | 19 | 20 | 21 | 22 | 23 | 24 | 25 | 26 | 27 |
| | M | T | W | T | F | S | S | M | T | W | T | F | S | S | M | T | W | T | F | S | S | M | T | W | T | F | S | S |
| Dr A | | | | | | | | | | | | | | | | | | | | | | | | | | | | |
| Dr B | | | | | | | | | | | | | | | | | | | | | | | | | | | | |
| Dr C | | | | | | | | | | | | | | | | | | | | | | | | | | | | |
| Dr D | | | | | | | | | | | | | | | | | | | | | | | | | | | | |
| Dr E | | | | | | | | | | | | | | | | | | | | | | | | | | | | |

**Figure 16.11** A blank out of hours rota.

| Doctor | MV | AV | EV | NV | MB | AB | EB | NB | Total |
|---|---|---|---|---|---|---|---|---|---|
| **Dr A** | 0 | 2 | 4 | 2 | 0 | 1 | 2 | 1 | 12 |
| **Dr B** | 0 | 1 | 2 | 3 | 2 | 0 | 1 | 2 | 11 |
| **Dr C** | 1 | 0 | 5 | 2 | 1 | 0 | 0 | 2 | 11 |
| **Dr D** | 1 | 0 | 3 | 6 | 0 | 0 | 0 | 5 | 15 |
| **Dr E (Part Time)** | 0 | 3 | 0 | 1 | 0 | 1 | 0 | 0 | 5 |
| **TOTAL** | 2 | 6 | 14 | 14 | 3 | 2 | 3 | 10 | 54 |

Statistics of number of sessions per doctor carried out

**Figure 16.12**  An out of hours cooperative. V, visit; B, base.

folders, letters have to be folded, cut or shrunk to a smaller size on a photocopier in order to fit neatly in the file.

Whichever you use letters and tests are always filed chronologically with the latest at the top. The continuation sheets or cards where the doctor writes down details of the consultation can be filed in the same way or in date order with the latest at the back. This will depend on the doctor's preference in your surgery.

## PRACTICE ROTAS

Practice rotas are essential for the smooth running of the practice. They are an effective method of communication to ensure that the participants and attached staff know where clinics are being held and the staff who will be manning them, where and when doctors will be holding surgeries and when they are away. There are many types of rota and you will come across several different variations and layouts of rota in your working life. It may be a rota that includes you or simply one for your reference to enable you to carry out your work in an efficient way by knowing the exact whereabouts of doctors and staff.

### Doctor rotas

Every doctor in any surgery will work by rotas or take part in some sort of rota. It may be purely as part of an out of hours service for patients in the case of a single-handed doctor but their surgeries and various clinics will be worked on a weekly or monthly basis. Several rotas may be in use at one time in larger surgeries, such as the daily surgery rota, the on call rota and the out of hours rota (Figs 16.10–16.12). These may also include or combine holiday rotas when doctors take it in turns to have certain school or bank holidays off. If the main surgery has branch surgeries, these will also have to be included and considered in the doctor and staff rotas.

### Staff rotas

Staff rotas for morning and afternoon shifts, Saturday morning surgeries and holiday cover will also be in existence. All surgeries and the many types of clinic sessions are usually worked out on a weekly basis and hence are also part of the rota system. A great deal of 'good will' goes on in general practice when it comes to emergency cover if staff are taken ill suddenly, or the doctors decide to hold an additional surgery over bank holidays. For good planning and avoiding the day-to-day stress of ensuring cover, rotas are an essential tool in the smooth running and effectiveness of the practice. Figures 16.13–16.15 provide some further examples.

As a medical secretary it may be one of your responsibilities to update and circulate the rotas. If it is, then accuracy and full knowledge of the surgery and advance notification of cancellations or holiday bookings will be vital.

| W/C 31st July | 31 July | 1 August | 2 August | 3 August | 4 August |
|---|---|---|---|---|---|
| Sue on hols | | Wendy | Wendy | Wendy | |
| Jane on hols | Wendy | Andrea | Andrea | Andrea | Wendy |
| | | Margaret C 1–3 p.m. | Margaret C 1–3 p.m. | Margaret C 1–3 p.m. | |

| W/C 7th August | 7 August | 8 August | 9 August | 10 August | 11 August |
|---|---|---|---|---|---|
| Jane on hols | Andrea | Andrea | Andrea | Andrea | Andrea |
| Val on hols | Wendy | Wendy | Wendy | Wendy | Wendy |
| | Pauline 6 p.m. | | | | Pauline 6 p.m. |
| | Margaret C 1–3 p.m. | Margaret C 1–3 p.m. | Margaret C 1–3 p.m. | Margaret C 1–3 p.m. | Margaret C 1–3 p.m. |

| W/C 14th August | 14 August | 15 August | 16 August | 17 August | 18 August |
|---|---|---|---|---|---|
| Val on hols | Pauline 8.30 a.m.–12 noon | Pauline 8.30 a.m.–12 noon | Pauline 8.30 a.m.–12 noon | Pauline 8.30 a.m.–12 noon | Pauline 8.30 a.m.–12 noon |
| | Pauline 2 p.m.–? | Pauline 2 p.m.–? | Pauline 2 p.m.–? | Pauline 2 p.m.–? | Pauline 2 p.m.–? |

**Figure 16.13** Holiday relief cover.

| W/C 31st October 1994 | MONDAY 31st | TUESDAY 1st Nov | WEDNESDAY 2nd | THURSDAY 3rd | FRIDAY 4th | SATURDAY 5th |
|---|---|---|---|---|---|---|
| MORNING | Veronica (C)<br>Judith<br>Joyce | Veronica<br>Judith<br>Sylvia (C) | Veronica<br>Lisa (C)<br>Sylvia | Veronica<br>Lisa<br>Helen (C) | Veronica<br>Joyce (C)<br>Helen | Judith (C) |
| AFTERNOON | Veronica<br>Lisa (C)<br>Sylvia | Veronica<br>Lisa<br>Helen (C) | Veronica<br>Joyce (C)<br>Helen | Veronica<br>Joyce<br>Judith (C) | Veronica<br>Sylvia (C)<br>Judith | |

| W/C 7th November 1994 | MONDAY 7th | TUESDAY 8th | WEDNESDAY 9th | THURSDAY 10th | FRIDAY 11th | SATURDAY 12th |
|---|---|---|---|---|---|---|
| MORNING | Veronica (C)<br>Helen<br>Joyce | Veronica<br>Judith (C)<br>Joyce | Veronica<br>Sylvia (C)<br>Judith | Veronica<br>Sylvia<br>Lisa (C) | Veronica<br>Helen (C)<br>Lisa | Joyce (C) |
| AFTERNOON | Veronica<br>Judith<br>Sylvia (C) | Veronica<br>Lisa (C)<br>Sylvia | Veronica<br>Helen (C)<br>Lisa | Veronica<br>Helen<br>Joyce (C) | Veronica<br>Judith (C)<br>Joyce | |

| W/C 14th November 1994 | MONDAY 14th | TUESDAY 15th | WEDNESDAY 16th | THURSDAY 17th | FRIDAY 18th | SATURDAY 19th |
|---|---|---|---|---|---|---|
| MORNING | Veronica (C)<br>Helen<br>Lisa | Veronica (C)<br>Helen<br>Joyce | Veronica<br>Judith (C)<br>Joyce | Veronica<br>Judith<br>Sylvia (C) | Veronica<br>Lisa (C)<br>Sylvia | Helen (C) |
| AFTERNOON | Veronica<br>Judith (C)<br>Joyce | Veronica<br>Judith (C)<br>Sylvia | Veronica 6.00 p.m.<br>Lisa (C)<br>Sylvia | Veronica<br>Lisa<br>Helen (C) | Veronica<br>Joyce (C)<br>Helen | |

| W/C 21st November 1994 | MONDAY 21st | TUESDAY 22nd | WEDNESDAY 23rd | THURSDAY 24th | FRIDAY 25th | SATURDAY 26th |
|---|---|---|---|---|---|---|
| MORNING | Veronica (C)<br>Sylvia<br>Lisa | Veronica<br>Helen (C)<br>Lisa | Veronica<br>Helen<br>Joyce (C) | Veronica<br>Judith (C)<br>Joyce | Veronica<br>Judith<br>Sylvia (C) | Lisa (C) |
| AFTERNOON | Veronica<br>Helen<br>Joyce (C) | Veronica<br>Judith (C)<br>Joyce | Veronica<br>Judith<br>Sylvia (C) | Veronica<br>Lisa (C)<br>Sylvia | Veronica<br>Lisa<br>Helen (C) | |

| W/C 28th November 1994 | MONDAY 28th | TUESDAY 29th | WEDNESDAY 30th | THURSDAY 1st Dec | FRIDAY 2nd Dec | SATURDAY 3rd Dec |
|---|---|---|---|---|---|---|
| MORNING | Veronica (C)<br>Sylvia<br>Judith | Veronica<br>Sylvia<br>Lisa (C) | Veronica<br>Helen (C)<br>Lisa | Veronica<br>Helen<br>Joyce (C) | Veronica<br>Judith (C)<br>Joyce | Sylvia (C) |
| AFTERNOON | Veronica<br>Helen (C)<br>Lisa | Veronica<br>Helen<br>Joyce (C) | Veronica<br>Judith (C)<br>Joyce | Veronica<br>Judith<br>Sylvia (C) | Veronica<br>Lisa (C)<br>Sylvia | |

*N.B.* *(C) by the side of the name of a person indicates that she is responsible, during that shift, for all repeat prescriptions, prescription updates and tea making and once this work is completed the usual filing and helping with the retrieving of files and checking of the boxes of files ready for the next surgeries.*

**Figure 16.14** Reception staff rota.

Page 1

**January table (Dec '96 – Feb)**

| | Dec '96 | | January 1997 | | | | | | | | | | | | | | | | | | | | | | | | | | | Feb |
|---|---|---|---|---|---|---|---|---|---|---|---|---|---|---|---|---|---|---|---|---|---|---|---|---|---|---|---|---|---|---|---|
| | 30 | 31 | 1 | 2 | 3 | 4 | 6 | 7 | 8 | 9 | 10 | 11 | 13 | 14 | 15 | 16 | 17 | 18 | 20 | 21 | 22 | 23 | 24 | 25 | 27 | 28 | 29 | 30 | 31 | 1 |
| | M | T | W | T | F | S | M | T | W | T | F | S | M | T | W | T | F | S | M | T | W | T | F | S | M | T | W | T | F | S |
| Veronica | d | d | d | d | d | o | d | d | d | d | d | o | d | d | d | d | d | o | d | d | d | d | d | o | d | d | d | d | d | o |
| Helen | pm | am | am | o | pm | o | pm | pm | am | d | d | o | pm | pm | am | am | am | o | o | pm | pm | pm | am | o | am | am | d | pm | pm | am |
| Lisa | am | am | o | pm | pm | am | am | am | am | o | pm | pm | pm | pm | am | o | pm | o | pm | o | am | pm | am | o | am | o | pm | pm | am | o |
| Sylvia | am | o | pm | pm | am | o | am | am | o | pm | pm | am | am | o | am | pm | am | o | am | pm | am | am | am | o | o | pm | pm | am | am | o |
| Judith | o | pm | pm | am | am | am | am | o | pm | pm | am | am | o | am | o | am | pm | am | pm | am | am | am | o | o | pm | pm | am | am | o | o |
| Joyce | pm | pm | am | am | am | o | pm | am | pm | am | am | o | am | pm | pm | am | am | o | am | am | am | o | pm | o | pm | pm | am | am | pm | o |

**February table (February – March)**

| February | | | | | | | | | | | | | | | | | | | | | | | | March |
|---|---|---|---|---|---|---|---|---|---|---|---|---|---|---|---|---|---|---|---|---|---|---|---|---|
| | 3 | 4 | 5 | 6 | 7 | 8 | 10 | 11 | 12 | 13 | 14 | 15 | 17 | 18 | 19 | 20 | 21 | 22 | 24 | 25 | 26 | 27 | 28 | 1 |
| | M | T | W | T | F | S | M | T | W | T | F | S | M | T | W | T | F | S | M | T | W | T | F | S |
| Veronica | d | d | d | d | d | o | d | d | d | d | d | o | d | d | d | d | d | o | d | d | d | d | d | o |
| Helen | pm | am | am | o | pm | o | pm | pm | am | am | o | o | pm | pm | am | am | o | o | pm | am | am | o | pm | am |
| Lisa | am | am | am | o | pm | o | am | am | o | pm | pm | am | am | am | am | o | pm | am | am | am | am | o | pm | o |
| Sylvia | am | o | pm | pm | am | o | am | o | pm | pm | am | am | am | o | pm | pm | am | o | am | o | pm | pm | am | o |
| Judith | o | pm | pm | am | am | am | o | pm | pm | am | am | am | o | pm | pm | am | am | o | o | pm | pm | am | am | o |
| Joyce | pm | pm | am | am | am | o | pm | pm | am | am | am | o | pm | pm | am | am | am | am | pm | pm | am | am | am | am |

**March table (March – April)**

| March | | | | | | | | | | | | | | | | | | | | | | | | April | | | | | | |
|---|---|---|---|---|---|---|---|---|---|---|---|---|---|---|---|---|---|---|---|---|---|---|---|---|---|---|---|---|---|---|
| | 10 | 11 | 12 | 13 | 14 | 15 | 17 | 18 | 19 | 20 | 21 | 22 | 24 | 25 | 26 | 27 | 28 | 29 | 31 | 1 | 2 | 3 | 4 | 5 | 7 | 8 | 9 | 10 | 11 | 12 |
| | M | T | W | T | F | S | M | T | W | T | F | S | M | T | W | T | F | S | M | T | W | T | F | S | M | T | W | T | F | S |
| Veronica | d | d | d | d | d | o | d | d | d | d | d | o | d | d | d | d | d | o | d | d | d | d | d | o | d | d | d | d | d | o |
| Helen | pm | am | am | o | pm | o | pm | am | am | o | pm | o | pm | pm | am | am | am | o | am | o | pm | pm | am | o | am | am | o | pm | pm | am |
| Lisa | am | am | am | o | pm | am | pm | pm | am | o | pm | o | pm | pm | am | am | am | o | o | pm | pm | am | am | o | pm | o | pm | pm | am | o |
| Sylvia | am | am | o | pm | pm | o | am | am | o | pm | pm | am | am | o | pm | pm | am | o | pm | pm | am | am | am | o | am | o | pm | pm | am | o |
| Judith | o | pm | pm | am | am | o | o | pm | pm | am | am | am | o | am | o | pm | pm | o | am | am | am | o | pm | o | pm | pm | am | am | o | o |
| Joyce | pm | pm | am | am | am | o | pm | pm | am | am | am | o | pm | am | am | o | pm | o | am | am | am | o | pm | am | pm | pm | am | am | pm | o |

Key: 'd' = DAYS; 'am' = MORNINGS (from 8.15 a.m. to 1.00 p.m., Saturday 8.30 a.m. to 12 noon); 'pm' = AFTERNOONS (from 1.15 p.m. to 6.00 p.m.).

**Figure 16.15** Receptionists' rota for 1997.

## CONCLUSION

From the contents of this chapter you can see that there are many areas to general practice. You may not have to know every detail of all the forms and procedures but a good general knowledge of all these aspects is essential. Knowing who deals with what, when people are available, where people are, etc., enables you to pass on doctor, patient, hospital queries to the right person quickly and efficiently. This will eliminate delays and give a good impression of the working efficiency of the surgery. It will also show you as a confident, capable and caring secretary.

 **Exercises**

An up-to-date procedure folder or book is a useful reference tool. Would you be able to work with the practice staff in producing one? What problems might you encounter?

List the rotas used at your practice. Are they helpful or confusing? Could you improve communications by implementing a set rota?

## FURTHER READING

Salisbury C, Sawyer T 1998 Handbook of practice nursing, 2nd edn. Churchill Livingstone, Edinburgh

Quinn NE, Simon P 1996 The GP's receptionist's handbook. Baillière Tindall, London

Pickersgill D 1992 The law and general practice. Radcliffe, Oxford

Jones T 1996 The structure of the NHS. Publishing Initiatives, Thetford

# 17 Clinical considerations

*Stephanie J Green*

## OBJECTIVES

- To promote an awareness of health and safety issues in general practice
- To describe procedures for infection control and disposal of waste
- To provide an understanding of sterilisation procedures
- To highlight the importance of safe handling of specimens
- To provide an outline of tests and investigations in common use.

## INTRODUCTION

This chapter is intended to make the medical secretary aware of their responsibilities within the general practice and of various important practical issues in relation to the clinical environment. It will refer in a more applied way to issues mentioned in previous chapters, especially Chapters 3 and 10. Because the medical secretary works as one of the team within the general practice environment means an understanding of the issues covered in this chapter is most important.

General practices need to provide safe and healthy working conditions with everyone able to work together in an informed and therefore confident manner. They should all know where problem areas might be and how they can be overcome safely and satisfactorily. When working in a medical environment in whatever capacity, it is important that the following issues are addressed by each member of the team. Whatever our role, none of us can work alone here.

In Chapters 3 and 10 reference has been made to health and safety legislation at work. In this chapter, we will look at the specific application to general practice, not forgetting that the responsibilities lie with both the employee and employer, as in any other workplace.

## HEALTH AND SAFETY

The aim of the Health and Safety at Work Act 1974 is to ensure the safety, health and welfare of both people at work and those who are not working but may be at risk from those who are – in the case of general practice this will be clients or patients. There are obligations laid down for employers, who should prepare a consultative policy for health and safety in their workplace. There are also requirements for the employee, these are:

◆ to take due care of themselves and others while at work
◆ to abide by agreed policies
◆ to make correct use of protective clothing
◆ to attend training
◆ to ensure that safety procedures are observed and maintained.

General practice will have particular concerns which will be addressed in this chapter, but it will do no harm to remember some of the day-to-day issues that are included within the health and safety legislation. These are the provision of eating facilities, heating, lighting and consideration for visitors, whether it is the postman or a patient. There will be more specific medical points to consider here, but there is a legal obligation to produce a safety policy if there are more than five employees – which will inevitably apply to most general practices. In hospitals there are special departments devoted to occupational health and infection control.

**Reflection point**

◆ As a medical secretary there will be specific health and safety issues which might affect your work. What do you think they are? What does health and safety legislation have to say about the management of these issues. If you do not know ... FIND OUT! As a clue, one of them might include the optician.

# ACCIDENTS

The responsibility for the prevention of accidents rests with every member of the workforce. Every member of the team should be safety conscious, from the safe cleaning of floors to the safe disposal

**Box 17.1   Procedure for accidents**

◆ Report any accident to the practice manager.
◆ Maintain an accident book. This should be available for recording any incidents. Each incident should be described fully, signed and dated.
◆ Serious incidents resulting in permanent damage or death should be reported to the Health and Safety Executive.

of contaminated waste. In general practice the points listed in Box 17.1 should be followed.

## Control of Substances Hazardous to Health – COSSH

These regulations state that any dangerous or hazardous substance which is being used in general practice should be:

◆ identified
◆ given a description of the precautions which are to be taken and the hazards they might present
◆ given a plan of use
◆ provided with a contingency plan, should an unplanned occurrence take place.

Likewise, staff who may come into contact with hazardous substances must understand any risks involved and the precautions which must be taken. New staff must be given adequate instruction and supervision.

In a clinical environment such as general practice, there are bound to be substances which could be hazardous to health and safety and in a small workforce these could involve staff other than the practice nurse. These are:

◆ phenols
◆ bleaches
◆ industrial methylated spirit
◆ formaldehyde.

These should all be stored in a locked cupboard and separated from other lotions.

# INFECTION CONTROL

## Hand care

One of the most important aspects of controlling infection is basic handwashing. Poor handwashing techniques have been found to be an easy source of cross-infection, as areas of the hands can be missed if this is hastily carried out.

### Reflection point

◆ How do you wash your hands? Make a list of the occasions you know you should use thorough handwashing as part of a procedure. Is this just theoretical or do you think you actually carry this out? Now consider the general practice – are there additions to make to your list?

Extra protection for hands needs to be considered. Staff should always cover cuts and abrasions with a waterproof dressing, which should be regularly changed. If you have a problem with chapped skin or dermatitis, gloves should be worn to protect you from infection. There are different types of gloves that may be used:

◆ the household variety are used for cleaning
◆ non-sterile single use are used for examination and may be made of thin polythene or latex. Single use gloves are manufactured to a Department of Health specification
◆ surgical gloves are of a different specification and withstand sterilisation.

Wearing gloves does not remove the need to wash your hands thoroughly before and after any task or patient contact. This will include cleaning instruments, handling specimens, disinfectants and for cleaning up any form of spillage.

Having considered the importance of hand care, we also need to look at other aspects of basic hygiene. It has been shown that bacteria can multiply on moist soap and fabric towels, so to reduce the risk of cross-infection, soap dispensers and paper towels should be provided and elbow taps fitted, especially in clinical areas, to reduce hand-to-hand contamination. In surgical areas hand disinfectant solutions, which are often a mixture of chemical disinfectants such as chlorhexidine and alcohol, will be used before invasive procedures are undertaken.

## Protective clothing

There are occasions when there is a further risk of contamination, including clothing. For these procedures, disposable plastic aprons, face masks and eye protection may be necessary. All staff need to be familiar with procedures for dealing with body fluids should accidents happen. We may well be aware of the risk that HIV infection poses, but we must not underestimate the risk from other serious infections, such as hepatitis B.

## Spillage

If you are required to clear up any spillage of blood or any body fluids, the following points must be observed:

◆ wear rubber gloves and apron
◆ use disposable towels to absorb the spill
◆ use domestic bleach or Milton 10 000 p.p.m. to treat the spill and leave for 10 minutes
◆ after 10 minutes, discard the towels into the standard yellow waste bag for disposal.
◆ alternatively, chlorine granules may be supplied to cope with these situations – these inactivate any infectious agent; follow the manufacturer's instructions on the container.

Spillage on carpets can be a problem – if it has had a protective treatment applied to it, it may be possible to clean it with hot soapy water once the spillage has been cleared. Check with the manufacturer's instructions first. Perhaps this should be a planning consideration in the first place!

Spillage of mercury from a broken sphygmomanometer or thermometer needs very different treatment. This requires special precautions as it can give off toxic fumes. It should be contained within the machine where possible or tipped into an airtight container and covered with water. There are special kits available to cope with mercury spillage and advice might be obtained from a local pharmacist.

## Injury

As part of infection control it is necessary to consider what is best practice in the event of injury (Box 17.2).

## Immunisation

Most practices will provide protection for their staff with immunisation against hepatitis B and all staff should make sure that they are up to date with protection against tetanus, polio and tuberculosis.

## Work surfaces

As already discussed in Chapter 10, general cleaning must be of a high standard. However, in clinical sit-

---

### Box 17.2   Dealing with injury

*Needle stick or sharps injury*

- Encourage free bleeding
- Wash with soap and water
- Do not suck the wound
- Report the incident to the practice manager and record in the accident book
- Seek further advice or treatment

*Splash injury in the eyes*

- Crying will help to wash substances out
- Wash out using copious amounts of cold water
- Seek further treatment

*Blood*

- On skin with no cut or abrasion, wash with soap and water
- In mouth, spit out, rinse and spit again

---

uations, extra care must be taken. Work surfaces and trolleys should be cleaned before and after any procedure. Either industrial spirit 70% or Milton 1:1000 spray is adequate for cleaning glass surfaces or any others used during a sterile procedure.

## DISPOSAL OF WASTE

Waste can be divided into

- clinical waste
- sharps
- general waste.

### Clinical waste

This is waste such as human tissue, body fluids, contaminated material, swabs and dressings. The Health and Safety Act 1974 and the Environmental Protection Act 1990 state that this type of waste must be disposed of in yellow plastic bags, sealed, labelled with its source and incinerated. In this way clinical waste is readily recognised nationwide. Many Local Health Authorities operate a service which will provide bags and ties and will collect and dispose of the waste.

### Sharps

Blades, glass ampoules, syringes and needles, which should be kept as one unit once assembled, should all be disposed of into a special 'sharps' box. The following points must be remembered:

- the box should be out of the reach of children
- do not force or overfill a box
- do not try to retrieve anything from inside it once deposited
- the box should be closed and sealed when three-quarters full.

Once sharps boxes are sealed they are disposed of in the same way as the yellow clinical waste sacks. These should all be stored in a locked cupboard or room, to which the public have no access, until the contractor collects the rubbish. Sharps boxes should not be put inside any bags. Each practice should nominate a procedure for the regular changing of yellow bags and boxes.

## General waste

This should be placed in disposable bags and put into the local authority waste bin. Remember to check which is your designated day for collection. Local authorities have rules about how they will collect and empty bins, arrangements for bank holidays, etc. – it is a good idea to check these should you move to a new area. It is important that cleaning staff regularly empty bins from all areas as well as re-stocking items such as paper towels in cloakrooms. Remember that cleaning staff must be carefully protected from any potential injury or contamination.

## STERILISATION PROCEDURES

Part of a comprehensive infection control must include the methods by which articles used in general practice, whether for treatment or diagnosis, are rendered safe for use. Although the practice nurse will be the main professional concerned in this area, the informed medical secretary should also have a working knowledge of accepted protocols and the methods used in each practice.

## Pre-cleaning

Each practice must develop safe practice for the collection of dirty/used instruments from consulting rooms. One procedure may be to provide a named collection box, containing soapy water to soak articles, in each consulting room or treatment area. The disposal of these articles is usually the responsibility of the practice nurse on a daily/twice daily basis. In any event, used instruments must be thoroughly cleaned before they can be sterilised. When cleaning instruments, remember:

- to use a separate 'dedicated' sink for the cleaning process – a dirty area
- to wear household rubber gloves
- to wear a plastic apron, used for that job only and disposed of after use
- to use detergent and hot water to clean instruments, taking care to remove blood or other organic matter and paying particular attention to the joints, hinges and serrations of instruments

- to rinse carefully
- not to use a brush unless you protect your face, especially your eyes.

If these points are not observed properly, not only will staff put themselves at risk of contamination, but the instruments may not be in a fit state to be sterilised. If contaminants are left on instruments, those areas will fail to be sterilised properly and microorganisms could then survive the sterilising process.

## Sterilisation

As discussed in Chapter 10, autoclaves are considered to be the most efficient method of sterilisation, and this is the method most safely used in general practice. It is necessary to understand how each machine works and to follow the manufacturer's instructions for use and packing. Separate instruments need to be placed open in the autoclave so that each surface is exposed to the sterilising process. Gallipots and receivers should be put on their sides.

Health and safety note: leave instruments to cool down in the autoclave once the cycle is complete.

Following completion of the cycle, sterilised instruments can be laid inside a sterilised bowl or pack for a limited amount of time prior to a procedure. Ideally, instruments should be sterilised immediately before use. Instruments which are clean but unsterile should be stored in a dust-free environment.

## Chemical disinfectant

This method of rendering articles safe for use may have to be used on some occasions, but only when an autoclave is unsuitable. This is because the heat or pressure used in the autoclave may damage a piece of equipment made from material which cannot withstand the process. These may include leads, thermometers, nebuliser masks and mouthpieces. In these instances the following may be used:

- hypochlorite solution such as Milton, used in a spray form or as a soaking solution for 30 minutes.

◆ alcohol/industrial methylated spirit 70% used to immerse instruments for 10 minutes. There are also 70% alcohol wipes which may also be supplied for consulting rooms to clean surfaces or to wipe low risk items such as ear syringe nozzles.

The use and regular changing of these substances will probably be the responsibility of the practice nurse.

Lotions used for cleaning skin before an invasive procedure such as with minor surgery or IUCD fittings come in sterile 'one use' sachets. Cetrimide or normal saline are the lotions commonly used.

## SAFE HANDLING OF SPECIMENS

It goes without saying that specimens of any form will only be taken by trained staff with experience. These are performed to aid diagnosis and to help with the management of disease. However, there are some principles to be observed in the case of any member of staff who might receive a specimen or be required to deal with the dispatch of a specimen at any time. First and foremost are the health and safety considerations we have already looked at such as:

◆ wearing protective gloves and aprons
◆ ensuring that the tops of containers are tightened and secure to prevent spillage.

Because samples of all kinds are dealt with in general practice, it is necessary for a well ordered system to be organised, in many cases with cooperation with the local laboratory staff. Many general practices have a computer networked system with the local laboratory, enabling them to receive information and test results much faster and more efficiently than previously, when postal systems were the only resource. In addition to this, some hospitals and laboratories have a collection system organised with many general practices, enabling specimens to be transported on a daily basis at a known time. This is of great benefit, especially in more rural areas, where transport can be a problem and normal postal services would take too long.

However, some specimens may still need to be sent by normal postal services, in which case, post office regulations requiring secure packing must be adhered to. It may also be necessary to use a 'Biohazard' sticker on any specimen sent for testing, whether to a laboratory or through the post. All specimens should be considered to be a potential risk but some may be known to be a high risk, for example infectious diseases such as hepatitis B or HIV. In these cases a unique code instead of the patient's name may be used in order to maintain confidentiality.

When specimens are to be sent for analysis:

◆ accompanying forms must be completed accurately – check that the correct date and time of collection is filled in and that it has been signed
◆ check that the specimen container is labelled with the correct patient details
◆ check that the form's details and the patient details match.

You may find that some practices ask patients to put their own specimens into the transporting bag, thus making it unnecessary for staff to touch anything which may constitute a hazard. Marsupial bags are used in some areas – this is a polythene bag which is designed to take a laboratory form, which has a smaller sealable bag attached to it for the specimen. This is to lessen the risk of forms and specimens being parted and lost, which is not only dangerous but extremely annoying to both patient and staff.

Specimens which are to be collected by internal transport systems will be put together in a marked box ready for collection at a stated time.

Some specimens are analysed in the practice. These should also have a proper collection point. This will probably be organised by the practice nurse.

Specimens which are spilt should be dealt with as described in the section on spillage. Any glass involved or bits of containers should be removed into a sharps container using forceps. Always wear gloves for your protection.

It is important that adequate stocks of both forms and the corresponding containers are kept in all the relevant consulting and treatment rooms, so that tests may be performed immediately without the need for another appointment.

It is also important that medical secretaries have a working knowledge of how tests are carried out in their particular practice, who collects them, whether patients are expected to transport a sample to the laboratory themselves and how long one might expect a test to take. This will vary from not only one practice to another but from one area to another. Rural practices may do many more tests on the premises than inner city practices, who may use hospital facilities more readily.

Some specimens require special storage until they are dispatched. They should all be kept in a cool place to lessen the likelihood of deterioration. Some samples may even change in some way, which could produce a false result. If a sample has to be kept for a longer period of time it should be refrigerated. If there is any doubt, the laboratory should be consulted for their advice on safe storage.

### Reflection point

◆ What do you think are the most common types of samples likely to be sent from general practice? When you go on work experience make a point of finding out how your practice organises these investigations.

## Test results

It is most important that any test taken in the practice is recorded in the patient's notes. Some practices also keep a record of tests taken so that late or mislaid results may be traced. This form of log or record may also be used to audit the number of tests for the practice. Fundholding practices will be particularly interested in this in view of budgeting.

Just as important as sending results is how results are dealt with on return to the practice. Normally test results will be returned to the prac-

tice via the internal system or post office services and also by computer link as a back-up. Facsimile machines should never be used for sensitive or confidential material. Staff should be aware of the time lapse that may be involved between sending and receiving a test result, so that patients can be accurately advised. Many practices have a firm policy on processing test results and may use a stamp to summarise the possible actions, which the secretary should use. Care should be taken so that the actual results are not obliterated! Test results, once stamped, should be circulated around the medical staff, who will tick the appropriate box for action. They may also give information to staff on instructions to be given to the patient. These may be:

◆ to make a further appointment – this may be urgent or as soon as possible
◆ to pick up a prescription
◆ to make an appointment for further tests with the practice nurse.
◆ no action necessary.

If a test result has been found to be very abnormal the laboratory staff may telephone the practice immediately to advise them of this. In this case, the patient's notes should be extracted straight away and the appropriate doctor informed. It might be a good idea to have relevant telephone numbers ready as well, should the doctor wish to speak to the laboratory and the patient.

Remember, too, that test results which are obtained in hospital will go firstly to the hospital doctors who requested them, and then to the general practice by letter. It is always possible to speed this up by speaking either to the consultant's secretary or to the laboratory directly. It may be important to know a test result before a patient keeps an appointment with a doctor, as treatment may well depend upon that result.

It is also important that each practice has a policy on giving the test results over the telephone. Obviously, staff must be conversant with the practical considerations as described in this section, but there are other issues to consider. Some practices will not give test results to patients over the telephone.

### Scenario

A patient, whose name you do not recognise, telephones for her test result. How would you guarantee that you are talking to the person they say they are?

How would you differentiate between patients with the same surname, or between members of the same family with the same initials?

This chapter has demonstrated the need for cooperation both within the primary health care team and with other professional staff working in other areas. Remember, patient care is at the centre of the activity here, not just the efficient circulation of paper!

## TESTS AND INVESTIGATIONS

This section provides a summary of the more usual tests that may be encountered while working in general practice. From time to time there will be others which you will need to find out about.

### Blood tests

#### Haematology

◆ Full blood count (FBC). This will include:
Hb – haemoglobin, to check for anaemia
RBC – red cell count, to check for abnormalities
WBC – white cell count, patients on certain drugs need regular checks. Also used for the investigation and treatment of disease such as leukaemia.
◆ ESR – erythrocyte sedimentation rate, indication of infection or inflammation.
◆ Plasma viscosity is also used in the same way as ESR.
◆ International normalised ratio (INR) – for the management of patients on anticoagulant therapy.
◆ Platelet count – to aid the diagnosis of infection, inflammation, malignancy and trauma.

◆ Clotting times – to check the clotting system. Used in the diagnosis of haemophilia and obstructive jaundice.
◆ Prothrombin times – used in the treatment of haemorrhagic disease.
◆ Paul–Bunnell – for the diagnosis of glandular fever (mononucleosis); also the Monospot test.
◆ Rose–Waaler.  ⎫ both used in the diagnosis
◆ Latex fixation. ⎬ of rheumatoid arthritis.
◆ Antinuclear fact/antibody (ANF/ANA) – for lupus erythematosus.

### Bacterial blood tests

◆ VDRL (Venereal disease reference laboratory), TPHA (Treponema pallidum haemoglutin assay), WR (Wasserman reaction), GCFT (Gonococcal complement fixation test).
◆ Widal reaction – to test for typhoid, paratyphoid and brucellosis.

### Biochemical blood tests

◆ Blood sugar – for the diagnosis and management of diabetes.
◆ Glycosylated haemoglobin (HbA1) also for the management of diabetes.
◆ Cardiac enzymes – to diagnose myocardial infarction (heart attack).
◆ Urea and electrolytes (U & Es) + creatinine – for the management of kidney disease and to monitor patients on diuretics. If potassium levels are particularly required this will need to be from a fresh sample, and may only be taken in the morning.
◆ Liver function tests (LFTs) – to measure enzymes and salts for a number of conditions.
◆ Thyroid function (TFTs) – for the diagnosis and management of thyroid disease and to check on the dosage of thyroxine in treatment.
◆ Cholesterol and lipid profile – to screen for cholesterol problems, especially hypercholesterolaemia.
◆ Serum lithium – patients who are on lithium treatment require 3-monthly tests to check that levels are correct.

## Other tests

◆ Guthrie test – a test performed on infants between the 6th and 14th day after birth to diagnose phenylketonuria.
◆ Serum electrophoresis – to analyse different proteins present in the blood.
◆ Hormone levels – e.g. oestrogen in pregnancy.
◆ Screening for drug abuse.

## Urine tests

Stix tests are simple tests performed commonly in general practice, these may be:

◆ glucose – for glucosuria found in diabetes and sometimes in pregnancy
◆ albumin/protein – for albuminuria/proteinuria, found in pregnancy and in renal disease
◆ blood – for haematuria, found in infection and renal disease.

## Laboratory tests

### Microbiology

One of the most common tests performed in this laboratory is *culture and sensitivity*. This is used to identify an infection and to find out which antibiotic will treat any identified infective organisms. These are said to be 'sensitive' to that particular antibiotic. If antibiotics appear to have no effect on an organism it is said to be 'resistant'. Culture and sensitivity is used to identify infections in specimens from the following sources:

◆ urine
◆ faeces
◆ sputum
◆ throat
◆ nose
◆ ears
◆ urethra
◆ vagina
◆ wounds.

### Histology

This laboratory studies tissue microscopically. One of the most common areas of study used in

general practice is *cytology*. Here specimens are examined for abnormal cells and the following tests will be performed.

◆ Cervical smears – to screen for carcinoma of the cervix. This process is subject to the achievement of targets for general practitioners to encourage high attendance from patients and to obtain adequate smears.
◆ Sputum analysis – to diagnose disease, especially malignant, usually taken in the early morning before eating or drinking.
◆ Urine – to test for abnormal cells.
◆ Oral – to diagnose abnormal cells from the oral mucosa.
◆ Semen analysis – after vasectomy to ensure successful surgery, or for investigation of infertility.

## Investigations

### X-ray

Many investigations will have to be performed in hospital, usually in the outpatient department. These are often within the X-ray department which now performs many new and different investigations (Box 17.3).

### Endoscopic examination

This is an examination using an instrument made of flexible tubing, which is lit and is able to inspect hollow organs. A list of some of the endoscopic examinations follows:

◆ gastroscopy
◆ bronchoscopy
◆ oesophagoscopy
◆ endoscopic retrograde cholangiopancreatography
◆ endoscopy.

### Sigmoidoscopy, colonoscopy, proctoscopy

These are all used to investigate the lower bowel. Proctoscopy may be performed in general practice.

## Box 17.3   X-ray investigations

- Plain film, e.g. chest and limb
- Using radio-opaque dye – intravenous pyelogram (IVP), for kidney function or damage
- Cholecystogram, to investigate the gall bladder
- Barium meal, to investigate the oesophagus, stomach and small intestine
- Barium swallow, to investigate the oesophagus
- Barium enema, to investigate the large bowel
- Ultrasound scan, to examine soft tissue. This process gives a structural image
- Computed tomography scan (CT scan), to scan soft tissue in cross-sections of whole areas of the body being scanned, e.g. brain
- Nuclear magnetic resonance imaging (NMRI), uses the magnetic field in tissue to create 3D images of whole areas of the body, e.g. brain, abdomen
- Radioisotope – nuclear medicine, uses radioactive tracers injected into the body to measure the function of an organ, e.g. thyroid function
- Mammography, infrared or radiographic examination of the breast
- Bone mineral density, to measure the loss or gain of bone density over time, e.g. osteoporosis

### Cardiology

- ECG – electrocardiogram – this shows the electrical activity of the heart, and may be performed either in hospital or general practice.
- Echocardiography – this uses ultrasound to show the movements of the heart.
- Angiography/arteriography – this also uses radio-opaque contrast medium to examine blood vessels.

### Neurological

- EEG – electroencephalograph, records the electrical activity of the cortex of the brain.
- Lumbar puncture (LP) – a procedure to withdraw cerebrospinal fluid from the lumbar spine for diagnostic purposes.

### Respiratory

- Spirometer, to measure the air capacity of the lungs. This may also be measured using a peak flow meter, and is often used in general practice.

## CONCLUSION

After reading this chapter, medical secretaries should be more aware of the dangers which may be involved in medical practice and will be better prepared to cope with some of the important health and safety issues. Understanding of physiological tests should also be improved. Make sure you understand any instructions you have been given when you have to deal with any of the issues discussed in this chapter, so that danger is minimised, and the working environment is as safe as possible for all staff and patients.

 **Exercise**

Make a list of all Health and Safety issues you might find in general practice. Some may be specifically medical, others may be of a more general nature.

## FURTHER READING

Hampson GD 1994 Practice nurse handbook, 3rd edn. Blackwell Scientific Publications, Oxford

Simons P, Quinn B 1996 The GP receptionist's handbook. Baillière Tindall, London

# 18

# Drugs

*Tracey Sweet*

## OBJECTIVES

◆ To look at the difference between generic and proprietary names for drugs

◆ To identify the reference sources on drugs used to access information relevant to the role of the medical secretary

◆ To increase understanding of major legislation governing supply of medicines to the public

◆ To familiarise readers with the documentation in common use when prescribing and supplying drugs, and the need for its accurate completion

◆ To identify the procedures for running manual and computerised repeat prescribing systems efficiently and accurately

◆ To outline the possible functions of a medical secretary in a dispensing practice

◆ To increase knowledge of prescription charges and exemptions.

## INTRODUCTION

The medical secretary needs to understand the range of responsibilities she may have relating to the prescribing and supply of medicines to patients, including:

◆ the ordering and storage of drugs
◆ the writing or printing of repeat prescriptions
◆ the submission of prescriptions to the Prescription Pricing Authority (PPA)
◆ advising patients on prescription charges, exemption categories, etc.

Before reading this chapter, it is advisable to obtain up-to-date copies of the following reference sources:

— the *British National Formulary* (BNF)
— *Monthly Index of Medical Specialities* (MIMS)
— the *Drug Tariff*
— the *ABPI Compendium*.

## DRUG NAMES – GENERICS AND PROPRIETARIES

It is important that the medical secretary understands the difference between generic and proprietary names for drugs.

### The generic name

When a pharmaceutical company discovers a new compound, it is allocated a 'chemical' name, giving a technical description. The patent is registered using the drug's chemical name, giving the company 20 years of exclusive use.

The drug is also given a *generic* name. The generic name is the drug's official medical name, and often indicates the therapeutic class to which a drug belongs. The generic name is sometimes referred to as the 'approved name'. It is the name used in most medical literature.

## The proprietary name

The drug is marketed using a *proprietary* name. The proprietary name is a brand name or trademark. The name is designed to sell, and is usually easy to remember.

Companies hope that when the drug is manufactured by other firms, the GPs will continue to prescribe the drug by its original brand name. Other firms may use the generic name with their firm's endorsement on the packaging and tablets, or market the generic under their own proprietary name.

A well known example is the generic drug *ibuprofen*. Ibuprofen was originally produced by Boots as Brufen, but is now manufactured by many other suppliers under a variety of proprietary names (e.g., Nurofen) as well as in a generic form.

**When typing drug names, it is usual to write the proprietary name with an initial capital letter, but not the generic name.**

## Advantages of generic prescribing

**Economy.** Companies manufacturing generics have not incurred development costs, and are, therefore, able to produce the drug at much lower cost. The Department of Health are encouraging GPs to increase their use of generic prescribing to cut costs.

**Recognition.** Medical students are taught pharmacology using generic names, most prescribing in hospitals is by generic name and scientific journals use generic names.

## Disadvantages of generics

**Compliance.** The pharmacist may supply any producer's generic when dispensing a generic prescription. The patient may, therefore, be confused by receiving medication which varies in size, shape, taste, colour or format. This may undermine the patient's confidence with their medication, eventually affecting compliance. (NB: There are plans to standardise the appearance of generics in the future.)

**Naming.** The names of generics are overall less memorable than proprietary names – and harder to spell!

**Reduced investment.** The pharmaceutical industry may invest less on research and development as a reduction in profits occurs.

The average level of generic prescribing by GPs in the UK was 55% in September 1995.

# REFERENCE SOURCES

In order to work efficiently, the medical secretary must have the ability to access further information or check spellings of drug names, etc., as and when required. **The basic references should be easily accessible to the medical secretary, and they should be up to date at all times.** Out-of-date information could be dangerous.

Information on medicines can be obtained from a variety of sources. The more important texts are unbiased and non-promotional. The basic texts the medical secretary should be using, and keeping up to date, are:

— *British National Formulary* (BNF)
— *Monthly Index of Medical Specialities* (MIMS)
— *Statement of Fees and Allowances* (SFA)
— *Drug Tariff.*

## British National Formulary (BNF)

All doctors and pharmacists receive, free of charge, copies of the BNF. The Department of Health publishes it and arranges distribution within the NHS. The publication is the most widely used primary reference source for information on medicines and prescribing in the UK.

It is published twice yearly, so it is always reasonably up to date.

The main text consists of notes on all the preparations that are available in the UK, divided into numbered chapters on the important organ systems (e.g. the gastrointestinal system) and other main topics (e.g. infections).

Common over-the-counter preparations are now also included. This information is useful for the GP when checking interactions with prescribed medication.

The BNF is written using generic names. Where proprietaries are available, they are summarised after the notes on the generic drug.

The main text is supplemented by several useful appendices, including recommended wording for labelling medicines, which will be particularly relevant to medical secretaries working in dispensing practices. The addresses and telephone numbers for all of the pharmaceutical companies with products detailed in the BNF are listed. The medical secretary may occasionally be asked to contact one of the companies with an enquiry regarding a product.

Inside the back cover is a table giving common Latin abbreviations with their recognised translation. This may be useful to a medical secretary faced with a handwritten prescription containing an unfamiliar abbreviation.

A computerised version of the BNF is now available on subscription to health care professionals. The computer screen format is identical to the pages of the pocket book version of the BNF, but provides additional facilities. For example, a click on an entry in the contents list or index immediately accesses the required page.

## Monthly Index of Medical Specialities (MIMS)

This commonly used prescribing guide is published by an independent company, and sent free to all GPs every month. It is, therefore, always up to date. MIMS contains details of all prescribable proprietary drugs, including prices. The index includes both proprietary and generic names for products.

Like the BNF, MIMS is arranged into therapeutic categories (e.g. cardiovascular system), and includes the names, addresses and telephone numbers of all the pharmaceutical companies with products entered in MIMS.

## Statement of Fees and Allowances (SFA)

The *Statement of Fees and Allowances* (SFA) is commonly referred to as the 'Red Book'. It is a loose-leaf, ring-bound book containing all of the information governing GPs' payments, and includes a section on payments for dispensing services, including the current fees.

The 'Red Book' is updated regularly via replacement pages from the Department of Health, which are fitted into the ring file. It is often the medical secretary's responsibility to keep the ring file up to date.

## Drug Tariff

The *Drug Tariff* is an essential reference source, particularly for dispensing practices. It is compiled by the Prescription Pricing Authority (PPA) for the Department of Health, and is updated each month. A copy is sent to all GPs.

Examples of the information it provides include:

◆ the information to be added to prescriptions (the 'endorsements') to enable the correct payments to be made to dispensing doctors and community pharmacists
◆ an up-to-date list of items which cannot be prescribed on an NHS prescription (the 'blacklist')
◆ prescription charge details
◆ a list of prescribable appliances (e.g. catheters and stoma bags).

## ABPI Compendium of Data Sheets and Summaries of Product Characteristics

Data Sheets and Summaries of Product Characteristics (SPCs) are documents prepared by pharmaceutical companies on their products. They are non-promotional, factual information sheets, conforming to a standard format.

The ABPI Compendium is a compendium of data sheets and SPCs containing the majority of products made by companies in the UK. It is issued free to all doctors and pharmacists by the Association of British Pharmaceutical Industry (ABPI).

Much more detailed information is available on drugs from this reference source, including storage requirements, legal category, treatment of overdosage, etc.

## Pharmaceutical representatives

Pharmaceutical representatives have access to a large database of up-to-date technical information and literature maintained by the companies for whom they work. Representatives can, therefore, be a valuable source of information, particularly on a new drug.

Some representatives provide resources and information for the practice, e.g.:

◆ posters for the waiting room (e.g. for flu vaccination campaigns)
◆ specialised record cards, printed by the company, for recording blood pressure checks, diabetic clinic attendances, etc.
◆ advice on storing vaccines.

The medical secretary may be responsible for making appointments for the representatives to see GPs to discuss new drug developments, etc. Appointments may also be made with practice or dispensary managers to discuss discounts on bulk orders, etc.

## THE MEDICINES ACT 1968

The Medicines Act 1968 is concerned with the manufacture, sale, supply, packaging, labelling, advertising, safety and use of medicines.

The Medicines Act requires each drug to be licensed before marketing. Product licences are considered on the basis of their safety, quality and efficacy.

Thalidomide was first marketed in 1956 for the treatment of insomnia and vomiting in early pregnancy. In 1961 there was a marked increase in the incidence of congenital birth defects, typically an absence or reduction of the long bones of the limbs. Unfortunately, the association with thalidomide was not recognised for several years with the result that thousands of babies were born worldwide with these deformities.

The legal framework governing the licensing of drugs results from the recommendations of a Committee set up as a direct result of the thalidomide disaster. (Before the Medicines Act came into effect, there was no legal requirement for approval or control of the development of new medicines on the grounds of their safety.)

Under the Act, the *Committee on the Safety of Medicines (CSM)* advises on the safety, quality and effectiveness of new medicines and collects and investigates reports on adverse reactions to all medicines on the market, issuing warnings about any newly identified hazards.

## The yellow card system

Under a voluntary scheme, introduced in 1964, GPs are requested to report *suspected* adverse drug reactions to the Committee on the Safety of Medicines on yellow, pre-paid report forms, found at the back of the BNF, as well as the back of prescription forms. In recent years, there have been several examples of drugs being withdrawn by the CSM as a result of adverse reaction reporting. The CSM may, alternatively, modify either the indications for use, contraindications to use or the recommended dose.

## 'Black triangle' requirement

Drugs annotated with an inverted black triangle in the BNF and MIMS carry a requirement to report all adverse reactions to the CSM, however minor. The symbol is used for the first 2 years of a product's life.

## Medicines classification

The Act legislates for three classes of medicinal products as shown in Box 18.1.

As prescription charges increase, more and more prescriptions cost less over the counter than the actual prescription charge. The medical secretary may, therefore, be asked by some patients whether their prescription can be purchased over the counter. The legal classification of each drug is

---

**Box 18.1    The three classes of medicines**

◆ *General Sale List Medicines (GSL)* – medicines which can, with reasonable safety, be sold or supplied at non-pharmacy retail premises, e.g. Rennie tablets

◆ *Pharmacy Medicines (P)* – medicines which can be sold at pharmacies, but *only* under the supervision of a pharmacist, e.g. Cerumol ear drops

◆ *Prescription Only Medicines (POM)* – medicines only available on prescription from a doctor, dentist or veterinary surgeon, e.g., amoxycillin

---

shown in the ABPI Compendium of Data Sheets and SPCs. The retail cost is shown in MIMS.

## Supply of medicines

A Prescription Only Medicine (POM) prescribed by a GP on a prescription must be provided in accordance with the Medicines Act 1968. For example, the drug must be supplied in a suitable container (as listed in the *Drug Tariff*).

The Medicines Act requires all medicine labels to include the following information:

— the patient's name
— the date on which the medicine is dispensed
— the dispensing GP or pharmacist's name, address and telephone number
— a reminder that medicines should be kept out of the reach of children.

Some warning labels, such as 'for external use only', if appropriate, are also a legal requirement.

Although not a legal requirement, labels also usually show:

— the name of the product
— the quantity
— directions regarding use.

## Dispensing of medicines

The Medicines Act 1968 gives GPs the right to dispense medicines when certain conditions are met.

Practice and community nurses with health visiting or district nursing qualifications are also able to prescribe a limited range of drugs, once they have undergone a programme of training.

## THE LIMITED LIST

In an attempt to control the cost of prescribed drugs, on 1 April 1985 the Department of Health created a 'blacklist' of products in certain therapeutic groups which should not be prescribed by GPs at NHS expense. Some drugs are barred from NHS prescribing completely, whilst others are excluded as proprietaries but accepted in their generic form. For example, Valium is blacklisted, but its generic version, diazepam, is still prescribable.

Should GPs prescribe blacklisted products the community pharmacist or dispensing doctor would not receive payment. The BNF shows blacklisted items with the symbol NHS. The *Drug Tariff* has a totally up-to-date list. (As the list occasionally changes, it is important to access an up-to-date list of blacklisted products.) Should a patient insist on a blacklisted drug, the GP could issue a private prescription and the patient would pay the full cost of the drug.

## DRUGS TO BE PRESCRIBED IN CERTAIN CIRCUMSTANCES UNDER THE NHS

A small number of drugs can only be prescribed under the NHS for *certain patients* for the treatment of *specific conditions*, as detailed in the *Drug Tariff*. The GP must add SLS (meaning selected list scheme) to the prescription form to confirm that the patient is being treated for the specified condition.

## BORDERLINE SUBSTANCES

In certain circumstances some foods and preparations have the characteristics of drugs. The Advisory Committee on Borderline Substances advises on the circumstances when such substances may be regarded as drugs, i.e. for the treatment of specified conditions. When prescribing borderline substances for an approved condition, the prescription must be endorsed 'ACBS'. Without this endorsement, the GP is likely to be questioned by the Health Authority on the prescribing of the item.

The BNF and *Drug Tariff* list borderline substances.

# MISUSE OF DRUGS ACT 1971

The Misuse of Drugs Act 1971 provides comprehensive control to prevent the misuse of *controlled drugs*.

## The schedules and classes of drugs

Controlled drugs are classified into five *schedules*, beginning with the most heavily controlled drugs. The schedules dictate the requirements with regard to import, export, production, supply, possession, prescribing and record-keeping.

*Schedule 1* drugs (e.g. cannabis and LSD) are not used medicinally. The possession and supply of such drugs is prohibited.

*Schedule 2* drugs include diamorphine, morphine and pethidine, and are subject to the full drug requirements relating to:

— prescription writing
— safe custody
— entries in controlled drugs register
— destruction.

Many Schedule 2 drugs are available in injection form, and are personally administered by GPs. All medical secretaries, whether working in an urban or rural dispensing practice, are, therefore, likely to be required to order controlled drugs and be responsible for maintaining an accurate controlled drugs register. It is important that the medical secretary is conversant with the legalities related to such functions.

*Schedule 3* drugs are subject to special prescription writing requirements only.

*Schedule 4* drugs include most benzodiazepines which are subject to minimal controls.

*Schedule 5* drugs include those, which because of their strength, are exempt from virtually all the controlled drugs requirements.

Preparations contained in Schedules 2 and 3 are marked CD in the BNF and MIMS. The ABPI Compendium of Data Sheets and SPCs gives the schedule for all controlled drugs.

## Security of controlled drugs

All controlled drugs in Schedule 2 must be kept in a locked safe or cabinet, with nothing on the outside to indicate its use. The number of keyholders should be limited. It is sensible to avoid fitting the cabinet where it can be seen by members of the public, for example opposite a reception hatch or window.

Safe custody requirements also apply to the following Schedule 3 drugs:

— buprenorphine (e.g. Temegesic)
— diethylpropion
— temazepam.

## Prescribing controlled drugs – prescription requirements

In addition to the usual information required when writing prescriptions, for drugs listed in Schedules 2 and 3 the prescription must also comply with the following legal requirements:

◆ be handwritten by the GP
◆ include the total quantity or number of dosage units written in *words and figures*.

Temazepam is the only Schedule 3 drug which is exempt from all the special prescription writing requirements. Phenobarbitone, another Schedule 3 drug, is exempt from the handwriting requirements only (except in relation to the date).

If the prescription given to the patient is incomplete, or incorrectly written, it cannot be dispensed, and will be returned to the GP for clarification.

## Invoices

All invoices for Schedule 3 and 5 controlled drugs must be retained for 2 years.

**Box 18.2** Information required in the Controlled Drugs Register

*For drugs received*

The date received

The name and address of supplying person/firm

The amount received

The form in which supplied

*For drugs supplied*

The date supply made

The name and address of person supplied

The name of the GP authorised to hold and supply the drugs

The amount supplied

The form in which supplied

## The Controlled Drugs Register

Every transaction, in relation to Schedule 2 drugs *received* and *dispensed*, must be recorded in the controlled drugs register. A separate register must be kept for each surgery.

The register must include the entries shown in Box 18.2.

The register must:

◆ be a bound book with ruled and headed columns
◆ be written in ink or indelible biro
◆ have separate sections for each class of drug
◆ have entries made on the day of transaction, or the following day
◆ have no cancellations or alterations (corrections must be made in the margin or as a footnote, and must be signed and dated)
◆ be kept on the premises to which the register relates
◆ be available for inspection at any time, e.g. by the Home Office drugs inspector
◆ be kept for 2 years from the date of the last entry.

Whilst not legal requirements, the following are considered to be good practice:

◆ A column to record the balance of stock. (This allows the actual stock to be reconciled with the entry recorded in the register, thus enabling any stock shortages to be identified and investigated.)
◆ Separate registers for each GP's bag.

## Destruction of controlled drugs

Once drugs have passed their expiry date, they must be destroyed. Controlled drugs in Schedule 2 may only be destroyed in the presence of a person authorised by the Secretary of State, e.g. a police officer or Home Office inspector.

Details including the name of the drug, the amount and date must be entered in the controlled drugs register, and signed by the person in whose presence the drug was destroyed.

This legal requirement does not apply to controlled drugs returned to a GP by a patient. The 'audit trail' of controlled drugs leads from their import, through every stage, and ends with supply to the patient.

## Security

The Misuse of Drugs Act covers security measures to help prevent users unlawfully obtaining supplies of drugs and prescription pads.

### Security of prescriptions

There are detailed instructions regarding writing prescriptions for controlled drugs in a way that reduces the opportunity to make unauthorised alterations. It is obviously good practice to apply the same procedures to all prescriptions.

Prescriptions should be regarded as security stationery. To improve security, in line with the requirements of the Misuse of Drugs Act, prescription forms now include serial numbers. Practice staff are required to record the serial numbers of prescription forms received from the Health Authority. In the event of a loss or suspected theft, the practice must inform the police and the Health Authority immediately of the missing serial numbers. Stolen prescription forms may then be detected if they are subsequently presented for dispensing.

Prescriptions also now have a coloured background to make photocopying more difficult, and contain anti-tampering devices within the ink and paper to make forgeries detectable. Forms also have a message which can be seen under UV lights to aid detection of counterfoiled forms.

However, to avoid losses or thefts, blank prescription forms:

◆ must not be pre-signed
◆ must be locked away when not in use
◆ must not be left unattended at a reception desk or in the consulting room
◆ must not be left in a car, particularly if displaying a DOCTOR ON CALL sign
◆ must not be used as notepads.

Prescriptions given to patients should have an oblique line below the last item to prevent the addition of items. A circle around the quantity to be supplied also helps avoid unauthorised alterations.

### Security of premises

It is important, particularly in the case of dispensing practices, that security for the whole premises is good. Addicts may break into a surgery if they feel able to obtain money, prescription forms or drugs. Good security measures will, therefore, act as a deterrent.

Measures can include:

◆ window locks for all windows
◆ window bars, particularly for dispensaries
◆ an intruder alarm system, preferably connected to the police station
◆ security lighting which activates when someone approaches the building.

Dispensing practices should consider storing their medicines other than alphabetically, as an addict would then have more difficulty in finding the drugs required.

Only limited amounts of cash should be kept on the premises, in a lockable tin, preferably in a locked drawer. Dispensing practices should ensure that the prescription charges collected are banked regularly.

## DOCUMENTATION

There are a variety of standard forms necessary for prescribing and dispensing. Most of them are available from the Health Authority. Many practices have also devised their own forms.

The medical secretary is often responsible for maintaining adequate stocks of both the standard Health Authority forms and those that are devised by the practice. They should be kept neatly in drawers and cupboards, easily accessible, e.g. prepayment certificates in the reception area.

**The medical secretary should be familiar with the forms, and know how to use them.**

### Standard documentation

#### NHS prescription forms

Prescriptions are produced by doctors as a request to a pharmacist or dispenser to supply specific items. NHS prescription forms in dispensing practices then become a record of supply, which are used as a request for payment to the PPA.

NHS prescriptions are:

— an order for medication
— an invoice for submission to the PPA.

The back of the prescription form provides a checklist for the patient to tick and sign if eligible for free prescriptions.

The vast majority of prescriptions in general practice are issued on a FP10C computerised prescription form or a FP10NC for handwritten prescriptions (Fig. 18.1). Both of these forms are green.

**Prescriptions are valid for 6 months.**

NAME

Age if under
12 years

yrs.    mths.    Address

*Pricing
Office
use only*

*Pharmacy Stamp*

| Pharmacist's pack & quantity endorsement | No. of days treatment N.B. Ensure dose is stated | NP |
|---|---|---|

Signature of Doctor

Date

For phar-macist No. of Prescns. on form

IMPORTANT:- Read the notes overleaf before going to the pharmacy

Form FP10 C
(Rev 98)

---

FP10 C

Do you (the patient) have to pay for this prescription?

NO ☒ fill in **Parts 1 and 3**    YES ☒ fill in **Parts 2 and 3**

Give all details we ask for    See notes at bottom of page

**Part 1**    For patients who do not have to pay

The patient does not have to pay because he/she :

A ☒ is under 16 years of age

B ☒ is 16, 17 or 18 *and* in full-time education

C ☒ is 60 years of age or over

D ☒ has a maternity exemption certificate

E ☒ has a medical exemption certificate

F ☒ has a prescription prepayment certificate

G- ☒ has a War/MoD exemption certificate    No:

H ☒ *gets Income Support    * Give details of person getting benefit. This may be your partner. Checks may be made with the DSS.

I ☒ *gets Family Credit    Name:

J ☒ *gets Disability Working Allowance    Date of birth: /  /

K ☒ *gets Income-based Jobseeker's Allowance

L ☒ *has a current HC2 charges certificate

X ☒ was prescribed a free-of-charge contraceptive

Now fill in Part 3

**Part 2**    For patients who have to pay

I have paid £ ___ for this prescription

Now fill in Part 3

**Part 3**    Your declaration

I am the ☒ patient ☒ patient's representative

I declare that the information is true and complete

**WARNING : FALSE INFORMATION MAY LEAD TO PROSECUTION**

Name
*In capitals*

Address
*If different from overleaf*

Postcode

Signed    Date    /  /

• Leaflet HC11 tells you if you are entitled to free prescriptions. It is available from most pharmacies and all main Post Offices. Medical conditions that entitle you to free prescriptions are listed in HC11.

• If you think you may be entitled to free prescriptions, pay *now* and get an NHS receipt (FP57). It tells you how to get your money back.

**Figure 18.1**    Prescription form FP10. (Reproduced by permission of the Department of Health.)

Drs. A. B. Smith & C. D. Jones. Tel: 01579 337744

```
Qty 21 AMOXYCILLIN CAPS 250MG (AAH)
ONE to be taken THREE TIMES daily

TAKE AT REGULAR INTERVALS-FINISH COURSE

13-09-1996 Mr Percy Patient
```
Keep out of children's reach

Drs. A. B. Smith & C. D. Jones. Tel: 01579 337744

```
13-09-1996              One item enclosed
Mr Percy Patient
19 The Road
St. Stephen St. Austell

PL26 1ZZ
```
Keep out of children's reach

**Figure 18.2**  Computer printed labels.

673

```
PLEASE TICK BOX FOR THE MEDICINE YOU
REQUIRE.

When requesting or collecting repeat
prescriptions please call after 11 am.
As from 2nd August 97 Saturday surgeries
will only be held at the Mile Road
surgery. Telephone No.

16.7.97
-----------------------------------------
THYROXINE TABLETS                 60  [ ]
100mcg, ONE TO BE TAKEN DAILY
-----------------------------------------




Review is due before 15.1.98
-----------------------------------------
```

**Figure 18.3**  A repeat prescription form.

**Prescriptions for controlled drugs are valid for 13 weeks.**

## Prescription writing requirements

The prescription form provides all of the information on which the prescription will be dispensed. It is important, therefore, that the patient and the medication are clearly identified with sufficient information to enable the correct drug to be dispensed with an accurate label to the correct patient (Fig. 18.2). The medical secretary is often involved in the printing of repeat prescription forms (Fig. 18.3). However, to be able to check computerised prescriptions include sufficient and appropriate detail, and to enable a service to be maintained when the practice computers are out of action, the medical secretary also needs to be familiar with the recommendations for prescription *writing*.

The prescription form should include the information shown in Box 18.3.

Handwritten prescriptions should be written in ink (legibly).

---

**Box 18.3  Information that should be included on a prescription**

◆ The date
◆ The full name and address of the patient
◆ The age of the patient (this is a legal requirement for children under 12 years of age)
◆ The name of the drug (preferably in capital letters) and its strength
◆ The form (e.g. tablets, capsules, syrup)
◆ The frequency (the number of doses in a day)
◆ The dose (how many are to be taken at each frequency)
◆ The quantity to be dispensed
◆ The GP's name, surgery address, telephone number and national index code and the name of his Health Authority
◆ The signature of the GP.

## Special markings

The name and strength of the drug should always appear on the label of a dispensed medicine unless the GP deletes the letters NP (nomen propium – Latin for proper name) from the prescription form. The name of the preparation will not then appear on the label. Instead, wording such as 'the sleeping tablets' would be used. The use of NP is a rare event, but occasionally the GP may not want the patient to know what is being prescribed, for example if the patient is able to relate the drug name to a particular disease or a placebo is being used.

## Abbreviations

All of the instructions on a prescription form should be written or printed in English and in full. The only acceptable exceptions to this rule are the commonly used Latin abbreviations, e.g.

| | |
|---|---|
| bd | twice a day |
| mane | in the morning |
| nocte | at night |

In addition, the following 'rules' should be observed:

◆ print/write quantities of less than 1 gram in milligrams, e.g. 500 mg, not 0.5 g
◆ print/write quantities of less than 1 mg in micrograms, e.g. 100 micrograms, not 0.1 mg
◆ add a zero in front of a decimal point when there is no other figure and decimals are unavoidable, e.g. 0.5 ml, not .5 ml.

## Computerised prescriptions

Computerised prescription forms (FP10C) are available from the Health Authority in continuous stationery form. They are double the width of a prescription, perforated between the two halves – the left side comprising the prescription, and the right side blank.

Computer software usually leaves it to the practice to decide on the content of the blank side. This tear-off section can provide a very useful source of information for the patient, and is often used to list current repeat prescriptions, thereby doubling as a repeat prescription request form. A practice message may be added – either on a prescribing matter or some other administrative function, e.g.

— a reminder that a review of repeat drugs is due
— simple health advice
— information on new arrangements for appointments.

It is illegal to computer print a prescription for a Schedule 2 or 3 controlled drug (except temazepam and phenobarbitone).

## Nurses' prescription forms

Practice nurses with a district nursing or health visitor qualification are allowed to prescribe from a limited list of drugs once they have undergone an approved nurse prescribers' course. The items which nurses are entitled to prescribe are published in the *Drug Tariff* and the BNF. The prescription form used is a lilac FP10 PN. The prescription form includes the nurse's UKCC PIN number, the practice identification number and the full address of the practice.

Similarly, community nurses and health visitors can prescribe from the same limited list on completion of an approved course. The prescription form used is a grey FP10CN.

## Form FP10(MDA)

This form is used by GPs to prescribe controlled drugs for the treatment of drug addiction for dispensing in instalments (usually on a daily basis). Supplies are obtainable from the Health Authority in pads of 10 numbered forms. The form is a light blue, double-sided, prescription form.

## Application for dispensing services

Form GMSI, the form used by patients to register with a GP, is also used to apply for dispensing services at dispensing practices, usually at the time of registration or following a change of address to a dispensing area of the practice.

### Invoice for drugs and appliances supplied – Form FP34D

Form FP34D is completed at the end of each month, and sent with prescription forms to the PPA to claim reimbursement of drug expenditure and dispensing fees.

### Receipt form – FP57

Form FP57, a receipt of prescription charges paid, should be issued to any patient seeking a refund. The form is only relevant to dispensing practices.

Patients requesting receipts include those on a low income, and those who have applied for, but not yet received, an exemption certificate.

### Prepayment certificates – Form FP95

Patients who need frequent prescriptions and who pay prescription charges can save money by purchasing a prepayment certificate (often referred to as a 'season ticket'). A prepayment certificate is cost-effective for patients who need more than five items in 4 months.

The medical secretary can help patients by drawing their attention to the availability of prepayment certificates.

The application form is available from practices, the Post Office and Benefit Agency offices. The application form and payment are sent to the Health Authority by the patient, and a prepayment certificate is then issued.

### NHS prescriptions – How to Get Your Prescriptions Dispensed – leaflet HC11

It is important that patients who might be entitled to exemption from charges or to help with costs on grounds of low income are informed accordingly. The HC11 leaflet should be displayed prominently for patients, as it explains who is eligible for free prescriptions, as well as information on prepayment certificates and refunds.

## Practice-specific documentation

### Private prescriptions

Private prescriptions should be written on headed notepaper, or on specially printed prescription forms. A private prescription has to include the same essential identifying information as an NHS prescription. In addition, it must specify the GP's qualifications.

Unlike NHS prescriptions, private prescriptions can be repeated. Most private prescription forms include a box for 'number of repeats'. The prescription can then be supplied the authorised number of times.

Private prescription forms must be presented and dispensed for the first time within 6 months of issue.

The same rules apply to the writing of both NHS and private prescriptions for controlled drugs. Repeat dispensing of private prescriptions for controlled drugs is not allowed. However, the GP can direct that a prescription be dispensed in instalments.

Private prescriptions are written for:

◆ medicines solely in anticipation of the onset of an illness abroad, e.g. drugs taken on holiday for possible illnesses such as diarrhoea and vomiting
◆ malaria prophylaxis
◆ private patients
◆ blacklisted substances
◆ overseas visitors (at the GP's discretion)
◆ patients unable to produce a medical card, where the GP has reasonable doubts that the patient is registered with the practice.

GPs are entitled to charge a patient for issuing a private prescription in the above circumstances, unless it is for a blacklisted product. The British Medical Association (BMA) publish a recommended fee each year.

## REPEAT PRESCRIPTIONS

A repeat prescription is an order for further supply of medication without a face-to-face contact with the GP. Repeat prescriptions are for patients who need replacement drugs more frequently than they need to see the GP, e.g. patients with hypertension, asthma and diabetes. Up to two-thirds of all prescriptions are issued as repeats.

Not all drug therapy is suitable for inclusion in a repeat prescribing system, e.g. some drugs are intended for short-term use only.

GPs differ on the quantity of drug they prescribe for patients on a repeat prescription. However, there is a generally held view that prescribing should be for a maximum of 28 days. This helps control drug misuse and reduce drug wastage, e.g. due to changes in medication, deaths, etc.

Patients may continue to receive medication unnecessarily or be using it inappropriately unless they are regularly reviewed by the GP, or sometimes the practice nurse. The patient may be suffering from a condition, such as hypertension, which needs regular review. The repeat prescription system will, therefore, limit repeats – either by the number of prescriptions or by a time interval. The review period will depend on the drug, the condition being treated and the individual patient. When producing repeat prescriptions, the medical secretary must ensure that the authorised number of repeats is not exceeded.

The medical secretary is often responsible for the production of repeat prescriptions, and should, therefore, be familiar with the following aspects of a repeat prescription system.

## Accepting repeat prescriptions

Various procedures have been developed for accepting repeat prescriptions, whether requested by letter, over the telephone or in person.

**Repeat prescription cards.** Listing the authorised repeats are handed in or posted to the surgery. The items requested should be clearly indicated by the patient.

**Telephone requests.** Some practices accept requests by telephone, particularly for the housebound and elderly. Other practices discourage telephone requests as errors can occur during transcription. Mistakes over drug names can be difficult to avoid. It is essential, therefore, that the person taking the request has access to the patient's prescribing records whilst on the telephone.

A separate telephone line for repeat prescription requests may be required to avoid congestion.

**Right-hand side of FP10C.** This can be used to request repeats. The print-out holds an up-to-date record of authorised repeat medication for the patient to tick and post or hand in to the practice.

## Producing prescriptions

From the various requests, the medical secretary must produce accurate repeat prescriptions.

By referring to the repeat prescribing records, the medical secretary should check that:

◆ the patient and the drugs are clearly identified
◆ the drug, dose and quantity correspond
◆ the item is authorised as a repeat
◆ a further issue is authorised
◆ the interval since the last issue is neither too early nor too late.

In the case of queries, the GP will usually need the medical records as well as the repeat prescribing records.

Each time a repeat prescription is issued, the date and drugs dispensed should be recorded, using manual or computerised records. There are two common systems.

**Repeat prescription sheets.** Separate record sheets can be tagged to the patients' records or filed alphabetically, separate from the main filing system.

**Computerised repeat prescribing records.** These are increasingly popular. They provide a fast and efficient recording system. A computerised repeat prescription system has the following advantages:

— The prescription forms are legible, typewritten and accurate.
— The computer gives the patient a printed record of their repeat medication.
— The patient is automatically informed if he/she is due for review before further repeats.
— The computer monitors the interval between prescriptions.

## Collection arrangements

Most practices ask for a minimum of 24 hours' notice for collection of repeat prescriptions. The secretary will need to ensure that the prescription forms are signed by the GP in time for collection. The forms are often stored alphabetically awaiting collection. The storage area must be a secure place away from the reception desk as signed prescriptions are open to abuse if stolen.

Arrangements can be made to post prescription forms to patients, particularly the infirm or housebound. (Practices often encourage patients to provide a stamped, addressed envelope.)

Prescriptions may be collected by a local pharmacist, so that the medication can be dispensed ready for the patient to collect later that day.

## The advantages of repeat prescribing

An efficient repeat prescribing system gives the patients easy access to medication when needed. The need to consult the GP is reduced, saving time for both the GP and the patient. Patients can plan when to collect their prescriptions or arrange for collection on their behalf.

Patients who are uncomfortable when asked to make frequent contact with health care workers find a repeat prescribing system suits them much better.

## Disadvantages of repeat prescribing

The patient does not see the GP as often. The patient may begin to take their medication incorrectly or may mix drugs inappropriately with over-the-counter medicines.

# DISPENSING OF DRUGS

It is not only medical secretaries working in dispensing practices who will be involved in dispensing matters. Almost all practices dispense a limited range of drugs to their patients. Some medical secretaries may be required to undertake dispensing duties, but this work requires specialist training and is, therefore, outside the remit of this textbook.

All practices dispense drugs to their patients if needed for their *immediate* treatment, as well as some *personally administered* drugs. The full list of drugs which may be personally administered is included in the *Statement of Fees and Allowances* (Red Book). The most commonly dispensed items for personal administration include vaccines, injections, intrauterine contraceptive devices and sutures.

Patients in rural areas may obtain all their medicines from a dispensing GP provided they live more than one mile from the nearest pharmacy.

Dispensing GPs can also dispense to all temporary residents (irrespective of where they live).

## Payments for dispensing services

To obtain payment for NHS prescriptions, each item dispensed must be recorded on an FP10 and sent to the PPA. The PPA then prices the prescriptions, and notifies Health Authorities of the payments due to dispensing GPs and community pharmacists.

Remuneration comprises the following elements:

- ◆ the *basic price* of the drug (as defined in the *Drug Tariff* for generic preparations and MIMS for proprietary products)
- ◆ an *on-cost allowance* (currently 10.5% of the basic price)
- ◆ a *container allowance* paid whether or not a container, medicine spoon, etc., is required
- ◆ a *dispensing fee* paid on a sliding scale according to the number of prescription items submitted each month
- ◆ a *VAT allowance* to cover VAT on purchases of drugs, appliances and containers – unless the practice is entitled to reclaim VAT from HM Customs and Excise.

Before payments are made to the practice a deduction is made from the basic price to allow for the discount that GPs are assumed to obtain from their suppliers.

The PPA no longer requires separate FP10s for eight high-volume personally administered vaccines, e.g. influenza and tetanus. Instead an Appendix to Form FP34D is completed each month, listing the number of each vaccine administered. (A list of the patients who received each vaccine is retained at the practice.)

## Submitting prescription forms to the PPA

It is often the medical secretary's responsibility to send the prescription forms to the PPA at the end of each month. The following procedure should be followed:

1. Form FP34D should be completed. Each GP's name and national index code is entered, along with the number of prescription forms and items being submitted on their prescription forms. The number of high-volume vaccines administered is recorded in the Appendix.

2. The secretary should check that the prescriptions have been correctly completed and signed. If a prescription form is not clear, the PPA will not be able to price the item, and the form will be returned to the practice for clarification, delaying payment.

3. The prescription forms for the month, along with a completed and signed FP34D, are parcelled up securely, and posted to the PPA using an address label supplied by the Health Authority. It is recommended that the parcel is sent by recorded delivery. The package must arrive no later than the 5th day of the month after the prescriptions were dispensed. For example, prescriptions dispensed during March should arrive by 5 April. If the secretary misses the deadline, the PPA may delay payment.

## Collecting prescription charges

Dispensing GPs are responsible for collecting prescription charges for each item supplied to those patients who pay. The total charges collected are either declared to the Health Authority each month, and deducted from drug payments received, or sent direct to the Health Authority.

The medical secretary may be required to collect prescription charges from patients. The cash received should be stored securely in a lockable cupboard, etc., and regularly transferred to the bank.

Some patients may pay prescription charges by cheque.

**Reflection point**

◆ If you are presented with a cheque, what information would you need to ensure that it had been completed correctly?

## Prescription charges

Over 80% of items are issued to patients who are exempt from paying prescription charges. The various categories of patients who are eligible for free prescriptions are shown in Box 18.4.

## Purchasing drugs

Drugs can be obtained from several sources:

— direct from drug companies (usually in bulk)
— through drug representatives
— from a wholesaler.

The majority of practices deal mainly with wholesalers. Bulk purchases from drug companies are usually reserved for drugs which are frequently prescribed. Some drug companies offer higher discounts than wholesalers, sometimes on a 'special offer' basis. Special offers are usually promoted by the drug representative. Practices occasionally combine their orders to reach the larger quantities required to obtain additional discount.

## Stock control

Stock control is a key element in the provision of a good dispensing service, as well as affecting profits.

Patients who have to return for some, or all, of their drugs because of inadequate stock are getting a poor level of service.

| Box 18.4 | Criteria for free prescriptions |

*Automatic exemption on age grounds*

◆ Children under 16

◆ Students under 19 in full-time education

◆ Men and women aged 60 and over

*Patients holding Health Authority exemption certificates*

◆ Pregnant mothers

◆ Women who have given birth in the last 12 months

◆ Patients suffering from specified medical conditions, e.g. diabetes and epilepsy (the full list is included in the *Drug Tariff*)

◆ War and service pensioners (only for prescriptions needed to treat their war disablement)

*Patients who have purchased a prepayment certificate (Form FP95)*

*People with DSS exemption certificates*, including people receiving income support or family credit

*Free prescriptions*

◆ Prescription charges are not made for items supplied under the *personal administration* arrangements

◆ *Contraceptive substances and appliances* are prescribed free of charge to women

◆ *Bulk prescriptions* are not chargeable. A bulk prescription is a single prescription form for two or more patients. It is only valid for schools or institutions of 20 or more people, where the GP writing the prescription is responsible for at least 10 of the residents. The prescription is made out in the name of the institution, instead of a patient's name. Only P and GSL products can be prescribed on a bulk prescription.

However, excess stock can be an expensive error as the drug may be superseded by newer versions or become out of date before there is an opportunity for use. The only patient using the drug may have moved out of the area or died. Excess stock also requires additional storage space. GPs are not reimbursed for the cost of drugs until they are dispensed. It is wise, therefore, to make the interval between purchase of drugs and reimbursement as short as possible.

A good system of stock control requires the setting of minimum stock levels and re-order quantities for each drug to ensure that enough of a product is held to meet demand without tying up money unnecessarily or risking wastage.

Appropriate stock levels are determined by:

◆ the number of prescriptions dispensed
◆ the average quantity prescribed per prescription
◆ the delivery intervals
◆ the shelf-life of drug
◆ the cost of the drug
◆ the requirement for immediate availability of some drugs.

Drug usage figures can be estimated by inspecting invoices. Alternatively, a fully computerised practice can access drug usage figures very quickly.

There are several computer packages offering electronic ordering facilities and electronic stock control, saving time spent monitoring stock levels and preparing order lists.

There are also several manual stock control systems, including the following:

1. An *order book* can be used to record the drugs stocked, along with minimum stock levels and re-order quantities. Tight stock control requires daily stock counts of the items used that day, noting where stock is below the minimum set. The supplies required are then ordered.

2. *Stock cards* can be used for each drug, and completed after dispensing each item. Each prescription quantity supplied is deducted from the current stock total, until a minimum is reached. The cards also carry the ordering details. (A file or ring binder could be used to serve the same purpose.)

3. The simplest system is to *label the shelves* with the minimum stock level and re-order quantities for each drug. However, a lot of time can be wasted checking that orders have been placed, particularly when several members of staff are involved in the process.

Adequate supplies of the various tablet and medicine containers, bags for dispensed medicines, prescription forms, labels, etc., also need to be maintained.

## Stock-taking

A stock-take is normally carried out at the end of the practice's financial year for inclusion in the practice accounts. A stock-take is also required on partnership dissolution. The drug stock is one of the main financial assets of the dispensing practice, and, therefore, needs to be accurately assessed. Stock-takes enable out-of-date stock to be identified and destroyed, excessive quantities of particular items to be highlighted and any stock shortages to be identified and investigated.

## Storage conditions

Storage conditions are detailed, as necessary, on the drug containers. Some drugs need to be kept in lightproof containers, some at certain temperatures and others need to be kept away from moisture. A maximum/minimum thermometer in the dispensary refrigerator is essential.

It is important that the storage instructions are followed. For example, if heat sensitive vaccines, such as polio, are stored at temperatures 6°C above the recommended range for just one day the vaccine would not be effective, and should not be used.

## Storage systems

Storage can be pull-out racks, drawers, open shelving or cupboards. Pull-out racks and drawers are secure, as well as space-saving. However, they are expensive. Shelves are more visible, but also more dusty, difficult to label and keep tidy.

Whichever storage system is used, the drugs should be stocked in a methodical manner. The most common methods are as follows:

1. *Alphabetical* storage ensures that all items are easily found. However, over-stocking in a particular therapeutic group will not be so obvious. Alphabetical filing can also increase the chance of selecting and dispensing a wrong, but similarly named, item.

2. Storing according to *drug groups* (as set out in MIMS and the BNF) enables the GP to choose a particular type of medication by looking at the range stocked. Over-stocking of a particular drug group is readily seen.

## Expiry dates

Drugs deteriorate with time. Stock with the shortest shelf-life should always be at the front, and used first. It is essential to check expiry dates regularly, and to remove and destroy out-of-date drugs promptly. Checks should include drugs in the GPs' bags. Stock should rarely need to be destroyed. Whenever it does, ordering and stock level decisions should be reviewed.

## SUMMARY OF KEY ISSUES

The *generic* name is a drug's official medical name, and often indicates the therapeutic class to which a drug belongs. The *proprietary* name is the brand name. When typing drug names, it is usual to write the proprietary name with an initial capital letter, but not the generic name.

The reference sources with which the medical secretary should be familiar are the *British National Formulary* (BNF), the *Monthly Index of Medical Specialities* (MIMS) and the *Drug Tariff*. It is important that information is accessed from up-to-date editions.

The *Statement of Fees and Allowances* ('Red Book') sets out the payment arrangements for dispensing GPs.

The *Medicines Act 1968* is concerned with the safety of medicines, and legislates for three classes of medicinal products:

◆ General Sale List medicines (GSL)
◆ Pharmacy medicines (P)
◆ Prescription Only Medicines (POM).

The Medicines Act also controls the supply of medicines, e.g. labelling requirements. It gives certain GPs the right to dispense medicines.

The *Misuse of Drugs Act 1971* provides comprehensive control to prevent the misuse of controlled drugs. Schedule 2 and 3 drugs are the most heavily controlled with special requirements relating to prescription writing, safe custody, entries in controlled drugs registers and destruction.

Prescriptions for drugs in Schedules 2 and 3 must be handwritten by the GP, with the total quantity or number of dosage units written in words and figures.

*NHS prescription forms* are an order for medication, and an invoice for submission to the PPA.

Prescriptions are valid for 6 months. Prescriptions for controlled drugs are valid for 13 weeks.

The medical secretary may be responsible for maintaining supplies of prescription forms and other documentation relating to the prescribing and supply of medicines.

The medical secretary is often responsible for producing *repeat prescriptions*. Prescriptions must be accurately prepared – either manually or using a computer. Checks to be made by the secretary include ensuring that the item is authorised as a repeat, that a further issue is authorised and neither too early nor too late. Accurate records of the drugs issued must also be made.

Patients in rural areas may obtain their medicines from a *dispensing practice* provided they live more than one mile from the nearest pharmacy. However, all practices dispense drugs to their patients if needed for their immediate treatment, as well as some *personally administered items*. It is often the medical secretary who is responsible for sending the prescription forms and Form FP34D to the Prescription Pricing Authority (PPA) each month.

The medical secretary may be responsible for ordering drug supplies, and maintaining an efficient stock control system. Manufacturers' storage instructions must be followed, and expiry dates checked regularly.

## CONCLUSIONS

The medical secretary is likely to be involved in several aspects relating to the prescribing and supply of medicines to patients, including:

◆ typing of letters including reference to drugs prescribed
◆ arranging appointments for pharmaceutical representatives to see the GP or practice manager
◆ making entries in the controlled drugs register
◆ arranging for destruction of expired controlled drugs
◆ maintaining supplies of the various documentation
◆ advising patients on prescription charges, exemption categories, etc.
◆ producing repeat prescriptions
◆ submitting prescription forms to the PPA
◆ collecting prescription charges from dispensing patients
◆ ordering drugs and maintaining an efficient stock control system.

All of these tasks must be carried out paying due regard to accuracy and security.

Accuracy is particularly important when accepting repeat prescription requests and producing the prescriptions.

Security of blank and signed prescription forms is essential if drug abuse is to be avoided. Complying with the Misuse of Drugs Act also requires practices to ensure that controlled drugs are securely stored.

It is clear that the medical secretary's responsibilities in relation to drugs should be taken extremely seriously to ensure that patients receive accurate prescriptions and drug abuse is minimised.

## Exercises

◆ A patient at the reception desk requests a repeat prescription for his 'blood pressure tablets'. What procedure would you follow, and to which reference sources may you refer?

◆ As a secretary working at a busy general practice, it is necessary for you to be aware of measures to prevent drug abuse. A new member of staff is joining the practice as a receptionist. Prepare an information sheet for her, explaining the special care that must be taken to prevent drug abuse.

◆ You are a medical secretary working in a dispensing practice. The computer is not working and the GP has written a prescription including the abbreviation tds. Use the BNF to check the meaning of this abbreviation.

◆ You are a medical secretary typing a referral letter. The GP has dictated the letter, and you want to check the spelling of a drug used for gout which sounds like Zylauric. Use the BNF to check the spelling. The GP has also asked you to contact the company manufacturing this drug with an enquiry. Use the BNF to find the name, address and telephone number of the company.

◆ Using MIMS, look up the generic names for these proprietary products:

Adalat
Inderal
Floxapen
Ventolin
Voltarol.

◆ Look up the following drugs in the ABPI Compendium of Data Sheets and SPCs, and enter their legal categories (P, POM or GSL).

Canesten cream
Frusene
Liquid Gaviscon

You will see that GSL products can be sold with reasonable safety from retail outlets, but self-administration of POM medicines could be dangerous.

Check the price of the GSL and P products in an up-to-date copy of MIMS.

◆ Refer to the *Drug Tariff* to identify which patients may be prescribed cyanocobalamin tablets under the NHS.

◆ Using the *Drug Tariff*, research the approved conditions for which sunflower oil may be prescribed.

◆ Find a recent edition of the BNF, and refer to the specimen prescription form for a controlled drug. Take a photocopy and file with your course notes.

BLANK

# Appendices

BLANK

# Appendix I

# 1 Prefixes and suffixes

A knowledge of the prefixes and suffixes used in medical terminology, and outlined below, will help the medical secretary to understand the meaning of a large number of commonly used words and phrases. In addition, a good medical dictionary is an essential tool.

| | | | |
|---|---|---|---|
| **a-, an-** not, without | **carp-** wrist | **cyst-** bladder | **flav-** yellow |
| **ab-** away from | **cata-, kata-** down, negative | **cyt-** cell | **galact-** milk |
| **acr-** extremity, peak | | **-cyte** cell | **gastr-** stomach |
| **ad-** towards | **cav-** hollow | **dacry-** tear | **-genic** producing |
| **aden-** gland | **-cele** swelling | **dactyl-** finger | **ger-** old age |
| **adip-** fat | **cent-** hundred | **de-** down, from | **gloss-** tongue |
| **-aemia** blood | **-centesis** piercing | **dec-** ten | **glyc-** sweet |
| **aer-** air | **cephal-** head | **demi-** half | **gnath-** jaw |
| **-aesthesia** sensation | **cerebr-** brain | **dent-** tooth | **-gram** tracing |
| **-algia** pain | **cervic-** neck | **derm-** skin | **-graph** tracing |
| **amyl-** starch | **cheil-, chil-** lip | **-desis** binding | **gynae-** female |
| **ana-** up | **cheir-, chir-** hand | **dextr-** right | **haem-** blood |
| **andr-** male | **chlor-** green | **di-, diplo-** two, double | **hemi-** half |
| **angi-** (blood) vessel | **chol-** bile | | **hepat-** liver |
| **ante-** before, in front | **chondr-** cartilage | **dia-** through | **hex-** six |
| **anti-** against | **chrom-** colour | **dis-** apart, away from | **hist-** tissue, web |
| **apo-** away, from | **-cide** killing | **dors-** back | **hom-** same, like |
| **arthr-** joint | **cine-, kine-** motion | **dys-** difficult, abnormal | **hydr-** water |
| **-asis** state of | **-cle** small | | **hyper-** above |
| **aut-** self | **co-, col-, com-, con-** together, with | **ect-** outside | **hypno-** sleep |
| **bi-, bis-** two | | **-ectasis** stretching | **hypo-** below |
| **bil-** bile | **colp-** vagina | **-ectomy** cutting out | **hyster-** womb |
| **bio-** life | **contra-** against, counter | **em-, en-, end-, ent-** in, inside, within | **-ia, -iasis** state, condition |
| **blast-** bud | | | |
| **blephar-** eyelid | **cortic-** bark, rind | **enter-** intestine | **idi-** peculiar, distinct |
| **brachi-** arm | **cost-** rib | **epi-** upon, over | **infra-** below |
| **brachy-** short | **cox-** hip | **erythr-** red | **inter-** between |
| **brady-** slow | **crani-** skull | **eu-** good, normal | **intra-** within |
| **bronch-** windpipe | **cryo-** cold | **ex-, exo-** out of | **intro-** inwards |
| **calc-** chalk | **crypt-** hidden, concealed | **extra-** outside | **iso-** equal |
| **carcin-** cancer | | **faci-** face | **-itis** inflammation of |
| **card-** heart | **cyan-** blue | **-facient** making | **kary-** nut, nucleus |

kerat- horn, cornea
-kinesis, -kinetic motion
lact- milk
laryng- windpipe
later- side
leuc-, leuk- white
-lith stone
-lysis destruction
macr- large
mal- bad, abnormal
-malacia softening
mamm- breast
mast- breast
medi- middle
megal- large
-megaly enlargement
melan- black
meso- middle
meta- after
metr- uterus
micr- small
milli- thousand
mono- single
-morph form
muco- mucus
multi- many
myc- fungus
myel- marrow
myo- muscle
narc- numb
naso- nose
necr- corpse
neo- new
nephr- kidney
neur- nerve
ocul- eye

odont- tooth
-odynia pain
-oid like
oligo- few
-ology study
-oma tumour
onc- mass
onych- nail
oö- egg
ophthalm- eye
-opsy looking
or- mouth
orchid- testis
orth- straight
os- mouth
os-, oste- bone
-osis pathological state
-ostomy opening
ot- ear
-otomy cutting
ovi- egg
pachy- thick
paed- child
pan- all
para- beside, beyond
path- suffering, disease
-pathy disease
-penia lack
pent- five
per- through
peri- around
-pexy fixing
-phagia swallowing
pharmac- drug
-phasia speech

phleb- vein
-phobia irrational fear
phon- sound
photo- light
phren- diaphragm, mind
-phylaxis prevention, protection
physi- form, nature
-plegia paralysis
pneum- lung
pod- foot
-poiesis formation
poly- many
post- after
prae-, pre-, pro- before, in front
proct- anus
pseud- false
psych- mind
pyo- pus, matter
pyr- fire, fever
quadr- four
quint- five
radi- ray
re- back, again
ren- kidney
retro- backwards
rhin- nose
-rrhoea discharge
-rrhaphy repair
rub- red
salping- (uterine) tube
sarc- flesh
sclero- hard
-scope viewing instrument

-scopy looking
semi- half
sept- seven
-sonic sound
sphygm- pulse
splen- spleen
spondy- vertebra
steat- fat
sub- below
super-, supra- above
syn- with
tachy- quick
tars- eyelid, instep
-taxia, -taxis arrangement, order
tetra- four
therm- heat
thorac- chest
thromb- clot
-tome cutting instrument
toxic- poison
trans- through, across
tri- three
trich- hair
troph- nourishment
-tropy turning
tympano- middle ear
ultra- beyond
uni- one
uri- urine
-uria urine
vas- vessel
xanth- yellow
xero- dry
zoo- animal

Reproduced with permission from Kasner K, Tindall DH 1984 Baillière's Nurses' Dictionary, 20th edn. Baillière Tindall, London

# 2

# Bones and organs of the human body

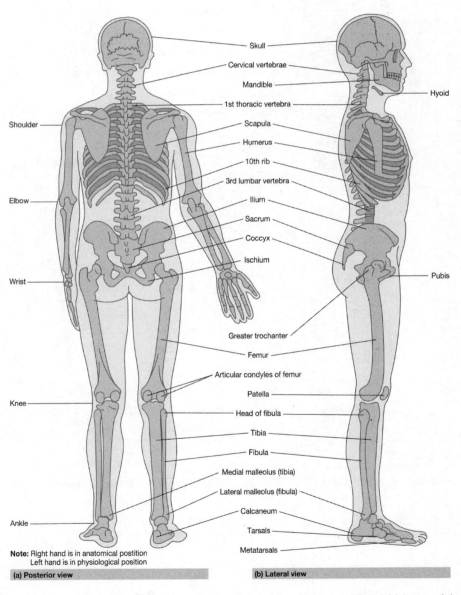

Skull
Cervical vertebrae
Mandible
Hyoid
1st thoracic vertebra
Shoulder
Scapula
Humerus
10th rib
3rd lumbar vertebra
Elbow
Ilium
Sacrum
Coccyx
Ischium
Wrist
Pubis
Greater trochanter
Femur
Articular condyles of femur
Patella
Knee
Head of fibula
Tibia
Fibula
Medial malleolus (tibia)
Lateral malleolus (fibula)
Calcaneum
Ankle
Tarsals
Metatarsals

**Note:** Right hand is in anatomical postition
Left hand is in physiological position

**(a) Posterior view**

**(b) Lateral view**

**Figure I** The human skeleton (a) posterior view, (b) right lateral view, (c) anterior view, (d) and (e) bones of the forearm. Reproduced with permission from Hinchliff SM, Montague SE, Watson R 1996 Physiology for nursing practice, 2nd edn. Baillière Tindall, London

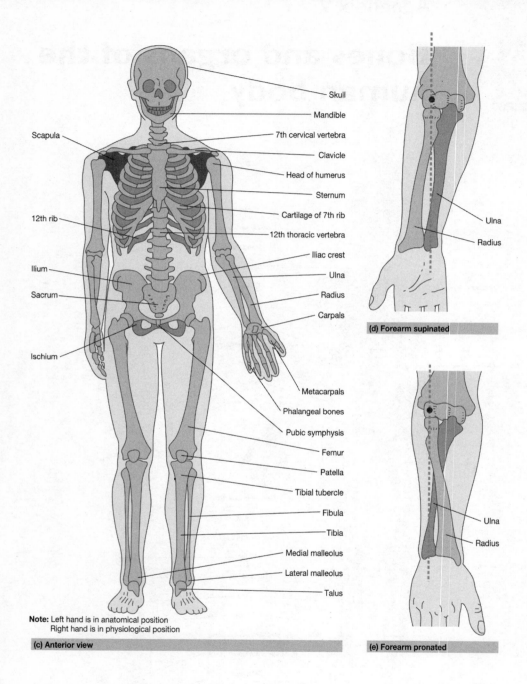

Skull
Mandible
7th cervical vertebra
Clavicle
Head of humerus
Sternum
Cartilage of 7th rib
12th thoracic vertebra
Iliac crest
Ulna
Radius
Carpals

Scapula
12th rib
Ilium
Sacrum
Ischium

Metacarpals
Phalangeal bones
Pubic symphysis
Femur
Patella
Tibial tubercle
Fibula
Tibia
Medial malleolus
Lateral malleolus
Talus

**Note:** Left hand is in anatomical position
Right hand is in physiological position

**(c) Anterior view**

Ulna
Radius

**(d) Forearm supinated**

Ulna
Radius

**(e) Forearm pronated**

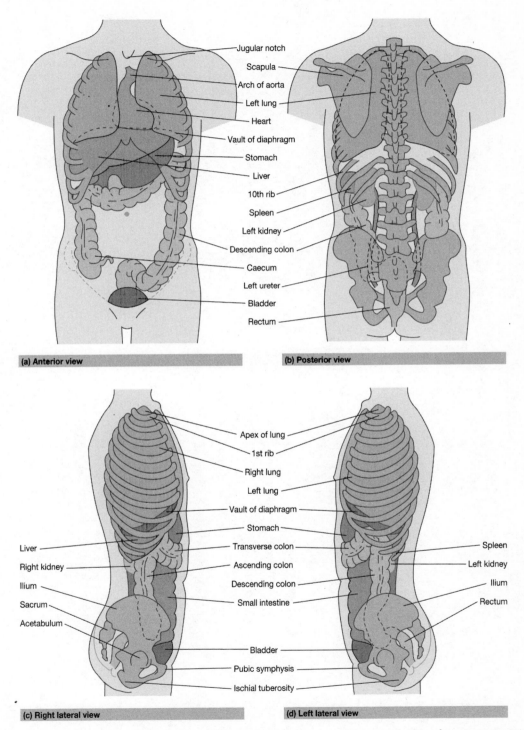

**Figure 2** Anatomical relationships between the organs of the trunk in anterior (a), posterior (b), right lateral (c) and left lateral (d) views. Reproduced with permission from Hinchliff SM, Montague SE, Watson R 1996 Physiology for nursing practice, 2nd edn. Baillière Tindall, London

# Appendix 3

**3**

# Useful Addresses

Action on Smoking and Health (ASH),
109 Gloucester Place,
London W1H 4EJ

Age Concern England
(National Old People's Welfare Council),
60 Pitcairn Road,
Mitcham,
Surrey CR4 3LL

Alcohol Concern
(The National Agency of Alcohol Misuse),
305 Grays Inn Road,
London WC1X 8QF

Alzheimer's Disease Society,
3rd Floor,
Bank Building,
Fulham Broadway,
London SW6 1EP

APEX Partnership,
22–24 Worple Road,
Wimbledon,
London SW19 4DD

Arthritis and Rheumatism Council (ARC),
41 Eagle Street,
London WC1R 4AR

Association of British Paediatric Nurses (ABPN),
PO Box 14,
Ashton-under-Lyne
OL5 9HH

Association of Carers,
First Floor,
21–23 New Road,
Chatham,
Kent ME4 4JQ

Association of Medical Secretaries,
Practice Managers, Administrators and
Receptionists,
Tavistock House North,
Tavistock Square,
London WC1H 9LN

Association of Radical Midwives,
c/o Haringey Women's Centre,
40 Turnpike Lane,
London N8

Association for Improvements in the Maternity
Services (AIMS),
163 Liverpool Road,
London N1 0RF

Asthma Society,
300 Upper Street,
London N1 2XX

Back Pain Association,
31–33 Park Road,
Teddington,
Middlesex TW11 0AB

Breast Care and Mastectomy Association,
26a Harrison Street,
London WC1H 8JG

British Association for Cancer United Patients
(BACUP),
3 Bath Place,
Rivington Street,
London EC2A 3JR

British Association for Counselling,
37a Sheep Street,
Rugby,
Warwickshire CV21 3BX

British Colostomy Association,
38–39 Eccleston Square,
London SW1V 1PB

British Council for the Rehabilitation of the
Disabled,
25 Mortimer Street,
London W1

British Deaf Association,
38 Victoria Place,
Carlisle,
Cumbria CA1 1HU

British Diabetic Association,
10 Queen Anne Street,
London W1M 0BD

British Dietetic Association,
Daimler House,
Paradise Circus,
Queensway,
Birmingham B1 2BJ

British Epilepsy Association,
Anstey House,
40 Hanover Square,
Leeds LS3 1BE

British Geriatrics Society (BGS),
1 St Andrew's Place,
London NW1 4LB

British Heart Foundation,
102 Gloucester Place,
London W1H 4DH

British Kidney Patients' Association,
Bonden,
Hampshire

British Medical Association,
Department of Ethics, Science and Information,
BMA House,
Tavistock Square,
London WC1H 9JR

British Nutrition Foundation,
15 Belgrave Square,
London SW1X 8PS

British Pregnancy Advisory Service,
Austry Manor,
Wooten Wawen,
Solihull,
West Midlands B95 6DA

British Red Cross Society (BRCS),
9 Grosvenor Crescent,
London SW1X 7EJ

Cancer Link,
17 Britannia Street,
London WC1X 9JN

Carers' National Association,
29 Chilwalk Mews,
London W2 3RG

Childline,
Royal Mail Building,
Studd Street,
London N1 0QW

Coeliac Society,
PO Box 220,
High Wycombe,
Buckinghamshire HP11 2HY

Committee on Safety of Drugs,
Finsbury Square House,
33–37a Finsbury Square,
London EC2

Compassionate Friends,
6 Denmark Street,
Bristol BS1 5DG

Coronary Prevention Group,
Central Middlesex Hospital,
Acton Lane,
London NW10

Cruse (National Association for the Widowed
and their Children),
Cruse House,
126 Sheen Road,
Richmond,
Surrey TW9 1UR

Department of Health,
Richmond House,
79 Whitehall,
London SE1 6LW

English National Board for Nursing, Midwifery
and Health Visiting (ENB),
Victory House,
170 Tottenham Court Road,
London WP1P 0HA

Family Planning Association (FPA),
Margaret Pyke House,
27–35 Mortimer Street,
London W1N 7RJ

Food and Drink Federation,
6 Catherine Street,
London WC2B 5JJ

Foresight – the Association for the Promotion of
Preconceptual Care,
The Old Vicarage,
Church Lane,
Witley,
Godalming,
Surrey GU8 5PN

Gamblers Anonymous and Gam-Anon,
17–23 Blantyre Street,
Cheyne Walk,
London SW10 0DT

General Medical Council (GMC),
44 Hallam Street,
London W1

Gerontology Nutrition Unit,
Royal Free Hospital,
School of Medicine,
21 Pond Street,
London NW3 2PN

Haemophilia Society,
123 Westminster Bridge Road,
London SE1 7HR

Health Education Authority,
78 New Oxford Street,
London WC1A 1AH

Health Visitors' Association,
50 Southwark Street,
London SE1 1UN

Help the Aged,
16–18 St James's Walk,
London EC1R 0BE

Hospice Information Service,
St Christopher's Hospice,
51–59 Lawrie Park Road,
Sydenham,
London SE26 6DZ

Hospital Caterers' Association,
43 Royston Road,
Penge,
London SE20 7QW

Ileostomy Association of Great Britain
and Ireland,
Amblehurst House,
Chobham,
Woking,
Surrey GU24 8PZ

Infection Control Nurses' Association (ICNA),
c/o Janet Roberts,
Clatterbridge Hospital,
Bebington,
Wirral,
Merseyside L63 4JY

Institute of Complementary Medicine,
21 Portland Place,
London W1N 3AF

International Council of Nurses,
37 rue Vermont,
1202 Geneva,
Switzerland

Invalids at Home,
23 Farm Avenue,
London NW2 2BJ

King's Fund Centre,
126 Albert Street,
London NW1 7NF

Lady Hoare Trust for Physically Disabled
Children (Associated with Arthritis Care),
7 North Street,
Midhurst,
West Sussex GU29 9DJ

Leukaemia Society,
28 Eastern Road,
London N2

London Food Commission,
PO Box 291,
London N5 1DU

MacMillan Cancer Relief,
Anchor House,
15–19 Britten Street,
London SW3 3TY

Malcolm Sargent Cancer Fund for Children,
14 Abingdon Road,
London W8 6AF

Marie Curie Memorial Foundation,
28 Belgrave Square,
London SW1X 8QG

Medic-Alert Foundation,
11–13 Alfton Terrace,
London N4 3JP

MIND (National Association for Mental Health),
22 Harley Street,
London W1N 2ED

Multiple Sclerosis Society of Great Britain and
Northern Ireland,
25 Effie Road,
Fulham,
London SW4 0QP

Narcotics Anonymous,
PO Box 246,
London SW1

National Advisory Centre on the Battered Child,
Denver House,
The Drive,
Bounds Green Road,
London N11

National Association for the Welfare of Children
in Hospital (NAWCH),
Argyle House,
29–31 Euston Road,
London NW1 2SD

National Board for Nursing, Midwifery and
Health Visiting for Northern Ireland,
123–137 York Street,
Belfast BT15 1JB

National Board for Nursing,
Midwifery and Health Visiting for Scotland,
Trinity Park House,
South Trinity Road,
Edinburgh EH5 3SF

National Childbirth Trust (NCT),
9 Queensborough Terrace,
London W2 3TB

National Council for One Parent Families,
255 Kentish Town Road,
London NW5 2LX

National Council for Vocational Qualifications,
222 Euston Road,
London NW1

National Federation of Kidney Patients'
Associations,
Acorn Lodge,
Woodsets,
Nr Worksop,
Notts S81 8AT

NHS Management Executive,
Quarry House,
Quarry Hill,
Leeds LS2 7EU

National Schizophrenia Fellowship,
79 Victoria Road,
Surbiton,
Surrey KT6 4NS

National Society for Epilepsy,
Chalfont Centre for Epilepsy,
Chalfont St Peter,
Gerrards Cross,
Bucks SL9 0RJ

National Society for PKU and Allied Disorders,
26 Towngate Grove,
Mirfield,
West Yorkshire

National Society for the Prevention of Cruelty to
Children (NSPCC),
67 Saffron Hill,
London EC1N 8RS

Neonatal Nurses' Association (NNA),
Room 7,
Milton Chambers,
19 Milton Street,
Nottingham NG1 3EN

Nursing and Hospital Careers
Information Centre,
121 Edgware Road,
London W2 2HX

Nutrition Society,
Grosvenor Gardens House,
35–37 Grosvenor Gardens,
London SW1W 0BS

Oxford Nutrition,
PO Box 31,
Oxford OX2 6HB

Parent's Friend,
c/o Voluntary Action Leeds,
Stringer House,
34 Lupton Street,
Hunslet,
Leeds LS10 2QW

Parkinson's Disease Society,
36 Portland Place,
London W1N 3DG

Pregnancy Advisory Service,
13 Charlotte Street,
London W1P 1HD

Primary Nursing Network,
Nursing Developments,
King's Fund Centre,
126 Albert Street,
London NW1 7NF

Renal Society,
64 South Hill Park,
London NW3 2SJ

Royal Association in Aid of the Deaf and Dumb,
27 Old Oak Road,
London W3 7SL

Royal College of Midwives (RCM),
15 Mansfield Street,
London W1M 0BE

Royal College of Nursing and Council of Nurses
of the United Kingdom (RCN),
20 Cavendish Square,
London W1M 0AB

Royal Institute of Public Health and Hygiene,
28 Portland Place,
London W1N 4DE

Royal National Institute for the Blind (RNIB),
224 Great Portland Place,
London W1N 6AA

Royal National Institute for the Deaf (RNID),
105 Gower Street,
London WC1E 6AH

Royal Society of Health,
13 Grosvenor Place,
London SW1X 7EN

Royal Society of Medicine,
1 Wimpole Street,
London W1M 8AE

Royal Society for the Prevention of Accidents
(RoSPA),
Cannon House,
The Priory,
Queensway,
Birmingham B4 6BS

St John Ambulance Association (StJAA),
1 Grosvenor Crescent,
London SW1X 7EF

Samaritans Incorporated,
17 Uxbridge Road,
Slough,
Berkshire SL1 1SN

SCOPE,
12 Park Crescent,
London W1N 4EQ

Sickle Cell Society,
Green Lodge,
Barretts Green Road,
London NW10 7AP

Standing Conference on Drug Abuse,
1–4 Hatton Place,
Hatton Garden,
London EC1N 8ND

Stillbirth and Neonatal Death Society (SANDS),
Argyle House,
29–31 Euston Road,
London NW1 2SD

Stress Syndrome Foundation,
Cedar House,
Yalding,
Kent ME18 6JD

Sue Ryder Foundation,
Cavendish,
Sudbury,
Suffolk CO10 8AY

Terrence Higgins Trust,
BM AIDS,
London WC1N 3XX

Tranquillizer Withdrawal Support,
160 Tosson Terrace,
Heaton,
Newcastle-upon-Tyne NE6 5EA

Twins and Multiple Births Association,
54 Broad Lane,
Hampton,
Middlesex TW12 3BG

UNISON (formerly COHSE, NUPE
and NALGO),
UNISON Towers,
137 High Holborn,
London WC1

United Kingdom Central Council for Nursing,
Midwifery and Health Visiting (UKCC),
23 Portland Place,
London W1N 3AF

Vegan Society,
47 Highlands Road,
Leatherhead,
Surrey

Vegetarian Society,
Parkdale,
Denham Road,
Altrincham,
Cheshire

Welsh National Board for Nursing, Midwifery
and Health Visiting,
13th Floor,
Pearl Assurance House,
Greyfriars Road,
Cardiff CF1 3AG

Women's Health Concern (WHC),
Ground Floor,
17 Earls Terrace,
London W8 6LP

Women's Royal Voluntary Service (WRVS),
17 Old Park Lane,
London W1Y 4AJ

World Health Organization,
Geneva,
Switzerland

Reproduced with permission from Weller BF 1997 Baillière's Nurses Dictionary, 22nd edn. Baillière Tindall, London

# 4

# Degrees, diplomas and organisations

ABPN    Association of British Paediatric Nurses

AIMSW    Association of the Institute of Medical Social Workers

APEX    Association of Professional and Executive Staffs

BA    Bachelor of Arts

BAO    Bachelor of the Art of Obstetrics

BAON    British Association of Orthopaedic Nurses

BC, BCh, BChir    Bachelor of Surgery

BDA    British Dental Association

BDSc    Bachelor of Dental Science

BHyg    Bachelor of Hygiene

BM    Bachelor of Medicine

BN    Bachelor of Nursing

BPOG    British Psychosocial Oncology Group

BRCS    British Red Cross Society

BS, ChB    Bachelor of Surgery

BSc (Soc SC-Nurs)    Bachelor of Science (Nursing)

CCHE    Central Council for Health Education

CM, ChM    Master of Surgery

CNAA    Council for National Academic Awards

CPH    Certificate in Public Health

CSP    Chartered Society of Physiotherapists

DA    Diploma in Anaesthetics

DCH    Diploma in Child Health

DCh    Doctor of Surgery

DCP    Diploma in Clinical Pathology

DDA    Dangerous Drugs Act

DDO    Diploma in Dental Orthopaedics

DDS    Doctor of Dental Surgery

DGO    Diploma in Gynaecology and Obstetrics

DHyg    Doctor of Hygiene

DIH    Diploma in Industrial Health

DipED    Diploma in Education

DipNEd    Diploma in Nursing Education

DLO    Diploma in Laryngology and Otology

DM    Doctor of Medicine

DMD    Doctor of Dental Medicine

DMR    Diploma in Medical Radiology

DMRE    Diploma in Medical Radiology and Electrology

DN    Diploma in Nursing

DNA    District Nursing Association

DNE    Diploma in Nursing Education

DO    Diploma in Ophthalmology

DObstRCOG    Diploma in Obstetrics of the Royal College of Obstetricians and Gynaecologists

DOMS    Diploma in Ophthalmologic Medicine and Surgery

DPA    Diploma in Public Administration

DPD    Diploma in Public Dentistry

DPH    Diploma in Public Health

DPhil    Doctor of Philosophy

DPhysMed    Diploma in Physical Medicine

DPM    Diploma in Psychological Medicine

DR    Diploma in Radiology

DSc    Doctor of Science

DSSc    Diploma in Sanitary Science

DTM&H    Diploma in Tropical Medicine and Hygiene

EN    Enrolled Nurse

ENB    English National Board for Nursing, Midwifery and Health Visiting

FACP    Fellow of American College of Physicians

FACS    Fellow of American College of Surgeons

FBPsS    Fellow of British Psychological Society

FCSP    Fellow of the Chartered Society of Physiotherapists

**FDS**   Fellow of Dental Surgery
**FETC**   Further Education Teaching Certificate
**FFA**   Fellow of Faculty of Anaesthetists
**FFHom**   Fellow of Faculty of Homeopathy
**FFR**   Fellow of Faculty of Radiologists
**FLS**   Fellow of Linnean Society
**FNIF**   Florence Nightingale International Foundation
**FPA**   Family Planning Association
**FRACP**   Fellow of the Royal Australian College of Physicians
**FRACS**   Fellow of the Royal Australian College of Surgeons
**FRCGP**   Fellow of the Royal College of General Practitioners
**FRCN**   Fellow of the Royal College of Nursing
**FRCOG**   Fellow of the Royal College of Obstetricians and Gynaecologists
**FRCP**   Fellow of the Royal College of Physicians of London
**FRCPath**   Fellow of the Royal College of Pathologists
**FRCPE***   Fellow of the Royal College of Physicians of Edinburgh
**FRCPS**   Fellow of the Royal College of Physicians and Surgeons
**FRCPsych**   Fellow of the Royal College of Psychiatrists
**FRCS**   Fellow of the Royal College of Surgeons of England
**FRCSE**   Fellow of the Royal College of Surgeons of Edinburgh
**FRES**   Fellow of the Royal Entomological Society
**FRIPHH**   Fellow of the Royal Institute of Public Health and Hygiene
**FRS**   Fellow of the Royal Society
**FRSanI**   Fellow of the Royal Sanitary Institute
**FRSH**   Fellow of the Royal Society of Health
**FSS**   Fellow of the Royal Statistical Society
**GMC**   General Medical Council
**GNVQ**   General National Vocational Qualification
**HSA**   Hospital Savings Association
**HV**   Health Visitor
**HVA**   Health Visitors' Association
**HVCert**   Health Visitors' Certificate
**ICN**   International Council of Nurses

**ICNA**   Infection Control Nurses' Association
**ICW**   International Council of Women
**IHF**   International Hospital Federation
**LAH**   Licentiate of Apothecaries Hall, Dublin
**LDS**   Licentiate in Dental Surgery
**LDSc**   Licentiate in Dental Science
**LM**   Licentiate in Midwifery
**LMS**   Licentiate in Medicine and Surgery
**LMSSA**   Licentiate in Medicine and Surgery, Society of Apothecaries
**LRCP**   Licentiate of Royal College of Physicians
**LRFPS**   Licentiate of Royal Faculty of Physicians and Surgeons
**LSA**   Licentiate of Society of Apothecaries
**LSSc**   Licentiate of Sanitary Science
**M-C**   Medico-Chirurgical
**MA**   Master of Arts
**MAO**   Master of the Art of Obstetrics
**MAOT**   Member of the Association of Occupational Therapists
**MB**   Bachelor of Medicine
**MBA**   Master of Business Administration
**MBIM**   Member of the British Institute of Management
**MC, MCh, MChir**   Master of Surgery
**MChD**   Master of Dental Surgery
**MChOrth**   Master of Orthopaedic Surgery
**MCPath**   Member of College of Pathology
**MCPS**   Member of College of Physicians and Surgeons
**MCSP**   Member of the Chartered Society of Physiotherapists
**MD**   Doctor of Medicine
**MDentSc**   Master of Dental Science
**MDS**   Master of Dental Surgery
**MFCP**   Member of the Faculty of Community Physicians
**MFHom**   Member of the Faculty of Homeopathy
**MHyg**   Master of Hygiene
**MIND**   National Association for Mental Health
**MMSA**   Master of Midwifery of Society of Apothecaries
**MPH**   Master of Public Health
**MPhil**   Master of Philosophy
**MRC**   Medical Research Council
**MRCGP**   Member of Royal College of General Practitioners

**MRCOG** Member of Royal College of Obstetricians and Gynaecologists

**MRCP** Member of Royal College of Physicians of London

**MRCPath** Member of Royal College of Pathologists

**MRCPsych** Member of Royal College of Psychiatrists

**MRCS** Member of Royal College of Surgeons of England

**MRSanI** Member of Royal Sanitary Institute

**MRSH** Member of the Royal Society of Health

**MS** Master of Surgery

**MSc** Master of Science

**MSF** Manufacturing Science and Health

**MSR(R)** Member of the Society of Radiographers (Radiography)

**MSR(T)** Member of the Society of Radiographers (Radiotherapy)

**MSRG** Member of the Society of Remedial Gymnasts

**MTD** Midwife Teachers' Diploma

**NAMCW** National Association for Maternal and Child Welfare

**NAMH** National Association for Mental Health

**NATN** National Association of Theatre Nurses

**NAWCH** National Association for the Welfare of Children in Hospital

**NHS** National Health Service

**NIB** Northern Ireland Board for Nursing, Midwifery and Health Visiting

**NNA** Neonatal Nurses' Association

**NNEB** National Nursery Education Board

**NUMINE** Network of Users of Microcomputers in Nurse Education

**OHNC** Occupational Health Nursing Certificate

**ONC** Orthopaedic Nurses' Certificate

**OND** Ophthalmic Nursing Diploma

**OT** Occupational Therapist

**PhD** Doctor of Philosophy

**PMRAFNS** Princess Mary's Royal Air Force Nursing Service

**PNA** Psychiatric Nurses' Association

**QARANC** Queen Alexandra's Royal Army Nursing Service

**QARNNS** Queen Alexandra's Royal Naval Nursing Service

**QIDN** Queen's Institute of District Nursing

**QNI** Queen's Nursing Institute

**RCM** Royal College of Midwives

**RCN** Royal College of Nursing

**RGN** Registered General Nurse

**RHV** Regional Health Visitor

**RMN** Registered Mental Nurse

**RN** Registered Nurse

**RNMH** Registered Nurse for the Mentally Handicapped

**RNT** Registered Nurse Tutor

**RSCN** Registered Sick Children's Nurse

**SCM** State Certified Midwife

**SEN** State Enrolled Nurse

**SNB** Scottish National Board for Nursing, Midwifery and Health Visiting

**SNNEB** Scottish National Nursing Examination Board

**SRN** State Registered Nurse

**SSStJ** Serving Sister of the Order of St John of Jerusalem

**StAAA** St John Ambulance Association

**StJAB** St John Ambulance Brigade

**TDD** Tuberculous Diseases Diploma

**UKCC** United Kingdom Central Council for Nursing, Midwifery and Health Visiting

**VSO** Voluntary Service Overseas

**WNB** Welsh National Board for Nursing, Midwifery and Health Visiting

**WRVS** Women's Royal Voluntary Service

*This may be written as FRCPEd, FRCP(Ed), FRCP(Edin) or FRCPE. It is correct to add the appropriate College after MRCP or FRCS of the Scottish Royal Colleges.

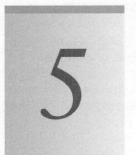

# 5

# Professional organisations and trade unions

## AMSPAR

The Association of Medical Secretaries, Practice Managers, Administrators and Receptionists was founded in 1964 (initially called the Association of Medical Secretaries). Its objectives were:

◆ to promote, encourage and support the education and maintenance of high standards amongst those engaged in these areas of work
◆ to promote, encourage and support research into administrative problems associated with medical practice
◆ to establish branches of the Association throughout the UK and elsewhere as a forum for support for members.

Membership is based on both formal qualifications or length of service. Currently membership is in excess of 5500.

AMSPAR has developed an educational system designed to provide specialist training which has been updated constantly to address the needs of the services. AMSPAR is registered with the DOE &E as an Examining and Validating Body. The courses are delivered by further education colleges. The qualifications at present are:

◆ Certificate in General Practice Reception
◆ Diploma in Health Services Reception
◆ Diploma and Certificate for Medical Secretaries
◆ Diploma and Certificate in Practice Management.

The Head Office is based in Tavistock House North, Tavistock Square, London and is run by the General Secretary. The Council of the Association is made up of the President, three Vice-presidents, Chairman, Treasurer and 18 Regional Members who meet quarterly, or more often if necessary.

The Association also publishes the AMSPAR Journal, which is distributed free of charge to members.

## APEX PARTNERSHIP

In 1989 the Association of Professional and Executive Staffs (APEX) merged with the GMB, Britain's general union. The Apex Partnership now represents members within the white collar section of the union, which has a membership of over 800 000. The GMB/Apex Partnership is committed to issues of equal pay and rights, and works for better pay and conditions of service and a healthier working environment. Through the GMB, it sponsors members of parliament (MPs) and is affiliated to the Trades Union Congress (TUC). The GMB/Apex Partnership is represented on the Nurses and Midwives General Whitley Council.

## BRITISH MEDICAL ASSOCIATION (BMA)

The British Medical Association is the most influential and powerful organisation set up to represent the interests of doctors in this country. It first started in 1832, under the name of the Provincial Medical and Surgical Association founded in Worcester by Charles Hastings. It exerted considerable pressure at the time to control the practice of unqualified practitioners by demanding a single licensing authority and a single qualification permitting practice in any branch of the medical profession.

Renamed the BMA in 1855, it has emerged as the largest medical association and the principal body representing British doctors. The BMA has representation on the Central Health Services Council, the General Medical Services Committee and the Central Consultants' and Specialists' Committee.

The BMA has a regional structure. The Executive body of the Association is the BMA Council which is made up of some 70 doctors elected annually and a few ex-officio members.

The work of the Association can be grouped under five headings:

◆ Representation – collective and individual
◆ Publishing – 18 journals including the *BMJ*
◆ Clinical conferences – organises clinical meetings and annual scientific meetings
◆ Benevolent – a number of charity events are organised
◆ Insurance – the Medical Insurance Agency was started in 1907 to obtain the best insurance terms for individual doctors.

## BRIDGES

Formerly the Association of Professions for Mentally Handicapped People (APMH), BRIDGES is a charity totally committed to working in partnership with people with learning disabilities to enable them to benefit from improved services and opportunities. It has no bias towards any profession or discipline, recognising that better services develop from effective working partnerships across all 'boundaries' in the promotion and dissemination of good practice.

## COMMUNITY AND DISTRICT NURSING ASSOCIATION (CDNA)

The CDNA is a professional organisation and trade union which addresses directly the needs of nurses and health workers in the community. It is the fourth largest nursing union and the fastest growing. The CDNA continually campaigns for improved working conditions for its members. It organises courses, workshops and conferences and publishes a quarterly magazine, *Nursing Care*.

## GENERAL MEDICAL COUNCIL (GMC)

The campaign calling for a single licensing authority in the middle of the 19th century resulted in the passing of the 1858 Medical Act. The Act created the General Council of Medical Education and Registration, now called the General Medical Council (GMC).

The Council is made up of members representing the Royal Colleges, the Universities, the Crown and the profession at large.

The GMC is responsible for the following:

◆ maintaining a register of practitioners
◆ supervising the educational standards of training institutions (in practice the GMC relies on the Royal Colleges for this)
◆ disciplining doctors – ultimate sanction being 'striking off' the name from the register, for example in cases of gross misconduct
◆ publication of the British Pharmacopoeia.

## HEALTH VISITORS' ASSOCIATION (HVA)

The HVA is the main professional organisation representing the interests of health visitors and school nurses while taking in those of practice nurses and district nurses as well; it has some 17 000 members. It was the first health organisation to affiliate to the TUC (in 1924) and combine the roles of trade union and professional association.

The HVA's professional service to members includes update and refresher education courses and the provision of a specialist library and information service. It is also closely concerned with professional development and standards of practice. It provides industrial advice to members through its labour relations department and network of local representatives. It publishes a monthly professional journal, *Health Visitor*, which is distributed free to all members.

## INFECTION CONTROL NURSES' ASSOCIATION (ICNA)

The ICNA is a registered charity, formed in 1970, whose primary objective is the advancement of education in infection control for the benefit of the whole community. The association also aims to meet the professional needs of infection control nurses and comprises a network of regional groups which acts as a support network and information source for members. The national executive committee manages the business affairs of the association and supports regional groups in organising study days and conferences. The association publishes the *Journal of Infection Control Nursing* as a supplement to *Nursing Times* six times a year. It is not affiliated to the TUC and does not sponsor MPs.

## INTERNATIONAL COUNCIL OF NURSES (ICN)

Founded in 1899, the ICN is the oldest international professional organisation in the health care field. ICN accepts into membership one association of nurses per country. There are 95 national nurses' organisations in membership. In addition, ICN works with approximately 50 other national associations or groups of nurses with a view to their future membership.

The governing body of the ICN is the Council of National Representatives (CNR) elected on the principle of one country, one vote. The CNR meets every 2 years to determine policy matters affecting the nursing profession. Every fourth year this meeting is held in conjunction with an ICN quadrennial congress, open to nurses throughout the world.

ICN is in official relationship with the World Health Organization (WHO), is included on the special list of non-governmental organisations maintained by the International Labour Organization (ILO), for consultative purposes is in relationship with the United Nations Educational, Scientific and Cultural Organization (UNESCO) and with the United Nations International Children's Emergency Fund (UNICEF), is on the Consultative Register of the Economics and Social Council (ECOSCO), and is in relationship with the International Committee of the Red Cross, the League of Red Cross Societies, the World Medical Association, the International Hospital Federation and the Union of International Associations.

## KING'S FUND

The King Edward's Hospital Fund for London (King's Fund for short) is an independent charity founded in 1897 and incorporated by Act of Parliament.

It seeks to encourage good practice and innovation in health care through research, experiment, education and direct grant.

The King's Fund operates through the three arms of its organisation

◆ The King's Fund College
◆ The King's Fund Centre
◆ The Fund's Project Committee.

The College provides facilities for courses run by the Fund – short day courses and residential courses. The college specialises in health services management courses.

The Centre provides an information service and a forum for discussion of hospital problems and is involved in the advancement of inquiry, experiment and formation of new ideas. The Centre provides an excellent reference library and publication facilities.

Allied to the Centre's work is the Fund's Project Committee, which sponsors work of an experimental nature. It offers grants and publication facilities to enable successful experimental work to become better known. Examples of these include the development of Nursing Development Units (NDUs) throughout the NHS, and 'SHARE' project aimed at improving services for minority ethnic populations.

## NEONATAL NURSES' ASSOCIATION (NNA)

The NNA was formed in 1977, bringing together nurses and midwives working in the field of neonatal care. The aim of the association as a registered charity and a professional organisation is the promotion of good standards of neonatal nursing for the benefit of babies, their families and the nurses and midwives involved in their care.

The NNA comprises a network of regional groups throughout the UK. It publishes a yearbook, biannual newsletter to all members and the *Journal of Neonatal Nursing*.

## ROYAL COLLEGES

The Royal Colleges are medical corporations mainly concerned with the education and post-registration training and development of doctors. Some of the Royal Colleges have a long history and have played a significant part in raising the profile and prestige of their particular branch of medicine. The oldest, the Royal College of Physicians, was founded in 1518 as the Royal College of Physicians of London. The prestige of surgeons grew later with the expansion of voluntary hospitals. The Company of Surgeons was founded in 1745; by 1800 it became the Royal College of Surgeons.

Other medical corporations subsequently established include:

the Royal College of Obstetricians and Gynaecologists (1929)
the Royal College of General Practitioners (1952)
the Royal College of Pathologists (1962)
the Royal College of Psychiatrists (1971).

The power and influence of the Royal Colleges are seen through the supervision of training posts and educational facilities. The Colleges have power to remove training approval from medical posts, thus making it impossible for the vacancy to be filled. Where this has happened it has been on the grounds that the following had not been met in part or whole:

◆ adequacy and availability of experience to sustain the terms of the syllabus for post-registration training
◆ adequacy of facilities, e.g. library, study leave, etc., to support training.

## ROYAL COLLEGE OF MIDWIVES (RCM)

The RCM functions as a trade union and professional organisation for 90% of the country's practising midwives (36 000 members). It is the only British organisation that represents all categories of midwife, and offers services to meet educational, professional and industrial relations needs. In recent years its membership has increased by 25%.

The RCM is a member organisation and is governed by an elected council of 27 members. It has board officers in each of the four countries of the UK and has over 230 branches. The interests of members at local level are served by a wide network of stewards and branch officers.

The organisation is committed to encouraging high standards of care in midwifery, and to the reduction of social deprivation and deficits in health.

The Royal College of Midwives is an independent trade union, is not affiliated to the TUC, and does not sponsor MPs.

## ROYAL COLLEGE OF NURSING OF THE UNITED KINGDOM (RCN)

The RCN is the largest organisation in the UK representing the interests of qualified nurses and students of nursing. It has in excess of 300 000 members. The organisation is committed to meeting the professional, educational and labour relations needs of its members through its board offices at country level and regional offices in each of the countries. The structure of the membership is based on local branches, members of which elect officers to represent their interests, and also elect to the council of the college on a regional basis. The college comprises departments that meet the specific needs of its membership: labour relations/legal, professional, international, welfare, students and education.

The Education Department is controlled by the RCN Institute of Advanced Nursing Education in London, Birmingham and Belfast, who offer a wide variety of educational programmes and courses for nurses.

The professional needs of its members are addressed by the Department of Nursing Policy and Practice. The diverse interests of nurses are reflected by the wide variety of professional associations, societies, forums and special interest groups run by the professional officers in this department.

The International Department liaises closely with nursing organisations in other countries, and with international organisations. Through this department, the RCN represents the interests of British nurses on the Standing Nursing/Midwifery Committee of the EU. The International Department is available to offer practical advice and help with contracts and conditions of service for those nurses wishing to work overseas. It can also help in arranging overseas study visits.

The Labour Relations/Legal Department offers a service to those experiencing difficulties in their place of work. It is concerned with salaries/conditions of service, health and safety at work and legal problems of nurses. The department coordinates a nationwide stewards' scheme and a network of health and safety representatives.

Nurseline is a confidential counselling service available to all nurses. The headquarters building of the RCN houses the largest nursing library in Europe with 40 000 volumes and 220 regular journals. The specialist collections of literature and nursing research (the Historical Collection and the Sternberg Collection) can be found here.

The RCN operates a wide range of membership services, has its own housing association for retired nurses, and confers fellowships upon nurses who are deemed to have made a significant contribution to the art and science of nursing.

The organisation is an independent trade union, is not affiliated to the TUC and does not sponsor MPs. The RCN represents UK nursing on the board of the International Council of Nurses.

## RED CROSS

The Red Cross is a humanitarian agency with national affiliates in almost every country. It was first established to care for the victims of battle in times of war. It is now involved in the prevention and relief of human suffering generally.

Its wartime activities are better known, its aims being to provide a neutral service for the care of the war wounded whether friend or foe. Its peacetime activities are very impressive; they include:

◆ first aid, and accident prevention
◆ provision and supply of aids (wheelchairs, walking frames, etc.).

In developing countries the list includes:

◆ water safety
◆ training of nurses' aids and mothers' assistants
◆ maintaining maternal and child welfare clinics and blood banks.

The establishment of the Red Cross is attributed to a Swiss, Henri Dunant, who was moved by the sight of the wounded at the battle of Solferino in June 1859. In a publication in 1862, he proposed the formation in all countries of voluntary relief societies; by 1864 the first societies were established.

In the UK, apart from the peacetime activities mentioned above, the Red Cross contributes actively in the NHS by providing volunteers who, in some hospitals, man the hospital shop, provide a tea and buffet service for outpatients and visitors, a library service, and a goods shopping trolley service to the wards.

The Red Cross is still active in tracing relatives separated by war, and maintains a parcel and befriending service for foreign veterans surviving in NHS institutions.

## ST JOHN AMBULANCE

The St John Ambulance Brigade was formed in 1887. It is a voluntary organisation which depends on public donations. The organisation aims to serve the community through the following:

◆ providing first aid training
◆ providing volunteer first aiders at sporting and public events
◆ maintaining a fleet of ambulance vehicles.

The Brigade has to fund the above as well as costs of uniforms, equipment such as wheelchairs, medical dressing and resuscitation equipment from money raised.

The Brigade has three categories of members:

◆ St John Badgers – children between 6 and 10
◆ St John Cadets – for those aged 10 to 18 and adult members.

Among some of the new schemes launched recently has been a project to attend to the primary care needs of the homeless, using National Lottery financial support for this (1997).

# UKCC

The United Kingdom Central Council for Nursing, Midwifery and Health Visiting (UKCC) was set up by the 1979 Nurses Act, replacing the General Nursing Council (GNC). With effect from 1 July 1983, it became responsible for the following:

◆ establishing and improving standards of training and professional conduct
◆ determining rules for the registration of nurses (HVs and Midwives)
◆ maintaining a single professional register
◆ giving guidance on professional conduct and protecting the public from unsafe practitioners.

The Council is made up of 45 members. Originally 17 of them were appointed by the Secretary of State and the remaining 28 were nominated by the four National Boards (seven each by the English, Welsh, Scottish and Northern Irish NBs)

Since 1992, members of the Council are elected by the members for a 5-year term.

The NBs are statutory bodies in their own right

and responsible for implementing policies and rules decided by the UKCC. In particular, they have to provide, or arrange for others to provide, courses of training leading to registration and further postgraduate training and carry out investigations on alleged professional misconduct prior to referral to the UKCC Professional Conduct Committee.

The Council headquarters is at 23 Portland Place, London, and is managed by the Council's Chief Executive.

Recent high profile cases of reinstatement of convicted nurses have provoked outrage amongst nurses themselves, with demands for powers to impose lifelong bans. Other issues under scrutiny include the future of nurse prescribing, the future of Project 2000, the future NVQ in nursing, and professional conduct in the fast expanding nursing and care home sector.

A review to last over 5 years on the role of the UKCC was launched by the government in 1997.

# UNISON

UNISON is the UK's biggest union with more than a million members. It was created on 1 July 1993 by the former Confederation of Health Service Employees (COHSE), the National and Local Government Officers' Association (NALGO) and the National Union of Public Employees (NUPE). In October 1993 the British Association of Occupational Therapy linked up with UNISON. One million UNISON members are women.

UNISON represents employees in health care, local government, higher education, water, gas, electricity and transport.

UNISON is the major union in the health service. Its health care service group represents over 400 000 employees in the NHS covering nursing, ancillary, professional, managerial, administrative, clerical and ambulance staff.

UNISON holds the majority of officership positions on national negotiating bodies and is the leading union of local level in the NHS.

Reproduced in part with permission from Weller BF 1997 Baillière's Nurses' Dictionary, 22nd edn. Baillière Tindall, London

# Drugs and the law

The main Acts governing the use of medicines are the Medicines Act 1968 and the Misuse of Drugs Act 1971.

## THE MISUSE OF DRUGS ACT 1971

This Act imposes controls on those drugs liable to produce dependence or cause harm if misused. The substances cited in Schedule 2 of the Act are known as 'Controlled Drugs' or 'CDs' and include:

| | |
|---|---|
| amphetamine | fentanyl |
| cocaine | methadone |
| codeine injection | methylphenidate |
| dexamphetamine | morphine |
| dextromoramide | pethidine |
| diamorphine (heroin) | phenazocine |
| dihydrocodeine injection | |
| dipipanone (diconal) | |

Note also the controls which apply to Schedule 3 drugs such as buprenorphine and, very recently, temazepam.

Registered medical practitioners and registered dentists may prescribe preparations containing controlled drugs. However, the Misuse of Drugs (Notification of and Supply to Addicts) Regulations 1973 state that medical practitioners may not prescribe, administer or supply controlled drugs to addicted persons as a means of treating their addiction, unless specifically licensed to do so. This is to ensure that addicts will be referred for treatment to a hospital or clinic.

A prescription involving controlled drugs must fulfil the following conditions:

1. Patient's name and address specified in ink.
2. Signed and dated by prescriber.
3. Dose and dosage form, e.g. tab, cap, etc. to be specified.
4. Total quantity to be supplied written in words and figures.

NB. All above in the doctor's handwriting (computer-generated prescriptions are not permitted).

Accurate records must be kept by general practitioners, dentists and hospital staff of all purchases, amounts of drugs issued and dosages given. In hospital the following controls are imposed:

1. Special double locked cupboard for controlled drugs alone.
2. Key kept and carried by ward sister or deputy.
3. Supplies can be obtained by prescription signed by a medical officer, and the drugs can only be given under such written instructions. Ward stocks of controlled drugs in frequent use can also be ordered in special Controlled Drugs Order Books. Each order must be signed by the sister-in-charge.
4. Written record of each dose is made stating date, patient's name, time administered and dosage. This record is signed by nurse giving drug and another nurse who has checked the source of the drug as well as the dosage against the prescription.

All containers used for controlled drugs must bear special labels to distinguish them clearly. The hospital pharmacist checks the contents of the CD cupboard at regular intervals against the record books. Any discrepancies require full investigation.

# THE MEDICINES ACT 1968

Under this Act, medicines are divided into three groups:

Prescription Only Medicines (POM) (apart from Controlled Drugs)
Pharmacy Only Medicines (P)
General Sales List Medicines (GSL)

The POM list includes most of the potent drugs in common use, from antibiotics to hypnotics. The list is too extensive to permit reference to individual drugs as it includes most medicines which should not be used without medical supervision.

Pharmacy Only Medicines are drugs supplied under control and supervision of a registered pharmacist. Representative drugs include ibuprofen, antihistamines and glyceryl trinitrate.

The General Sales List includes commonly used drugs such as aspirin and paracetamol, available through any retail outlet.

These distinctions of POM, P and GSL medicines do not apply to hospitals where it is accepted practice that medicines are supplied only on prescription.

Reproduced with permission from Churchill Livingstone's Dictionary of Nursing, 17th edn, 1996. Churchill Livingstone, Edinburgh

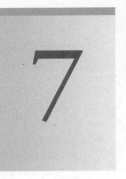

# Prescription abbreviations

These are abbreviations that are used extensively in writing prescriptions.

**a.c.**  before meals
**Amps.**  Ampoules
**b.d.**  twice daily
**b.i.d.**  twice daily
**c.**  with
**Caps**  capsules
**Gtt**  Drops
**Liq**  Solution
**mitte**  dispense
**mane**  in the morning
**mcg**  micrograms
    (there are 1000 mcg in one milligram)
**mg**  milligram(s)
    (there are 1000 mg in one gram)
**Mist**  mixture
**ml**  millilitre(s) (there are 1000 ml in one litre)

**nocte**  at bed-time
**o.d.**  once daily
**o.m.**  each morning
**o.n.**  each night
**o.p.**  original pack
**p.c.**  after meals
**prn**  as required
**q.i.d.**  four times daily
**q.d.s.**  four times daily
**Rx**  supply
**Sig**  let it be labelled
**s.o.s.**  when required
**stat**  to be taken immediately
**Syr**  Syrup
**Tabs**  tablets
**t.d.s**  three times daily
**t.i.d.**  three times daily
**Ung**  ointment
**ut dict**  as directed

8

# Medical abbreviations

In order to produce concise notes and instructions quickly, doctors and other health care practitioners are forced to use a large number of abbreviations. This can cause problems for medical secretaries as there is little standardisation of medical abbreviations and they are easy to misinterpret. Care should be taken in their use.

The following list contains only those abbreviations which are widely used and are not specific to one hospital or practice. Where abbreviations have a Latin origin they appear in italics with the Latin words following in brackets.

*aa (ana)*   of each
*a.c. (ante cibum)*   before meals
*ad*   to; up to
*ad lib. (ad libitum)*   as much as needed
*aet. (aetas)*   aged
**A/G ratio**   albumin/globulin ratio
**alb.**   albumin
*alt. dieb. (alternis diebus)*   every other day
*alt. hor. (alternis horis)*   every other hour
*alt. noct. (alternis noctibus)*   every other night
**AN**   antenatal
*ante (ante)*   before
**AP**   anteroposterior
**APH**   antepartum haemorrhage
**APT**   alum-precipitated toxoid
*aq. (aqua)*   water
*aq.-dist. (aqua distillata)*   distilled water
**ARM**   artificial rupture of membranes
**Ba.E**   barium enema
**Ba.M**   barium meal
**BBA**   born before arrival
**BCG**   Bacille Calmette–Guérin
*b.d.* or *b.i.d. (bis in die)*   twice daily
**BI**   bone injury
*bib. (bibe)*   drink
**BID**   brought in dead
**BMR**   basal metabolic rate

**BNF**   British National Formulary (with date)
**BO**   bowels opened
**BP**   blood pressure or British Pharmacopoeia (with date)
**BPC**   British Pharmaceutical Codex (with date)
**BS**   breath sounds
**C** *(centum gradus)*   centigrade
*c. (circa)*   about
*c. (cum)*   with
**Ca.**   carcinoma
*caps (capsula)*   capsule
**CCF**   congestive cardiac failure
**cf.**   compare
**circ.**   circumcision
**CF**   cystic fibrosis
**cm**   centimetre
**CNS**   central nervous system
**c.o.**   complains of
*Crem (cremor)*   cream
**CSF**   cerebrospinal fluid
**CSOM**   chronic suppurative otitis media
**CSU**   catheter specimen of urine
**CVS**   cardiovascular system
**Cx**   cervix
**D&C**   dilatation and curettage
*dil. (dilutus)*   dilute
**DNA**   did not attend

**DOB**    date of birth
**DT**    delirium tremens
**D and V**    diarrhoea and vomiting
**DU**    duodenal ulcer
**DXR**    deep X-ray
**ECG**    electrocardiogram
**ECT**    electroconvulsive therapy
**EDC**    expected date of confinement
**EDD**    expected date of delivery
**EEG**    electroencephalogram
**ENT**    ear, nose and throat
*e.s. (enema saponis)*    soap enema
**ESN**    educationally subnormal
**ESR**    erythrocyte sedimentation rate
**EUA**    examination under anaesthesia
*ext. (extractum)*    extract
**F**    Fahrenheit
**FB**    foreign body
**FH**    fetal heart or family history
**FHH**    fetal heart heard
**FHNH**    fetal heart not heard
**Fib.**    fibula
*fl. (fluidum)*    fluid
**FMF**    fetal movements felt
*ft. (fiat)*    let there be made
**FTM**    fractional test meal
**g**    gram
**GA**    general anaesthetic
**G and O**    gas and oxygen
**GB**    gall bladder
**GC**    gonorrhoea
**GCFT**    gonorrhoea complement fixation test
**GI**    gastrointestinal
**GP**    general practitioner
**GPI**    general paralysis of insane
**GTT**    glucose tolerance test
**GU**    gastric ulcer
*gt. (gutta)*    drop (eye-drops)
**Gyn.**    gynaecology
*h. (hora)*    hour
**Hb**    haemoglobin
**HP**    house physician
**HS**    house surgeon
*h.s. (hora somni)*    at bed-time
**HV**    health visitor
*id. (idem)*    the same
*i.e. (id est)*    that is
*in d. (in dies)*    daily

**IP**    inpatient
**IQ**    intelligence quotient
*ISQ (in statu quo)*    without change
**IV**    intravenous
**IVP**    intravenous pyelogram
**IZS**    insulin zinc suspension
**KJ**    knee jerk
**KP**    keratitis punctata
**l**    litre (should be written in full)
**LA**    local anaesthetic or local authority
**Lab.**    laboratory
**LE cells**    lupus erythematosus cells
**LIF**    left iliac fossa
**LIH**    left inguinal hernia
*liq. (liquor)*    a solution in water
**LMP**    last menstrual period
**LOA**    left occipitoanterior
**LOP**    left occipitoposterior
**LSCS**    lower segment caesarean section
**LV**    left ventricle
*M. (misce)*    mix
**m.**    minim
**mCi**    millicurie
**MCD**    mean corpuscular diameter
**MCH**    mean corpuscular haemoglobin
**MCHC**    mean corpuscular haemoglobin concentration
**MCV**    mean corpuscular volume
**mEq**    milliequivalent
*mist. (mistura)*    mixture
**mm.**    millimetre
**mmHg**    millimetres of mercury
**MMR**    mass miniature radiography
**MS**    multiple sclerosis
**MSU**    midstream urine
**NAD**    no abnormality detected
**NBI**    no bone injury
**neg.**    negative
**NG**    new growth
*no. (numero)*    number
*noct. (nocte)*    at night
*n.p. (nomen proprium)*    give proper name
**NPU**    not passed urine
**OA**    osteoarthritis
**Ob.**    obstetrics
**OE**    on examination
*Omn. hor. (omni hora)*    every hour
*Omn. noct. (omni nocte)*    every night

**Op.** operation
**OP** outpatient
**PA** pernicious anaemia
**Path.** pathology
**PBI** protein bound iodine
*p.c. (post cibum)* after meals
**PCO** patient complains of
**PID** prolapsed intervertebral disc
**PMH** previous medical history
**PN** postnatal
**POP** plaster of Paris
**PP** private patients
**PPH** postpartum haemorrhage
*p.r. (per rectum)* rectal examination or by the rectum
*p.r.n. (pro re nata)* whenever necessary
**PY** physiotherapy
**PU** passed urine
**PUO** pyrexia of unknown origin
*p.v. (per vaginam)* vaginal examination or by the vagina
**PZI** protamine zinc insulin
*q. (quaque)* every
*q.h. (quaque hora)* every hour
*q.i.d. (quater in die)* four times a day
*quotid. (quotidie)* daily
*q.s. (quantum sufficiat)* sufficient quantity
*Rx (recipe)* take
**RA** rheumatoid arthritis
**RBC** red blood corpuscle
**Rh.** rhesus factor
**RIF** right iliac fossa
**RIH** right inguinal hernia
**RLL** right lower lobe
**ROA** right occipitoanterior

**ROL** right occipitolateral
**ROP** right occipitoposterior
**RS** respiratory system
*s̄. (sine)* without
**SB** stillborn
**SG** specific gravity
*sig. (signetur)* let it be labelled
**SMR** submucous resection
*sol. (solutis)* solution
*s.o.s. (si opus sit)* if necessary
**sp. gr.** specific gravity
*ss. (semis)* half
*stat. (statim)* at once
**SWD** short wave diathermy
*syr. (syrupus)* syrup
**T and A** tonsils and adenoids
**TAB** typhoid and paratyphoid A and B
**TB** tuberculosis
**TCA** to come again
**TCI** to come in
*t.i.d. (ter in die)* three times a day
**TPR** temperature, pulse and respiration
*tr. (tinctura)* tincture
*Ung. (unguentum)* ointment
**VD** venereal disease
*vi (virgo intacta)* virgin
*Vin. (vinum).* wine
**VV** varicose vein
**Vx** vertex
**WBC** white blood corpuscle
**WR** Wasserman reaction
**wt** weight
**XR** X-ray
**YOB** year of birth

---

Symbols that are commonly used include: ♂ male; ♀ female; # fracture; −ve negative; +ve positive; △ diagnosis.

# 9

# Personal profiles

Personal profiles or portfolios have become a recognised method of summarising personal achievement, interests and progress. These were brought into the school environment through the National Record of Achievement. This is in order to give you an individual record of experience and achievements to which you can add personal statements, examination results and records, which may provide valuable material for a future CV. You will no doubt remember that your school record of achievement was presented in a special folder with space allocated to different aspects of development. It is useful to consider how this can be extended for future use.

## PERSONAL STATEMENT

This is expected to contain information about activities you have been involved in, whether they are clubs, sports, musical activities, drama, etc. It should include activities which you took part in out of college or school hours. Once you have left training, interests may change or even be extended; there is every reason to update your personal statement in this area from time to time.

## QUALIFICATIONS AND EXAMINATION RESULTS

It is most useful to keep an accurate and up-to-date record of qualifications gained and when these were achieved. It is very easy to forget the year that particular examinations were taken, especially when many secretarial examinations take place at several points during each year. To keep a track on these, there should be space allowed to record all successes or re-takes accurately, so that a true record is always there for reference. Whether you wish to include examination slips within the plastic wallets provided is up to you, but it should be stressed that actual certificates and examination slips should be kept together carefully for future reference. Some places of employment may require actual evidence of your success and ask to see official documents.

When making a record of results, always state:

◆ the type of qualification, e.g. Medical Secretarial Diploma
◆ the subject area
◆ the awarding body, e.g. AMSPAR
◆ the level/result/grade, e.g. Diploma or Certificate
◆ the date of achievement.

## ACHIEVEMENT AND EXPERIENCE

You may have copies of tutors' reports or work placement evidence you would like to include in this section. Other experience you may like to add here are those recognised today as 'key skills'. These are:

◆ Planning and presentation of information. This may be through listening, reading and using it to present ideas to others whether by speaking, writing or using images.
◆ Using information technology to process, prepare and present material in different contexts.

◆ Using application of number to enable calculation and presentation of data.
◆ Effective personal skills when working as a team or in a one to one situation.
◆ Problem solving.
◆ Personal skills, developing and improving skills in order to improve personal performance.

You may also like to add some thoughts of your own on what you think your particular strengths or qualities are. These may be things such as determination or an ability to work under pressure. You may like to include evidence from particular employment to illustrate this.

## EMPLOYMENT HISTORY

This is an important section to keep updated. Again, it is all too easy to forget exact dates of jobs you have taken in the past. Keep a record here of:

◆ job title
◆ name of employer
◆ address and telephone number.

It might also be useful to keep a note of any other details connected to work, such as:

◆ National Insurance number
◆ Pay roll number.

## INDIVIDUAL ACTION PLANS

From time to time it might be useful to sit back and assess where your career is taking you, whether you envisage any change or progress in your job, or indeed, do you want a change at all! A change might be inevitable at some time as circumstances change. In order to develop plans or to just assess where you are at the moment, it might be useful to think in terms of

◆ a review
◆ long- or short-term goals – and therefore . . .
◆ targets to achieve
◆ methods to achieve them.

It is always useful to ask someone else whom you trust and respect to read your personal statements and letters first. Always compose them in a rough form first, before producing a well word-processed version.

Whatever you choose to include in your personal profile, try to make sure that the statements and records will create a positive picture of you.

# 10 Career prospects for the qualified medical secretary

*Dilys Jones*

The medical secretary needs a wide range of skills and abilities. She requires compassion and a concern for people, and the ability to prioritise and to work with great accuracy. She must apply the rules of confidentiality and be aware of the legal aspects. If she makes a mistake, a patient's health may suffer.

AMSPAR stands for the Association of Medical Secretaries, Practice Managers, Administrators and Receptionists. It was established in 1964 and is recognised by the Department of Education and the BMA. It is the largest association for administrative staff in the field of health care and exists to promote, encourage and support the education and maintenance of high standards.

For the medical secretary AMSPAR offers Diploma and Certificate training courses. A list of colleges offering these qualifications is available from head office*. In addition to full training courses, some colleges offer short courses in one or more subject areas aimed at the medical secretary. If you do not possess any AMSPAR qualifications you are still eligible to apply for membership. If you have worked in a health care environment for at least 10 years you are eligible for full membership; 5 years you are eligible to become an associate member and under 5 years you are eligible for affiliate membership. Some of the benefits of membership are: a free legal helpline, participation in local and national conferences, free subscription to the AMSPAR Journal and use of designated letters, e.g. MAMS.

Most medical secretaries find their first job in an NHS hospital, a private hospital, health centre or a general practice. However, there are many other organisations keen to employ qualified medical secretaries, for example in clinical audit, the various medical research bodies, pharmaceutical companies, social services, community-based agencies and medical publishers.

The range of job opportunities in these organisations should not be overlooked. In the largest hospitals, for example, in addition to the whole range of medical specialties, there may be a great deal of education and training in the attached medical school, schools of nursing, physiotherapy and radiography, etc., in which a medical secretary could support a teaching team. The names and addresses of all hospitals in England, Scotland, Wales and Northern Ireland can be found in the back of the Medical Directory (published annually) with details of the consultants in the various specialties. The Medical Directory is available in the reference section of public libraries.

Most of the medical specialties are supported by a college offering information, training and publications, for example The Royal College of Physicians and The Royal College of Surgeons. All these colleges would be interested in employing a qualified medical secretary – though you will find that most have their headquarters in the London area.

Many of the voluntary and community-based agencies advertise medical secretarial posts. A particularly good example is the hospice providing care for the terminally ill. There are a great many

*AMSPAR, Tavistock House North, Tavistock Square, London WC1H 9LN
(Tel: 0171 387 6005; Fax: 0171 388 2648).

charities such as the British Red Cross, Help the Aged, MIND, Save the Children Fund, Shelter and SCOPE. Details of these and many others are in *The Voluntary Agencies Directory* published annually by NCVO Publications and *Charities Digest* published annually by The Family Welfare Association and available in the reference section of public libraries. Details of research organisations are also included, for example British Heart Foundation, Imperial Cancer Research Fund, Institute of Cancer Research and Medical Research Council.

Some newly qualified medical secretaries may be unsure in which area of the medical field their future lies. Temping can be an interesting way of looking inside a number of organisations and might help you decide on your career path. For those returning to work after a long family break, temping can provide some flexibility before committing to a permanent appointment. Contacting your local hospital can be a good starting point as hospitals like to have a 'bank' of secretarial staff to call on to cover holidays and periods of sickness.

The AMSPAR Medical Secretarial Diploma course requires full-time students to spend a minimum of 25 days on field work. Work experience placements should be in hospital departments and general medical practice. Group visits to the health authority and community-based agencies can also be included. A work placement is a unique opportunity to observe the routine procedures and the communication links between staff and between the different departments. However, work experience is not provided for observation only, but for the student to learn and assist with a variety of duties. If this role is carried out successfully and the student fits in well with the other members of the team, it is worth bearing in mind that there may be the possibility of a job offer as a result of the work placement.

If you think you might be interested in medical publishing, you will find that the Royal Colleges publish weekly and monthly medical journals, pamphlets and books, and there are several medical publishers.

Recent changes in the structure of the health service have resulted in new administrative posts, and a motivated medical secretary willing to undertake further training may progress to a supervisory or management role.

# 11

# Applying for a job

*Dilys Jones*

## JOB ADVERTISEMENTS AND WHERE TO LOOK FOR THEM

Outside of London jobs for medical secretaries will be published in local newspapers. In the London area jobs may be advertised in local as well as national daily and evening newspapers. *The Times* newspaper advertises senior secretarial opportunities on a Wednesday. *The Times* also publishes a major secretarial supplement in the summer in conjunction with a job fair. *The Guardian* and *The Daily Telegraph* advertise relevant posts on a Thursday and *Daily Express* and *The Mail* advertise on a Tuesday.

If you are not finding that suitable jobs are being advertised you may decide to use an employment agency. These organisations are paid by employers to find suitable candidates for specific jobs and some agencies specialise in particular fields such as nursing or secretarial work. Make sure you choose an agency that will work for you in a field relevant to the type of job you want or you may find yourself attending interviews which are unsuitable. There are recruitment agencies in London that specialise in medical appointments, such as Medical & General Employment and Wren Bureau, and these agencies may be present at job fairs.

If you are out temping, keep a close eye on any staff notice boards. Whole careers have been founded on information stumbled across in such a manner.

When you see a job advertised in which you are interested, there is likely to be a contact name and address for you to write and obtain an application form and/or job description. Alternatively, there may be only a name and telephone number, and

you are invited to telephone for a job description. If you have to telephone at this stage, plan what you want to say before making the call as your telephone manner will be important.

A job description will usually include:

- the job title
- where the vacancy occurs
- the duties and responsibilities of the job, listed in some detail
- who the job holder reports to
- any special conditions of the job.

Study the job description carefully. If you decide to apply you will need to prepare a letter of application, to be accompanied by either a completed job application form or a curriculum vitae. Follow any instructions exactly; if you are asked to handwrite the covering letter, you must do so.

Consider the job advertisement on page 324.

## CURRICULUM VITAE

The letters CV are an abbreviation of curriculum vitae, which is Latin for 'course of life'. A CV is a summary of your career, educational and personal life relevant to the job you are applying for.

There is no single 'correct' way of writing a CV. Presenting a good CV is an opportunity to shine over the opposition, and it is worth spending some hours preparing your first one. Your CV must be word processed and printed on the best paper and printer available to you.

When you use your CV, it is important to tailor it to an advertised position or organisation. It may be just a matter of emphasising some experience or qualities you have that are particularly

---

*South London NHS Trust*
**FULL-TIME MEDICAL SECRETARY**
*required in the Orthopaedic Department*

*The ideal candidate will be well organised and possess good
communication skills and excellent medical secretarial skills.
Shorthand desirable but not essential.
Would suit AMSPAR qualified college leaver.*

*Good interpersonal skills needed for liaising with 2 consultants,
nursing staff and other members of the team. Up-to-date
hardware and software packages – training provided.*

*Hours: 37 per week. Salary: Grade 3 plus proficiency allowances.
For further details and a job description please contact
Sally Lang, Human Resources Department,
South London NHS Trust,
Fulham Road, Chelsea, London SW3 6LJ. Tel: 0171 352 8111*

---

relevant to the job you are applying for. If you are already working, your CV should show your present duties and responsibilities. Better still, also try to show evidence of your achievements in your current post. By keeping your CV on disk, it is easy to make a few amendments and keep it up to date.

It is usual to supply the names, addresses and telephone numbers of two referees at the end of your CV. If you are a college leaver one of your referees should be your course tutor. In addition, consider asking:

◆ a leader of a club you belong to
◆ a professional person who knows you well
◆ your supervisor at your Saturday job.

Do check with these people first that they are willing to write a reference for you.

If you are already employed and do not want your manager to know that you are applying for other jobs, you can mention this in your letter of application by saying something like 'Please do not contact my employer for a reference unless a job offer is to be made'.

On the CV itself, the guidelines are clear:

◆ No more than two pages
◆ Well laid out, with clear headings and plenty of white space
◆ A well chosen typeface (not too fancy)
◆ Make sure essential information is included (address, telephone no., etc.)
◆ Previous posts in reverse date order, focusing on achievements.

If you are just completing your college training course and are applying for your first job, your CV may look something like the example on page 325.

If you have held previous jobs, then your CV should list these with the latest or present job first. If you are now looking for a full-time job after taking a family break, your CV might look something like the example on page 326.

## JOB APPLICATION FORMS

Some organisations ask you to complete a printed job application form. These forms vary as each organisation designs its own.

CURRICULUM VITAE

**ALISON SMITH**

| | |
|---|---|
| 14 Stuart Rise | Date of Birth: 12 April 1978 |
| Burgess Hill | Marital Status: Single |
| West Sussex | Nationality: British |
| BN12 2RX | |
| Tel: 01444 871452 | |

EDUCATION AND QUALIFICATIONS

| | |
|---|---|
| 1987–1994 | Fairways Comprehensive School, Burgess Hill |
| GCSE | English (B), Mathematics (C), Biology (C), Geography (C), Art (D), French (D) |
| 1994–1996 | Brighton College<br>AMSPAR Medical Secretarial Diploma<br>RSA Medical Word Processing Stage II<br>RSA Medical Audio Transcription Stage II<br>RSA Medical Shorthand Speed 80 wpm |

WORK EXPERIENCE

| | |
|---|---|
| 1996 | 2 weeks assisting the medical secretaries in the Surgical Unit at Brighton Hospital (as part of my course) |
| | 2 weeks assisting the medical secretary/receptionists at the Thorpe Medical Centre, Burgess Hill (as part of my course) |
| 1995/96 | Saturday job – cashier at J Sainsbury plc, Burgess Hill |

INTERESTS

Bronze Duke of Edinburgh Award – I enjoyed the physical challenges and planning for the expedition

Computers – I am enthusiastic about computers and enjoy looking at software packages with my friends

Tennis – I play regularly at my local club and take part in local competitions

Riding – I help at sessions of Riding for the Disabled

REFEREES

| | |
|---|---|
| Mrs Jane Adams | Mr John Williamson |
| Business Department | Practice Manager |
| Brighton College | Thorpe Medical Centre |
| Southern Road | High Street |
| Brighton | Burgess Hill |
| East Sussex BN3 4RE | West Sussex BN16 2EY |
| Tel: 01273 644644 | Tel: 01273 532288 |

CURRICULUM VITAE

**ROSEMARY BROWN**

50 Hyde Road                          Date of Birth: 20 June 1962
Brighton                              Marital Status: Married
East Sussex                          Nationality: British
BN3 6BX
Tel: 01273 660342

EDUCATION AND QUALIFICATIONS

| | |
|---|---|
| 1971–1978 | St Mary's School, Brighton |
| GCSE | English (C), Mathematics (C), Biology (C), History (C), Art (D) |
| 1978–80 | Brighton College AMSPAR Medical Secretarial Diploma RSA Medical Audio Transcription Stage II RSA Medical Shorthand 100 wpm RSA Typewriting Stage III |
| 1995 | Brighton College – Evening Class RSA Word Processing Stage II |

WORK EXPERIENCE

| | |
|---|---|
| 1995–1996 | Medical Receptionist (part-time, 20 hours per week) Burgess Hill Health Centre |
| 1985–1995 | Family break to care for my 2 children |
| 1982–1985 | Senior Medical Secretary to the Director of the Paediatric Unit, Guy's Hospital, London. Duties included providing secretarial support to the consultants, maintaining the Director's diary, servicing committees, organising staffing rotas and recording statistical and financial information. |
| 1980–1982 | Medical Secretary to Consultant Surgeons. Responsible for providing efficient secretarial support to the surgical team, and dealing with patients and relatives in a friendly and reassuring manner. |

INTERESTS

Sailing – this is a hobby enjoyed by all the family
Reading – I enjoy a variety of books, but particularly biographies
School Governor at Mannington School since 1994

REFEREES

Mr Anthony Bryden                    Mr Robert White
Practice Manager                     Headmaster
Burgess Hill Health Centre           Mannington School
High Street                          West Road
Burgess Hill                         Brighton
West Sussex BN19 6ST                 East Sussex BN10 8XX
Tel: 01444 678954                    Tel: 01273 882365

Some advantages to completing forms are:

◆ the form tells you what information to provide
◆ the amount of space provided may indicate how much you are expected to write.

Some disadvantages are:

◆ it is very difficult to complete an application form using a word processor
◆ some organisations use the same form for all appointments so it may be difficult to give the information you feel is important.

When you receive an application form, read the instructions very carefully. It is likely that you will be asked to write in your own hand. A useful hint: photocopy the form before you start and draft your answers on the copy, remembering to match what you say to the job description. When you feel you have presented the information about yourself as effectively as possible you can copy your answers clearly and neatly on to the original.

## LETTERS OF APPLICATION

There are several types of letter that you may need to send when applying for a job. For example:

◆ a simple letter asking for an application form
◆ a letter of application to accompany a CV
◆ a covering letter with a completed application form
◆ a speculative letter.

You may put your letter of application on the word processor unless instructed otherwise. Whether typing or handwriting your letter, the advice is the same:

◆ use good quality white paper – it may have to be photocopied
◆ use size A4 so that it matches your CV
◆ use 1 inch margins
◆ the letter should be neat and well spaced
◆ quote the job reference number
◆ check for errors in spelling and grammar

◆ make sure the beginning and ending are correct for each other (e.g. Yours faithfully with Dear Sir, and Yours sincerely with Dear Mrs Williams).

Your letter is as important as your CV. It is an opportunity to further sell yourself as a person, as well as to highlight skills or experience that are particularly relevant to the job. Remember – your application may need to catch the reader's attention in the first 20 seconds in order to ensure that you are shortlisted for a job you really want.

Consider the following:

*Dear Sir*

*I would like to apply for the post of Medical Secretary you are advertising.*

*I have just passed the Medical Secretarial Diploma at College. I enclose a copy of my CV.*

*Yours faithfully*

This is a poor example of a letter of application. Even though the candidate has the right qualification for the job, the letter does not catch the reader's attention and encourage him/her to read the CV. Also, try and avoid the use of 'I' as the first word of each sentence!

A good letter of application needs to include:

◆ a heading – quoting the job reference number if there is one
◆ an introductory paragraph which says what the letter is about and what documents you are enclosing
◆ one or more paragraphs
  — drawing attention to any skills, qualifications or work experience particularly relevant to the job
  — giving additional details about yourself which are pertinent to the job
◆ a closing paragraph rounding off the letter.

As a college leaver who has just achieved the Medical Secretarial Diploma, your letter of application for the above post might look something like the example on page 328.

14 South Drive
BRIGHTON
East Sussex
BN1 4TW

5 July 1996

Mrs Ann Williams
Personnel Manager
Brighton Hospital
High Street
BRIGHTON
East Sussex
BN1 6AP

Dear Mrs Williams

**<u>Ref JP/476 – Medical Secretary in the Paediatric Unit</u>**

I would like to apply for the above post advertised in the Brighton Gazette of 2 July 1996. I attach my CV.

For the last 2 years I have been attending a full-time AMSPAR Medical Secretarial Diploma Course at Brighton College. I am optimistic that I have achieved the full qualification.

The course was very interesting and enjoyable. It has given me a broad picture of the structure of the health service and a good working knowledge of medical terminology, communication and office skills.

During my course I visited your hospital for 2 weeks in March 1996. I was attached to the medical secretaries in the Surgical Unit and assisting with the routine administrative procedures was a valuable learning experience.

I think of myself as hardworking and cheerful and look forward to achieving my aim to be part of a health service team.

If you wish to call me for interview I am available at any time.

Yours sincerely

Angela Smith

Enc

# SPECULATIVE APPLICATION LETTERS

As well as replying to advertisements, you may decide to approach organisations directly. Large organisations are bound to have vacancies from time to time.

If you have good qualifications and/or experience, you have every reason to be hopeful. You may be lucky and be offered an interview quickly. More likely the organisation will write and tell you that they are holding your details on file until a suitable vacancy occurs.

Before writing your speculative letter, find out who would be the best person to address your letter to. Phone the organisation and ask for the correct spelling of the person's name and his or her job title.

Your speculative letter is similar to your covering letter of application:

◆ a short opening paragraph explaining why you are writing
◆ specify your qualifications and experience for this kind of job
◆ give a reason for wanting to work with this organisation
◆ enclose your CV.

# LETTER OF ACCEPTANCE

Having been offered a job it is very important to conclude the process with a letter of acceptance straight away. You should reply by return of post.

A suitable letter of acceptance might be:

---

Dear Mrs Williams

**Ref JP/476 – Medical Secretary in the Paediatric Unit**

Thank you for your letter of 25 July concerning the above post. I write to confirm that I shall be delighted to accept the offer made in that letter.

As requested I will report to your office at 9.00 a.m. on Monday 2 September.

Yours sincerely

---

# FURTHER READING

Berry S 1997 Write a perfect CV in a weekend. Ward Lock

McGee P 1995 How to write a CV that works. How to Books Ltd

# 12

# How to present yourself at interview

*Dilys Jones*

If you have submitted a good letter of application and an effective CV for a specific job, you will be hoping that you are going to be shortlisted.

If you are shortlisted for a job the next stage is the interview. Most interviewees would confess to feeling nervous about the interview. The best way to combat nervousness is to prepare as thoroughly as possible.

Consider the following in relation to the job you have applied for.

- What are the employers looking for?
- What form will the interview take?
- What should you expect to be asked?
- What questions should you ask?

It is important that you go to the interview with a 'picture' of the organisation. If the interview is to take place in a hospital, visit the reception area and look for leaflets that might give you background information on the work of the hospital. If there do not appear to be any suitable leaflets, then the personnel department may be able to help with information on the structure of the organisation. Ask the reception staff how to get to the exact location of your interview so that you can feel confident of finding the room in good time on the interview day. This visit will also have given you the opportunity to check your route and travelling arrangements.

If your interview is in a general practice, you could visit the premises and ask the reception staff for a copy of the practice leaflet. This will give you a good day-to-day picture of the work of the practice.

Any information you have about the organisation will assist you to answer questions with more understanding and with more confidence.

## PLANNING FOR THE INTERVIEW

- Check your route and travelling arrangements.
- Decide what you are going to wear at least 3 days ahead of time. A suit would give a serious and professional first impression. Ensure that all accessories are clean. You will want to be comfortable in your outfit and to feel you look right for the interview.
- Prepare some questions that you may wish to ask at the end of the interview.
- Rehearse your answers to the most common questions beforehand.
- Remember to let your referees know that you have been shortlisted. You might want to give them some details so that they understand what the employer is looking for.

## QUESTIONS YOU MIGHT BE ASKED

If an initial interview is being set up by the personnel department, it is likely that a standardised list of criteria will be used to assess the candidate. Be prepared to talk about some or all of the following:

- why you want the job
- work experience, including your last job and previous jobs
- your training and qualifications relevant to the job
- flexibility
- long-term career plans
- leisure interests.

## WHAT TO TAKE TO THE INTERVIEW

- a copy of your CV, record of achievement, certificates, portfolio
- any information supplied about the job
- name and telephone number of the interviewer in case of delays
- a list of questions to ask at the end of the interview
- a notepad and pen
- everyday things:
  - glasses – if you need them
  - money
  - any travel or parking instructions
  - handkerchief or clean tissues
  - umbrella – if it looks like rain
  - women might want to carry a spare pair of tights.

Find something appropriate to carry things in. Try and borrow an envelope file or briefcase. Avoid using a plastic bag.

## THE INTERVIEW

Arrive well before the interview time. Nothing looks more unprofessional than being late.

Remember that you are there because you have impressed the person who is hiring. Whether you have a good CV, wrote a good letter of application or spoke well on the phone, you have made a positive first impression.

At interview it is your task to show that you can do the job effectively. You must be positive and show you can communicate well verbally. Use active words to describe your skills, experience and achievements. You might find it helpful to think about the following active words to use in some of your responses:

| | | |
|---|---|---|
| achieve | coordinate | improve |
| capable | create | manage |
| control | develop | organise |

If asked a general opening question such as 'Tell me something about yourself', you might give the best impression by enquiring what aspects the interviewer would like to know about other than those mentioned in your CV.

Asked why do you want this job, you do not have to go into great detail. Something about your interest in the job, the service or the people, and the fact that you feel you have the necessary skills will often suffice.

Self motivation equals enthusiasm. If you want a job, and know why you want it, it is not difficult to show it. Your enthusiasm should shine through, and if you follow this by asking interesting questions, you will leave a favourable impression in the interviewer's mind. You should be able to demonstrate your motivation to achieve. If you have succeeded in achieving all the examinations for the Medical Secretarial Diploma your self motivation is evident.

## QUESTIONS YOU MIGHT WANT TO ASK

- Who would I be working with?
- What computer software do you use?
- What is the most demanding aspect of the job?
- Are there opportunities for further training and development?
- Are you able to tell me when a decision will be made?

There are many observers of the recruitment field who suggest that interviewers make up their minds about a candidate in the first four minutes of the interview, so first impressions of your appearance, manner, facial expression and attitude are most important.

It is likely that your interview is with more than one person. Greet each panel member with a firm handshake and smile. When asked to take a seat, sit well back in the chair and place your legs together, not crossed. Look the interviewer in the eye when you are speaking. Experienced interviewers appreciate that almost all candidates will be slightly nervous. Do not be surprised if the beginning of the interview is made up of small talk to break the ice.

Concentrate on the questions you are being asked. If necessary, pause to think before you answer. It is unlikely that a simple 'yes' or 'no' will suffice. Be prepared to expound on any question to the best of your ability. It may be that 30 seconds is the average length of your answers. Stop when you have said all you want to – do not ramble on in order to fill the silence.

Do not criticise any past employers. One of the things you have got to prove is that you are loyal. Find something good to say about previous jobs. You gained additional skills, but now you are looking for more responsibility.

Let the interviewer discuss salary first. The salary can be negotiated at a later stage. It is important to be offered the job first.

The interviewer will indicate that the interview is over. It is acceptable to ask when a decision is likely to be made. On leaving, smile and thank the interviewer(s) for seeing you. It is not necessary to shake hands again.

## KEY POINTS TO REMEMBER

**Do not:**

◆ interrupt the interviewer
◆ criticise past employers
◆ answer with a simple yes or no
◆ be jokey/flippant/sarcastic – not everybody has the same sense of humour
◆ smoke
◆ accept a cup of coffee – unless you can see somewhere to put it down.

**Do:**

◆ dress appropriately
◆ allow plenty of time to reach the interview in comfort
◆ look at the interviewer(s)
◆ smile occasionally – it relieves the tension
◆ think about likely questions and decide on your answers
◆ have questions ready beforehand – it does not go down well if you have none!

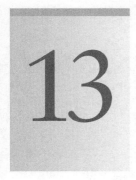

# 13 Guidelines for the preparation of material for publication in books and journals

## BOOKS

### Manuscript preparation (general)

- The manuscript should be printed on good quality A4 paper, on one side only.
- Text (including references, tables, figure legends, etc.) should be double-spaced.
- Generous margins should be left on all sides (at least 1″/2.5 cm at the side and 1.5″/3.75 cm top and bottom).
- Pages should be numbered sequentially from 1 to X000 throughout the manuscript.
- Copy your manuscript! Ensure the top copy goes to the publisher, a copy goes to your editor (if you are contributing to a multi-author work) and keep one copy for yourself.
- Include with your completed manuscript the full names and details of all authors for inclusion in the contributors' list. This includes full name, degrees, position, affiliations, and full address.
- The submitted manuscript for each chapter should include:
  - chapter title page (bearing title, authors' names, mailing address, telephone and fax numbers, book title, editors)
  - completed text
  - tables (each on a separate sheet)
  - figure legends (all listed together, separate from text)
  - figures (*plus* photocopies of all figures)
  - reference list/bibliography
  - permissions (for figures, tables, etc.).
- Intended positions of illustrations and tables should be clearly marked in the text.

## Preparing the text

- Do not justify the right-hand margin – leave text ragged.
- Use single spaces only between words, and between sentences.
- Do not indent the beginning of paragraphs – use a line space to separate them from the text or heading above.
- Do not use returns within the text, between lines. Use only to end paragraphs or headings, or to separate items in a list.
- Do not try to make paragraphs fit pages exactly by adding line spaces. If the last word of a sentence ends up on the next page, leave it.
- Use formatting commands as you would normally (italic, superscript, etc.).
- Do not use l (ell) for 1 (one) or O (oh) for 0 (zero).
- Use hyphens only where you would normally in a word (e.g. non-specific), and not at the end of lines.
- If possible, distinguish between opening and closing inverted commas.

### Headings

- Use simple different styles of text for headings, to denote level of importance, but be consistent!

### Artwork

- Mark the position of artwork, tables, etc. clearly with labels in the text,
  e.g. <Figure 1.1 near here>.

## Supplying your disk

Always supply a hard copy of your manuscript with a disk.

◆ Remember to keep a copy of the electronic version of your manuscript on your PC or on disk.
◆ Print out the text double spaced.
◆ Highlight on your hard copy any special coding or symbols you have used (e.g. if you have used ^B instead of the beta symbol) and include a list of their meanings at the front of the manuscript.
◆ List any styles of headings you have used, and their intended hierarchy.
◆ Supply the text as a series of files, one file for each chapter. Label files clearly, preferably with the chapter number and an abbreviation of the chapter author's name.
◆ Supply only the final version of each chapter.
◆ Label disks clearly with the name of the book and the author, the operating system and programs used, and what is on the disk.

## Style guide

◆ Use SI units (mm, kg, Pa, J, etc.).
◆ Abbreviations should be spelt out in the first instance, with the abbreviation in brackets following. Thereafter, use the abbreviation only. Abbreviations should be in capitals with no full points between, e.g. NSAID, USA.
◆ Numbers one to nine should be spelt out in full, unless with units, e.g. five patients, 5 mm.
◆ Single spaces should be used instead of commas in numbers of 10 000 and over (but remember 9999 and under are closed up).
◆ Avoid footnotes, except to tables.
◆ Lists should take the following form:

    1
    2
    3 (a)
      (b)
      (c) (i)
          (ii)

They can also run on in the text: (a) for the first; (b) for the second; (c) for the third, and so on.

## Figure legends

◆ Type as a list on a separate sheet and include at the back of the manuscript.

## References

### Vancouver

◆ Indicate references in the text with a number in square brackets [1] to [X00], sequentially, as they occur.
◆ Provide a corresponding numbered reference list. This list should not be alphabetised, but be in the sequence of occurrence in the text, e.g.

7 Barnes PJ & Holgate ST. Pathogenesis and hyperreactivity. In: Brewis RAL, Gibson GJ & Geddes DM (eds) *Respiratory Medicine*, 2nd edn. London: WB Saunders 1990: 558–9.
8 Sasson CSH, Hassell KT, Manutte RT *et al.* Hyperoxic induced hypercapnia in stable chronic obstructive disease. *Am Rev Resp Dis* 1987; **185**: 758–60.

### Harvard

◆ Cite references in the text by name and date: (Smith 1992), (Smith & Smith 1985), (Smith et al. 1987).
◆ The reference list should be in alphabetical order by name of author. Where several papers are by the same author, list the single author publication first, then two authors, then three or more. If there is more than one single author reference (for example) use date order (most recent first).

e.g. Brown J & Hughes L (1993)
     Jones B (1993) [*Note the initial*]
     Jones D (1992)
     Jones D & Thomas T (1993 *a*)
     Jones D & Thomas T (1993 *b*)

Barnes PJ & Holgate ST (1994) Pathogenesis and hyperreactivity. In: Brewis RAL, Gibson GJ & Geddes DM (eds) *Respiratory Medicine*, 2nd edn, pp. 558–60. London: WB Saunders.

Sassoon CSH, Hassell KT, Manutte RT *et al.* (1987) Hyperoxic induced hypercapnia in stable chronic obstructive pulmonary disease. *Am Rev Resp Dis* 135: 747–8.

## Journals

### Submission of manuscripts

Manuscripts should be submitted as A4 double spaced typescript with generous margins, complete in all respects, including a title and a suggested running head. The name and address of the author should appear in the exact form required for publication; the author's phone and fax number should also be included.

### Style

Papers should be structured conventionally: summary (≤200 words), introduction, materials and methods, results and discussion. Brevity without loss of precision will enhance all sections, particularly materials and methods. Footnotes should be avoided and acknowledgements, or grant sources, given at the end of the text.

### Units and abbreviations

The Royal Society of Medicine has published *Units, Symbols and Abbreviations – A Guide for Biological and Medical Editors and Authors* 4th ed. (Ed.) Baran, D. N. You should follow these, or similar, recommendations (e.g. IUPACIUB Commission on Biochemical Nomenclature), use metric units and, wherever possible, adopt the International System of Units (SI). Where SI units have not been universally accepted it is advisable to give values in traditional units in brackets. If abbreviations are used, the terms should be written out in full when first used, the abbreviation then being given in parenthesis. Where abbreviations are adopted, capitals are preferred, for example ECG, BMR (not ecg, bmr) without full stops.

### Tables

Tables should be numbered in Arabic numbers, given adequate titles or headings, typed on sepa-rate sheets of paper, attached to the manuscript, and should be cited in the text.

### Illustrations

Three high quality photographic prints of each illustration should be submitted, one of which must be fully labelled; if the other two prints are unlabelled, they should be accompanied by photocopies of the labelled prints. Do not send negatives or photocopies on their own. Mounting is undesirable. Indicate lightly in pencil, on the reverse side, permissible lines of cropping, your name, the figure number, optimal size, and the 'top' of the illustration. Labelling should be consistent with the text and must be large enough to be legible when reduced to page size.

Illustrations should be given adequate legends, typed up as a list separate from the text. The illustrations should also be cited in the text.

### Permissions

If illustrations are borrowed from published sources, written permission must be obtained from both publisher and author, and a credit line giving the source added to the legend. If text material totalling 250 to 300 words, or any tables, are borrowed verbatim from published sources, written permission is required from both publisher and author. With shorter quotations, it is sufficient to add a bibliographic credit. Permission letters for reproduced text or illustrations must accompany the manuscript. If you have been unable to obtain permission, please point this out.

### References

References in the text must correlate with the reference list and should be cited by name and date, not numbers, thus: Smith (1963); Smith and Jones (1965); Smith, Jones and Brown (1967). Where a reference has four or more authors it should be cited in the text thus: Smith et al. (1972). If there are two references for Smith and Jones (1965) these should be designated a and b. The same will apply to Smith et al. (1972), even if the co-authors in these references are different.

The reference list at the end of the paper should include the names of all the authors. References are listed alphabetically. Where several papers by the same author are cited these should be arranged in single-author, double-author, treble-author, and multi-author groups (in that order), the references being arranged chronologically within each group, the earliest first. Groups of references within the text are arranged in chronological order.

**Reference examples:**

1. *Journals*
Taylor PE, Almeida JD, Zuckerman AJ & Leach JM (1972) Relationship of Milan antigen to abnormal serum lipoprotein. *American Journal of Diseases of Children*, 123, 329–331.

2. *Books*
Zuckerman AJ (1970) *Virus Diseases of the Liver*. London: Butterworths. 168 pp.

3. *Extracts from books*
Evans AS (1972) Infectious mononucleosis. In *Communicable and Infectious Diseases* (Ed.) Top FH & Wehrle PF pp. 105–135. St Louis: CV Mosby.

4. *Conference reports, proceedings, etc.*
Stalder GA, Schultheiss HR & Allgower M (1970) The effects of i.v. 2-deoxy-D-glucose on the serum enzymes, serum potassium and the electrocardiogram and its clinical side-effects in humans. *Abstracts of the World Congress of Gastroenterology, Copenhagen, 1970.* p. 20.

5. *Reports and theses*
Murphy CT (1973) *An In Vitro Study of the Factors Affecting the Growth of Micro-organisms on the Skin.* PhD Thesis, University of London.

# Index